A Nurse's Survival Guide to General Practice Nursing

A Nurse's Survival Guide to General Practice Nursing

Karen Storey, RN, MSc, QN
Primary Care Nursing Lead
NHS England & NHS Improvement

Rhian Last, RN, PGC Quality Improvement, UCPPD, PGC Primary Care Education
Former Head of The Academy
Education for Health
Warwick
Immediate Past Editor-in-Chief
General Practice Nursing Journal

ELSEVIER

ELSEVIER

Executive Content Strategist: Robert Edwards
Content Development Specialist: Denise Roslonski
Publishing Services Manager: Shereen Jameel
Senior Project Manager: Umarani Natarajan
Design Direction: Amy L. Buxton

Printed in India

Last digit is the print number: 9 8 7 6 5 4 3 2 1

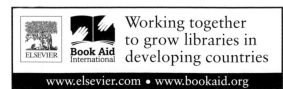

Dedication

To Emily, Hannah, Rebecca and Gordon, my wonderful family, who have been there during the hours spent getting this book from an idea to publication.
To my wise and dear friend, Brian Dolan, whose mentoring support brought about this opportunity to write a book.
To all those fabulous general practice and primary care nurses and professionals I've worked with over the years, you know who you are.

Karen Storey

To my family, whose support and enthusiasm for this book has been boundless.
To Dr Stewart Manning, Dr Howard Last, the staff and, above all, the patients at Oakley Medical Practice, Leeds with heartfelt thanks for a long and fulfilling career in general practice nursing.
To the students and primary care nurses I have had the privilege to teach, you are the future!

Rhian Last

Contents

Contributors

Gill Boast, RN, BSc (Hons), V300, PGCE, Senior Lecturer, Community Nursing, University of Wolverhampton, Wolverhampton County, England; GPN Lead/Facilitator, Primary Care, East Staffs CCG, Burton-on-Trent

Beverley Bostock, BSc, MSc, MA, Advanced Nurse Practitioner, Mann Cottage Surgery, Four Shires Medical Centre, Moreton-in-Marsh, Gloucestershire

Ruth Chambers, MD, FRCGP, OBE, Clinical Lead, Staffordshire Sustainability and Transformation Partnership, Stoke-on-Trent CCG, Stoke-on-Trent

Jane Chiodini, MSc, RGN, RM, FFTM, RCPS, Dean, Faculty of Travel Medicine, Royal College of Physicians and Surgeons of Glasgow, Glasgow

Lisa Clarke, GPN, PGCE, PG Dip, MA Education, Senior Lecturer, Faculty of Health, University of Wolverhamptom, Wolverhampton

Anne Connolly, MB, ChB, DFSRH, MRCGP, PG Dip Gynae (Hons), Bevan Healthcare, Bradford

Georgina Craig, MA (Hons), Director, The Experience-Led Care Programme, Georgina Craig Associated Limited, Abbots Langley, Hertfordshire

Helen Crowther, RN, QN, Clinical Nurse Advisor, Digital Primary Care, NHS X

Brian Dolan, OBE, FFNMRCSI, FRSA, RMN, RGN, Director, Health Service 360 UK, Visiting Professor of Nursing, Oxford Institute of Nursing, Midwifery and Allied Health Research (OxINMAHR), Honorary Professor of Leadership in Healthcare, University of Salford

Helen Donovan, MEd, BSc (Hons), RN, RM, RHV, Professional Lead, Public Health Nursing, Royal College of Nursing, London

Rachel Hatfield, BA (Hons), National Programme Manager, Technology-Enabled Care Services, Staffordshire STP

Heather Henry, RN, BSc (Hons), Queen's Nurse, MBA, Nurse Entrepreneur, Owner, Brightness Management Limited, Sale, Greater Manchester

Ann Hughes, RN, National digital nurse support, Telehealth facilitator

Jan Procter-King, RGN, RM, MA, Practice Nurse, The Ridge Medical Practice, General Practice, Bradford England, Lead Tutor, Primary Care Education, Leeds

Michael Kirby, MBBS, LRCP, MRCS, FRCP, Professor, Centre for Research in Primary and Community Care, University of Hertfordshire, Hatfield, Hertfordshire

Rhian Last, RN, PGC QI, PGC Primary Care Education, Former Head of The Academy, Education for Health, Warwick, Immediate Past Editor-in-Chief, *General Practice Nursing Journal*

Louise Newson, BSc (Hons), MBChB (Hons), MRCP, FRCGP, GP and Menopause Specialist, Newson Health, Winton House, Stratford-Upon-Avon

Alison Oldam, DClinPsy, BSc (Hons), Trainer, Et Al Training, Bradford

Clare Simpson, BA, ILM7, OD and Change Consultant, Chief Executive, Employment Matters Consulting Limited, Banbury, Oxfordshire

Paula Spooner, DPSN, BSc, MSc, PGCE, Nurse Consultant, Wakefield Clinical Commissioning Group, Wakefield West, Yorkshire

Sheinaz Akhtar Stansfield, MBA, Primary Care, Oxford Terrace and Rawling Road Medical Group, Gateshead

Karen Storey, RN, MSc, QN, Primary Care Nursing Lead, NHS England & NHS Improvement

Preface

We are delighted to present to you this first edition of *A Nurse's Survival Guide to General Practice Nursing* at a time when general practice nursing is in the spotlight and is recognised as essential to the future development of primary care.

It fills us with great pride to present to you this book, a collaboration amongst nurses and other health care professionals working in the field of general practice and primary care who have given freely of their time to provide essential knowledge to nurses new to general practice nursing.

This book epitomises the principles of interprofessional collaboration, bringing multidisciplinary professionals together to share their expert knowledge to benefit the development of nurses in general practice. All proceeds and royalties from sales of this book will be donated to the Cavell Nursing Trust to benefit nurses in general practice who encounter hardship during their nursing careers. The funds raised from this book will leave a legacy for nursing in this, the Year of the Nurse.

A few words on interprofessional collaboration as an approach for this book. Interprofessional collaboration increases team members' awareness of each other's roles, and the knowledge and skills that each have, leading to improvement in professionals' knowledge and decision-making, and increases patient satisfaction, improves health outcomes and improves patient care (Spicer et al., 2019). Applied in practice, collaboration can benefit and improve working for the whole workforce and can help to address some of the workforce pressures, as well as putting joy back into work. It breaks down professional barriers, prevents isolated working and is fundamental to multidisciplinary team working, which is at the core of Primary Care Networks (PCNs).

A nurse working in general practice today will experience a faster pace and an increased complexity of care compared with the norm 20 years ago. Population demographics have changed considerably, and there are more people in the population who are older and living longer with more complex health conditions. Demand on the system, a 24-hour culture and a requirement for instant access to consumables means that the demand for health care and primary care is ever increasing.

The general practice nursing workforce is changing too, from a predominantly older profile to a mixed-age profile, and the number of younger newly qualified nurses in the profession has increased since 2015 when students first began having placements in general practice. Historically, general practice nursing was often perceived as a profession for older, white, middle-class women at the end of their nursing career (Ipsos Mori, 2017). The General Practice Nursing Ten Point Plan (NHS England, 2017) aimed to change this perception by recruiting more nurses into the profession. The intent is to encourage nurses from more ethnically and diverse backgrounds and to provide support and development for General Practice Nurses (GPNs).

The requirement for nurses to be able to 'hit the ground running' is becoming a thing of the past; this might have been considered the norm 10 to 20 years ago as more older, experienced nurses transferred to general practice from secondary care, bringing with them their skills from many years learned on the job in other settings. For the new generation of nurses choosing general practice as a first-destination career, who will not have these experiential skills learned though years on the job, accredited education and training are essential. Many universities across England now deliver 'Fundamentals of General Practice' programmes, and this book will complement those programmes and provide essential information to assist nurses new to general practice.

The role of the GPN has evolved organically over the past decades and has moved away from being a task-orientated position to being a key role within an integrated, multidisciplinary primary care team (Redsell et al., 2007). GPNs have considerable autonomy in decision making, can take a history, make a diagnosis and decide on treatment options in conjunction with the patient and can prescribe medication. Having knowledge and access to up-to-date education is crucial if nurses are to have fulfilling careers in general practice and patients are to receive quality care.

Learning new skills while meeting the demand and the pace of general practice and the need for complex care, means that new GPNs need to have a number of resources to hand to help them survive in the fast-paced, highly pressurised area of work that general practice has become. This book, *A Nurse's Survival Guide to General Practice Nursing,* contains essential information about clinical, organisational and communication skills provided by key professionals in the field of primary care and will enable GPNs to thrive, not just survive. Not all of the traditional work carried out by nurses in general practice has been included in this book; however, we have included what we as editors consider essential for the modern GPN.

The clinical knowledge and skills pertaining to long-term condition management, sexual health, prevention and screening, as well as women's and men's health and some treatment room skills, have been included in this book. We have also taken the view that other skills such as communication, managing a consultation, caring for patients with mental health issues and being able to consider patients' holistic health and wellbeing are valuable survival skills, and have therefore included them in this book.

Understanding how general practice operates as an organisation that sits outside of the National Health Service (NHS) system but delivers NHS care has not previously been clear to nurses who work in general practice. This can lead to much confusion and frustration for nurses who may expect the same employment conditions as the rest of the NHS. We have therefore included a chapter which explains how general practice as an independent business operates, which will help new nurses to be clear from the outset regarding the benefits and limitations of this system.

A dedicated chapter on leadership written by one of the editors, who were both previously GPNs, is included. Developing leadership skills, managing a team, understanding the management of the practice and the wider health system and influencing for results are opportunities and priorities that previously were not considered priorities that nurses needed to focus on. There is a chapter focused on quality improvement, also written by one of the editors, including theories and tools that will equip GPNs with the knowledge and skills to facilitate change that will lead to improved and safer care. The lack of attention in previous years to these areas of professional development, leadership and organisational development has left GPNs feeling isolated and disconnected from their teams, the wider nursing profession and the wider health care system. This disconnect from the system often results in feelings of frustration because GPNs are unable to influence to make positive changes for themselves, their nursing teams, patients and populations. Understanding health care policy and how general practice functions and operates in the wider health care system, the direction of travel for primary care nursing and primary care itself is as essential as having clinical expertise, knowledge and skills.

The NHS Long Term Plan (2019) suggests that primary care has a key role to play in delivering essential changes to improve the quality of patient care and health outcomes. The plan sets out how PCNs will achieve the ambitions of the Long Term Plan by enabling general practices and their staff to work more collaboratively across population of 30,000 to 50,000 patients. Nurses are crucial to the success of achieving the aims of the PCNs and the Long Term Plan, and a dedicated chapter on PCNs has been included, with examples of how some PCNs are achieving this.

Key policy drivers such as the NHS Five Year Forward View (NHS England, 2015), the Health Education General Practice Nursing Workforce Plan (HEE, 2017), the NHS General Practice Nursing Ten Point Plan and other policy drivers have changed the face of general practice nursing over the last 5 years. Included in this book are chapters relating to policy, organisational development and quality improvement, which discuss in detail how GPNs can be part of the transformation of general practice and primary care. It is only recently that policy has focused on general practice nursing and recognised GPNs as enablers of change that has led to many improvements in general practice nursing. Some examples of these policy changes include the introduction of student nurses into general practice placements, the employment of newly qualified nurses in general practice and the introduction of new opportunities for experienced nurses to become mentors and supervisors; these types of changes have enabled transformation of the GPN workforce.

Throughout the book there will be opportunities for readers to take time out to reflect on their current and future practice as they read each chapter. This book will provide essential knowledge for meeting continuing professional development requirements for registered nurses, as well as essential knowledge for students experiencing general practice for the first time.

This book recognises that nurses working in general practice often work autonomously, and as a result the nature of work can be isolating; so the need for up-to-date knowledge is essential. This book will provide essential knowledge and resources for nurses new to general practice, some essential fundamental clinical skills and new ways of working to consult and communicate with patients and suggested ways to improve care delivery.

Karen Storey
Rhian Last

References

Health Education England. (2017). *The General Practice Nursing Workforce Development Plan.* https://www.hee.nhs.uk/.../The%20general%20practice%20nursing%20workforce%20.

Ipsos Mori. (2017). *General practice — developing confidence, capability and capacity. A ten point plan for general practice nursing, The recruitment, retention and return of nurses to General Practice Nursing in NHS England.* NHS England.

NHS England. (2015). *Five Year Forward View.* https://www.england.nhs.uk/five-year-forward-view/.

NHS England. (2017). *General Practice — developing confidence, capability and capacity. A ten-point action plan for general practice nursing.* https://www.england.nhs.uk/publication/general-practice-developing-confidence-capability-and-capacity/.

NHS England. (2019). *The NHS Long Term Plan.* https://www.longtermplan.nhs.uk/.

Redsell, S., Stokes, T., Jackson, C., Hastings, A., & Baker, R. (2007). Patients' accounts of the differences in nurses' and general practitioners' roles in primary care. *Journal of Advanced Nursing, 57*(2), 172–180. doi: 10.1111/j.1365-2648.2006.04085.x. PMID: 17214753.

Spicer, J., Ahluwalia, S., & Storey, K. (2019). *Collaborative Practice in Primary and Community Care.* Caipe Routledge.

Foreword

The great British philosopher Bertrand Russell once wrote that 'In all affairs, it's a healthy thing now and again to hang a question mark on all you take for granted'. Around 25 years ago, when I worked at the A&E (accident & emergency) primary care service in the Dept of General Practice and Primary Care at King's College Hospital in London, general practice nurses (GPNs) were not only becoming more prevalent, but their roles were also being reimagined in ways that at the time were so exciting, extending beyond immunisations and vaccinations to long-term condition management, men's and women's health and with a growing emphasis on people's mental health needs. It was a question mark on the then relatively narrow scope of practice to a much broader one about the complexity of peoples' lives and how to enhance the health of nation(s).

Just as emergency care has significantly evolved over that time, so too has general practice with the twins of greater acuity and more complex, older patient presentations becoming more prevalent. In many ways, nurses in both emergency care and general practice are generalist specialists who see patients across the whole span of life and need to know something about everything, while being sufficiently specialised to be recognised as subspecialties within the nursing family.

This book is the first of its kind and edited by two outstanding nurse leaders, Karen Storey and Rhian Last, who are generously donating all the proceeds to the Cavell Nurses' Trust to support nurses, midwives and healthcare assistants who face personal or financial crisis. It traverses the rich terrain of general practice nursing, which is increasingly recognised as central to ensuring the NHS continues to keep people in their own homes longer, values their time by ensuring so-called 'upstream' support of health promotion and illness prevention and/or mitigates long-term condition problems later.

The relationship that GPNs have with patients is guided by three elements that Dill and Gumpert (2012) call emotional connection, partnership and guided discovery. While universal to healthcare delivery, they lie at the heart of great primary care in particular, where there is time to build long-term relationships, understand the context of peoples' lives and work in a triumvirate of the head, heart and hands. True patient-centred care puts the patient where they belong – at our shared centre, as our raison d'être and in our hearts.

It is not enough to care for patients, it's about caring for them too, and GPNs have the privilege of building long-term, and even life-long, relations with extended families. Every moment is a teaching moment because while the public may look up to doctors, they look nurses in the eye. Because it's a relationship framed around greater equality and equity, the dynamics, disclosures and sense of feeling safe to raise things that may be perceived as 'too trivial' to bother the doctor about is so much of the precious added value that GPNs bring. When nurses, GPs and allied health work together in mutual trust, respect and understanding of each other's contributions, they are so much more than the sum of their parts.

In a Foreword that is being written at the end of 2020 – the International Year of the Nurse and the Midwife, a year dominated by COVID-19 – few would dispute the confluence of these events has put healthcare and nursing in particular on the global map. The importance and value of GPNs will be amplified even further now thatthe much hoped for vaccine has arrived on scene; it is an opportunity like few before to show how critical GP nurses are to the health and safety of nations, not least when it comes to the longer-term effects of COVID-19 on patients and their families.

COVID-19 has given us all an opportunity to examine all we took for granted. It has provided us with the gift of rethinking how and where healthcare is delivered. General Practice Nursing is no longer about buildings; it's about delivering services for patients in creative ways that values their time, experience and safety by not asking them to come to the surgery instead using technology to take services into their own homes.

What an amazing time to be a GPN, when new graduates cannot wait to join the ranks of their more seasoned nursing colleagues. While the anatomy (the structures) of general practice may change periodically, for instance through the introduction of primary care networks, the physiology, or if you prefer, the processes of care and desire to make it better and/or more tolerable for patients and their families, is immutable in time no matter how long one has practised as a GPN.

This book is both timely and timeless. As a survival guide, it answers many questions and hopefully stimulates questions in you like 'How do we acknowledge our past, respect our present and build on both to an even better future for general practice nursing'? This book is an outstanding building block to enable these hopes, dreams and ambitions to be realised and the editors and authors deserve all the plaudits this wonderful new book will surely bring.

Brian Dolan OBE, FFNMRCSI, FRSA, RMN, RGN
Director, Health Service 360, UK
Visiting Professor of Nursing, Oxford Institute of
Nursing, Midwifery and Allied Health Research (OxINMAHR)
Honorary Professor of Leadership in Healthcare, University of Salford

Reference

Dill, D., & Gumpert, P. (2012). What is the heart of health care? Advocating for and defining the clinical relationship in patient-centred care. *Journal of Participatory Medicine, 254*, e10.

Cavell Nurses' Trust transforms the lives of nursing professionals. The nurses, midwives and healthcare assistants we help say they are often happier, healthier and able to stay in or return to work.

We are the charity supporting UK nurses, midwives and healthcare assistants, both working and retired, when they are suffering personal or financial hardship often due to illness, disability, older age and domestic abuse.

We offer a tailored package of support to help everyone who gets in touch ranging from emotional support for those in crisis and signposting to specialist services, to one-off grants to quickly relieve financial hardship and even rapid emergency funding for those at great risk.

It's so wonderful therefore that this fantastic book not only gives nurses in primary pare such a broad range of thoughtful approaches to help them thrive and survive, but it will also help nurses in primary care know that Cavell Nurses' Trust is here to help.

And with the royalties from this book being donated to support our work, nurses in primary care have better than ever access to our help. So I must say a huge thank you on behalf of those we help to Karen Storey and Rhian Last to each author and contributor. Thank you so much.

John Orchard
Chief Executive, Cavell Nurses' Trust

Chapter 1

The role of the general practice nurse

Gill Boast, Lisa Clarke

Learning outcomes

After reading this chapter you should be able to:

1. Understand the development of the general practice nursing role
2. Relate the nine dimensions of the National Health Service Leadership Academy model (2013) to the issues and challenges of nursing in the general practice setting
3. Critically explore the concepts of care delivered by General Practice Nurses from preconceptual care to end of life

Introduction

General Practice Nursing is unique in that it spans all age groups throughout the life course and across all fields of nursing. The role of the General Practice Nurse (GPN) is very diverse with a wealth of opportunities to deliver high quality personalised care across the practice population. As a GPN working as part of a multidisciplinary team, it is a privilege to be part of some of the happiest and saddest times in people's lives. Within a single clinic setting a GPN can be managing the care of a vast range of patients, for example childhood and adult immunisations, cervical screening, contraception and sexual health, clinical review for those with a long-term condition, or providing holistic care for a person coming towards the end of their life. The clinical knowledge, expertise and skills required for the role are vast and complex. In addition, an understanding of the social determinants of health, influenced by the lifestyle that is adopted and the community that is lived in, is essential. Brown (2010) suggested that an ever-changing mix of skills and knowledge are required for the general practice nursing role and that nurses must constantly assimilate new information and keep abreast with changing guidelines. Keeping up with the demands of nursing across the lifespan in such a broad role can certainly be a challenge, but it is also what makes the role so interesting. At the time of writing this chapter the Covid-19 pandemic had just struck but it was clear in those early days of the pandemic the role of the GPN was undergoing further change and development to keep pace with the rapid development and release of national policy to support healthcare delivery in primary care during the pandemic. GPNs continued to see patients face to face, by telephone and virtually using technology to enable virtual consultations via video link. This rapid adaptation of technology has enabled a new way of reaching patients and improving access to care both patients and GPNs. The agile, adaptive and flexible GPN response to the many challenges that the pandemic presented for Primary Care epitomises the very best of General Practice Nursing.

Development of the general practice nurse role

The GPN role has grown, adapted and changed to include more advanced and specialist work to enhance patient care and reduce the pressures on General Practitioners (GPs); however, until recently, the GPN role has been poorly understood (Queen's Nursing Institute (QNI), 2015). To understand how the role has developed in this way, it is worth considering what has influenced this. When the National Health Service (NHS) was formed in 1948, GPs were appointed as independent contractors to provide medical care to all patients registered on their practice list. However, it was not until 1966 that a formal contract between the NHS and GPs was agreed, which included funding for ancillary staff and nurses (QNI, 2016). At that time, nurses who worked in general practice completed a limited range of tasks which could have been undertaken by any qualified nurse, and they acted as 'assistants' to GPs. Nurses in general practice were and still are employed by GPs who are independent contractors, which means that pay and terms and conditions of employment are independent of the NHS and not aligned to the NHS Agenda for Change (NHS Employers, 2019). The challenges associated with this have been acknowledged throughout the system and necessitate a review, although it will take new Primary Care Networks (PCNs), Local Medical Committees or GPs themselves to consider this in the long term as long as the current employment model exists. It is also worth noting that GPNs only became eligible to join the NHS Pension Scheme in 1997. Useful advice for GPNs regarding their pension arrangements can be found in the case study below. General practice remains the 'gatekeeper', which means that every individual must register with a GP to access health care across the United Kingdom (QNI, 2016).

Case study

Capital Nurse, in North Central London, has produced a guide, Taking Personal Responsibility for your NHS Pension–A Guide for General Practice Nurses, with helpful advice for GPNs: http://www.crosspathconsulting.co.uk/wp-content /uploads/2020/11/Practice-Nurse-Pensions-V1.pdf. (NB. At the time of writing, this guide is in draft format.)

Further changes to the GP Contract in 1990 and 2004 brought more emphasis to health promotion, screening and long-term condition management, and with that, a wider range of work and autonomy for GPNs. Some GPNs also expanded their role further and undertook the Specialist Practitioner Qualification (SPQ) or became Advanced Nurse Practitioners and developed their skills in the management of urgent or unscheduled care. Historically, GPN education, training and development were *ad hoc* and variable (Health Education England [HEE, 2017a]). The Royal College of General Practitioners produced a General Practice Nurse Competency Framework in 2015 (RCGP, 2015). Recently, the introduction of postregistration structured education programmes such as postgraduate Fundamentals of General Practice Nursing and other focused initiatives such as the NHS England and NHS Improvement GPN ten-point plan, HEE training hubs and the GPN career framework, aimed to standardise education for GPNs. This compares with GPs' training, which has benefited from a more structured Vocational Training Scheme (HEE, 2019). GPN training by comparison has been less formalised, and yet the GPN role is vital in so many ways for the population's health. At the time of writing, developments are ongoing, and 2021 will see a new career framework launched by NHS England/NHS Improvement in collaboration with Health Education England.

Policy affecting general practice nursing

GPNs are employed by small independent organisations owned by GPs. Access to training for GPNs is dependent upon the support offered from these individual employers. This has resulted in variation in the education and development offered to GPNs, and there is much variation between individual general practices (QNI, 2015). The requirement to standardise education and training for GPNs has led to several policy changes in recent years that have positively affected the profession.

There has been an acknowledgement that the role of the GPN is complex and has many facets. Specialist, up-to-date postregistration education is required for any new nurse entering the profession, as much of the undergraduate nursing curriculum historically focused on secondary care rather than primary or community care. Up-to-date clinical knowledge is essential for the role, as clinical advancements mean that health care delivery is forever changing and there is a requirement to keep abreast of these changes. GPNs are very aware of the Nursing and Midwifery Council (NMC) Code of Professional Standards to keep up to date and fulfil the requirements of the Code (NMC, 2018a); however, many GPNs are not aware of the policy that governs and determines general practice nursing.

In the last 5 to 10 years there have been several policy documents published by key organisations that have helped shape the future of general practice nursing. In 2014, NHS England published the Five Year Forward View (NHSE, 2014), which suggested that the GPN role would need to change to meet the demands and challenges of an ageing population with increasingly complex health care needs. GPNs are constantly required to take resourceful and innovative approaches to their consultations with patients, using a variety of ways to update and extend their knowledge and skills.

The General Practice Nursing Workforce Development Plan (HEE, 2017a) acknowledged this variation in GPN education, leadership and development. HEE also acknowledged that GPN training was often *ad hoc*, in-house and non-accredited and may not compare with training offered in organisations such as Higher Education Institutes that offer accredited education (HEE, 2017a). GPNs often work in isolated roles and may also be professionally isolated (Coventry University, 2016). Professional nursing support in general practice can be variable, depending on the number of nurses employed in the practice and whether there is any formalised leadership from a GPN lead. Often, professional development and advice can be sought from a GPN lead nurse employed by a Clinical Commissioning Group (CCG), and this is an important role that provides professional, clinical and leadership support and skills to GPNs.

Within the general practice nursing profession, there are significant workforce challenges. It has been acknowledged the lack of succession planning means that the GPN workforce is mainly made up of older individuals, with approximately 55% over the age of 50 years and only 10% under the age of 35 years. It has been estimated that one-third of GPNs are planning retirement in the next 5 to 10 years (NHSE, 2016a; QNI, 2015). The medical workforce in general practice is in a similar situation, and national organisations are focusing on finding new ways of working to address these workforce issues today and in the future to sustain and strengthen the general practice model (NHSE, 2016a; HEE, 2017a).

The QNI has advocated for the GPN role, which led to it producing a report in 2015 (QNI, 2015). This report, entitled 'General Practice Nursing in the 21st Century', helped to provide a focus on the GPN role and put forward evidence regarding the challenges and opportunities for GPNs. It was a call to action from which the QNI online resource 'Transition to General Practice Nursing' was developed (QNI, 2016).

The General Practice Forward View (NHSE, 2016a) pledged to increase investment and significantly expand the entire general practice workforce. Following this, Professor Jane Cummings launched a 5-year ten-point plan for general practice nursing (NHSE, 2016b) to raise the profile of the GPN role, and promote it as a first destination and viable career. The plan covered ten key actions that were designed to recruit, retain and return nurses to the profession to address the workforce challenges. The GPN ten-point plan has been further endorsed and prioritised by Ruth May, the current Chief Nursing Officer for England. The ten-point plan has produced many resources to support GPNs in their roles; one that is especially relevant to nurses new to general practice is the GPN induction template, which provides structure and support for nurses who are new to the role (NHS England, 2019a).

The NHS Long Term Plan (LTP) was published in 2019 and set out ambitions for the next 10 years to improve the quality of care delivered to patients, as well as health outcomes, to address some of the complex and challenging needs of the population (NHS England, 2019b). It introduced different ways of working in the form of PCNs, which encourage general practices to work together in groups of practices across a population of approximately 30,000 to 50,000 individuals. PCNs aim to provide opportunities for the nursing workforce to be involved and to plan and lead on the ambitions of the LTP, as well as bringing about much-needed change within the GPN profession to address many of the cultural, professional and workforce challenges. For these changes to be made, it is essential that nurses in general practice become aware of and involved in policy within the profession to bring about this essential change and to make general practice nursing fit for the future.

Specialist practitioner qualification

For many years, there has been an NMC recordable SPQ specifically for general practice nursing (NMC, 2001). Specialist practice involves higher levels of clinical judgement and decision-making, as well as improvement in the standards of care through skilled professional leadership, clinical audit, clinical research, teaching and support of colleagues (NMC, 2001). The NMC reviewed the educational standards relating to this and other postregistration programmes in 2020. In recent years, the SPQ has not been widely promoted or used in general practice nursing for many complex reasons. To promote the uptake of the SPQ, the QNI has introduced the Ellen Mary Award (QNI, 2019) to try to raise the profile of the SPQ and recognise the achievement of the most outstanding SPQ GPN students.

Advanced practice

The opportunity for GPNs to work at an advanced level exists, although the pathway to this outcome is currently poorly defined. The GPN ten-point plan aims to produce a more defined career pathway and framework to enable nurses who are new to the profession to understand the steps that need to be taken to progress their careers into advanced-level roles. In 1997, the United Kingdom Central Council missed an opportunity to set standards for advanced practice (NMC, 2001), and whilst there has been further educational development in an Advanced Clinical Practitioner (ACP) role (HEE, 2017b), there are no agreed standards for advanced practice, and this has led to variation in practice. In 2017, Health Education England produced an Advanced Clinical Practice framework to ensure that there is a national consistency in and understanding about what the ACP role is. In addition to this, the GPN ten-point plan produced a core capabilities framework (HEE, NHSE, Skills for Health, 2020) to assist GPNs working at an advanced level to map themselves against the ACP framework.

There are many similarities between the SPQ, which is recognised by the NMC, and the Advanced Clinical Practice educational programme, as they both cover core capabilities across clinical practice, health assessment, leadership and management, education and research. The Royal College of Nursing (RCN, 2018) has offered credentialing as a way forward and has stated that advanced practice is not about job titles but more about a level of practice (RCN, 2018). Furthermore, the NMC recognises the need to consider its role in regulation and plans to look at advanced practice as part of its wider review of nurse education and the development of its strategy for 2020 and beyond. In 2017, the QNI launched voluntary standards for general practice nursing education and practice for senior GPNs. These standards have been adopted by some universities and used as part of the SPQ GPN programme (NMC, 2001). Voluntary standards for nurses new to general practice nursing were also launched by the QNI in 2020 (QNI, 2020).

Aspects of the general practice nurse role

To look further into the many aspects of the GPN role, the nine dimensions of the NHS Leadership Academy Health Care Leadership Model (Fig. 1.1) have been used and applied to general practice nursing.

Inspiring shared purpose

Improving the population's health is a core component of general practice nursing. Inspiring patients to take responsibility for their own health and to be motivated to self-manage their condition is a vital skill as a GPN. The GPN could be seen as the lynchpin bringing many different sectors and agencies together for the benefit of the population, and this may become more evident as PCNs become more established (Penfold, 2019). GPNs are key members of the multidisciplinary team (MDT), and their unique holistic skills are beneficial to PCNs, to inspire a shared purpose and support inclusivity. As mentioned at the start of

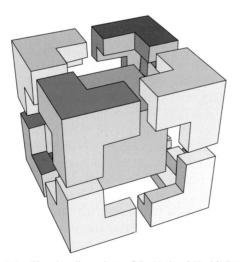

1. Inspiring shared purpose
2. Leading with care
3. Evaluating information
4. Connecting our service
5. Sharing the vision
6. Engaging the team
7. Holding to account
8. Developing capability
9. Influencing for results

Fig. 1.1   The nine dimensions of the National Health Service Leadership Academy Health Care Leadership Model. (From NHS Leadership Academy. (2013). *Healthcare Leadership Model: The nine dimensions of leadership behaviour.* http://www.leadershipacademy.nhs.uk/wp-content/uploads/2014/10/NHSLeadership-LeadershipModel-colour.pdf.)

this chapter, general practice nursing is unique in that it spans all age groups. 'From cradle to grave' is a term frequently used to identify the population served by GPNs; however, the role goes beyond this to incorporate preconceptual care that includes conversations with patients who are considering starting a family and involves the sharing of information and discussion that aims to empower individuals to make positive, healthy lifestyle changes. The Public Health Outcomes Framework sets out a vision that aims to improve the health of the nation (Public Health England, 2019a). With a target to increase healthy life expectancy and reduce differences in life expectancy and healthy life expectancy between communities, GPNs play an integral role in understanding the needs of their practice population and how to empower patients to make healthy life choices. The uniqueness of the GPN role is defined by the scope of practice and the specialism as an expert generalist. This requires knowledge and skills across a wide spectrum, from preconceptual care to end of life.

The areas of preconceptual care and frailty will be covered in this chapter, whilst health conditions relating to other age groups are covered in specific chapters within this book.

Preconceptual care

The provision of biomedical, behavioural and social health interventions to women and couples before conception occurs.

World Health Organisation (2012)

The National Institute for Health and Care Excellence (NICE, 2019a) recognises that preconceptual advice should be offered to all women from age 16 to 45 years. Within general practice, this requires a focused approach, with GPNs developing their knowledge, skills and competency to feel confident to undertake these discussions. The Office for National Statistics (2019) recently identified a decrease in conceptions amongst women below 40 years of age. Comparatively, conceptions in women over 40 years of age have increased for the second year running, and women over 35 years of age are often referred to as having 'advanced maternal age'. Evidence indicates that women who fall into this age group have an increased risk of poorer maternal outcomes from miscarriage, chromosomal abnormalities and obstetric complications.

It is recognised that poor nutritional intake, smoking, drug use and alcohol consumption are lifestyle choices that can have a major impact on the health of a woman and her baby (NICE, 2019a). To prevent this, preconceptual care should be routinely available for all women of reproductive age in primary care. To improve future pregnancy outcomes, a preconception consultation can open a discussion on the benefits of a healthy lifestyle that supports the development of a healthy baby, while acknowledging a woman's personal beliefs. GPNs are in an ideal position to use every opportunity to support patients in making positive changes to physical and mental health and wellbeing. Resources that support 'Making Every Contact Count' (NHS England, 2020a) are readily available at the following link: https://www.makingeverycontactcount.co.uk/media/1015/mecc_implementation_guide.pdf.

These conversations can be started opportunistically or at planned intervention appointments, for example, at cervical screening appointments, health check or sexual and reproductive health consultations, which are all ideal opportunities to discuss preconceptual care. An initial question of risk or intent of pregnancy can be a way to open the dialogue to reviewing personal aspects of health that may have an impact on fertility or future pregnancy. Skills and knowledge in undertaking this type of consultation can be gained by reviewing current evidence and best practice information, which can be found at: https://www.gov.uk/government/case-studies/preconception-and-pregnancy-opportunities-to-intervene.

The consultation should include discussion on:

- Physical health, including identification of past medical history and existing conditions
- Nutrition, including advice on nutritional supplements
- Consideration of over-the-counter, prescription and recreational drugs, alcohol and smoking
- Advice on genetic disorders if appropriate
- Contraception and cervical cytology screening history
- Psychosocial aspects

Dietary advice

Women should be encouraged to eat a healthy, balanced diet throughout their lives; however, for those women who wish to conceive, the GPN can have a discussion on the most up-to-date recommendations from NICE (2019a). This discussion can empower women to consider commencing nutritional supplements of folic acid and vitamin D, which support the growth of a healthy baby. Information regarding noncomplicated antenatal care can be accessed at: https://www.nice.org.uk/guidance/cg62/chapter/1-Guidance#lifestyle-considerations.

NICE (2019b) recommends taking 400 µg (0.4 mg) of folic acid supplements daily. This can reduce the risk of the baby developing neural tube defect (e.g., anencephaly or spina bifida) if taken at least a month before conception and for up to 12 weeks of the pregnancy. Folic acid is a vitamin which is found naturally in some foods such as spinach, sprouts, potatoes, green beans, cereals and bread, but this will not reliably supply adequate folic acid during pregnancy, when a good supply of folic acid is needed to aid the development of a healthy baby. Women can be advised to purchase folic acid supplements from their local pharmacist. However, for some women, it may be recommended to take 5 mg/day, and this will require a prescription as indicated in Box 1.1.

As a population, we all need vitamin D for development and maintenance of healthy bones. Many foods like oily fish, eggs, red meat and fortified cereals and spreads contain vitamin D. Sun exposure also promotes the generation of

---

Box 1.1 Indications for folic acid 5 mg

Previously affected pregnancy

Woman or partner (or family) with spinal cord defect

Currently taking medication for epilepsy

Body mass index >30 kg/m²

Woman affected by coeliac or diabetes

Woman affected by sickle cell or thalassaemia

From National Institute for Health and Care Excellence. (2019a). *Pre-conception – advice and management.* Clinical Knowledge Summary [online]. Available at: https://cks.nice.org.uk /pre-conception-advice-and-management#!scenario:1.

---

vitamin D, but in the United Kingdom, sunlight is more limited between October and April. Health professionals have a duty to recommend vitamin D supplements to specific population groups. NICE (2017a) recommends that, during pregnancy and whilst breast feeding, vitamin D supplements (10 μg/day) are prescribed to women, usually at the time of booking their first antenatal appointment.

Alcohol advice

Women should be advised to avoid alcohol consumption in the prenatal and pregnancy stages to reduce the chances of complications from alcohol use, as there are no known safe drinking limits (NICE, 2019a). Drinking alcohol has been linked to preterm birth and low birth weight, as well as more serious complications such as foetal alcohol spectrum disorder, an umbrella term used to describe a range of physical, learning and behavioural problems (Centers for Disease Control and Prevention, 2019).

Smoking advice

NICE guidance (2019a) advocates that all women planning a pregnancy or already pregnant who are smokers should be referred to stop smoking services. It has been found that women are four times more likely to quit with specialist support (NHS Smokefree, 2020). Smoking during pregnancy increases the risk of premature delivery, low birth weight, miscarriage, stillbirth and sudden infant death (NICE, 2019a). Immediate benefits can be seen from stopping smoking. The NHS Smokefree service offers women helpful tips and advice for a healthy pregnancy, with specialist support over the phone and through virtual platforms.

Pre-existing conditions

Many pre-existing medical conditions can adversely influence a woman's chances of conceiving (Harding, 2016). It is advisable that the woman continues with her usual form of contraception and any disease-specific medication until specific advice can be sought from a specialist team.

Preconceptual care for men

Preconceptual care should not only be isolated to women, as men will also benefit from a discussion about optimising their health (Manzoor, 2019 in Men's Health Forum, 2019). Aiming to empower men to increase control over their health and make positive changes will support development of a healthy baby. Advice on ways to improve male fertility is an important step to a successful pregnancy (Manzoor, 2019 in Men's Health Forum, 2019). However, this is a discussion that men may be reluctant to have with a GPN, so using 'Making Every Contact Count' can be a way of opening the discussion. It is known that men generally take more risks with their health than women (Baker, 2016), and therefore discussions should highlight weight management, use of alcohol within the recommended limit of 14 units per week, stopping smoking and avoiding recreational drugs. Encouraging exercise, a balanced diet, relaxation and mental wellbeing can assist in promoting health and fertility. Consideration must also be made for any underlying medical conditions and medications being taken, as some medicines may affect fertility (e.g., treatment of hypertension or depression). With the availability of helpful health-related advice on social media (Men's Health Forum, 2019), men can be guided to relevant websites that will offer support on many health-related issues while being supported by the GPN to make healthy lifestyle changes.

Termination of pregnancy

Because the percentage of conceptions leading to a termination of pregnancy has increased over the last 20 years (Department of Health, 2019), it is imperative that GPNs have an awareness of the local referral pathways that are available so that they can support women effectively. Legislation that governs termination of pregnancy dates to the Abortion Act (1967), which was later updated to the Human Fertilisation and Embryology Act (1990) (Legislation.gov.uk, 2020). By law, it is the responsibility of two doctors to agree that the woman meets the criteria for induced abortion, and that onward referral would need to be made. RCN (2017) offers clear guidelines for the professional role of the nurse who is involved in the care of women who reach a decision to terminate a pregnancy; this guidance can be found at the following link: https://www.rcn.org .uk/professional-development/publications/pub-005957.

Primarily, it is important to ensure that the woman is advised of all the options available to her so that she can make an informed decision and be provided the opportunity to discuss the risks and benefits of continuing or not continuing with her pregnancy. Supporting services for termination of pregnancy are offered by doctors, nurses, midwives and specialist community public health practitioners within a variety of settings. Most induced abortions can be carried out before 24 weeks of pregnancy, with those presenting later being considered if there is a risk (Legislation.gov.uk, 2020).

The general practice nurse's role in prevention and population health

The NHS LTP (NHS England, 2019b) suggests that primary care will be supported with funding, improved technology and improved ways of working to improve the health of the local population. The plan aims to move away from a model of just treating illness to preventing illness, identifying illness earlier and helping people earlier, using a comprehensive model of universal personalised care, which means that patients will have more choice and control over their mental and physical health, similar to that which they have come to expect in every other aspect of their life. Universal personalised care resources can be found here: https://www.england.nhs.uk/publication/universal -personalised-care-implementing-the-comprehensive-model/.

Person-centred care

There is no single definition of person-centred care; nonetheless, person-centred care emphasises health care quality and patient safety and means that patients are listened to and shown respect regarding how they want to be treated, taking into account their full range of physical, psychological and social needs. Patients become central to their own care pathway, with the ability to make informed decisions to effectively manage their health care needs (NHS England, 2020b). Person-centred care has not traditionally been considered an intrinsic aspect of health care quality, but over the last 20 years, it has increasingly become a prominent ambition within health care. Recent policy documents emphasise the value of patients' views (Five Year Forward View, NHS England, 2014). However, a survey by National Voices (2017) reported variation across the country depending upon what services were used and called for person-centred care to be given greater priority.

Recognising the challenges that the NHS faces in the current climate, the Health Foundation (2016) recommended that the health sector reconsider the relationship between the patient and services on offer. This would ensure a tailored and coordinated approach to care that incorporates the four principles of person-centred care (Fig. 1.2). Consideration for each element of the framework empowers patients to develop knowledge and become leaders in their own health care and treatment. For the therapeutic relationship to develop, the patient's wishes are explored to set goals and key priorities of care. The process recognises the patient's existing skills and experiences and the things that matter to them the most (NHS England, 2020c).

Personalised care benefits from an integrated approach and requires effective communication across health and social care.

Social prescribing

Person-centred care can be achieved by introducing social prescribing (NHS England, 2019c), which is when health professionals refer patients to support in the community to improve their health and wellbeing. Referring patients to

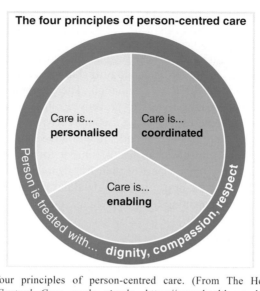

Fig. 1.2   The four principles of person-centred care. (From The Health Foundation. (2016). *Person-Centred Care made simple.* https://www.health.org.uk/sites/default/files /PersonCentredCareMadeSimple.pdf.)

a link worker in the practice can give patients more time to focus on 'what matters to them' and help them connect to community groups and statutory services for practical and emotional support. The King's Fund (2017) recognises that this approach and similar approaches have been used by the NHS for many years, and that people's health is determined by a range of factors, including social, economic and environmental issues. Social prescribing schemes therefore aim to address these issues in a holistic way, to maximise personalised care and realise the LTP.

All our health

Public Health England (PHE) has produced 'All Our Health' e-learning resources (PHE, 2019a), which aim to increase the knowledge, confidence and skills of health and care professionals in terms of preventing illness, protecting health and promoting patient wellbeing by embedding prevention into everyday practice. These resources also help clinicians to maximise health outcomes and reduce health inequalities (PHE, 2019a) and can be found at: https://portal.e-lfh .org.uk/Catalogue/Index?HierarchyId=0_41737_42670&programmeId=41737.

GPNs develop long-lasting professional relationships with their patients and are well-placed to understand individuals' specific difficulties. PHE has produced specific information regarding personalised care and population health, which focuses on lifestyle risk factors and making healthy choices; these resources can help GPNs within their consultations with patients (PHE, 2019b). The RCN (2019a) has also developed a range of webpages to help nurses access information in a quick and easy way; for example, information on cardiovascular

disease (CVD) prevention (PHE, 2019c) can be found here: https://www.rcn
.org.uk/clinical-topics/public-health/cardiovascular-disease-prevention.

Motivating people to reduce their risks and inspiring them to make lifestyle
changes is very much part of the GPN role. For example, GPNs have a vital role
to play in the achievement of the cardiovascular ambitions launched by PHE in
February 2019 (PHE, 2019d). The current focus is on atrial fibrillation, hypertension and hypercholesterolaemia, and more information can be found at the following site: https://www.england.nhs.uk/ourwork/clinical-policy/cvd/. CVD is still a
leading cause of death worldwide, and in England, accounts for one in four deaths
(PHE, 2019d). Poor cardiovascular health is linked to atrial fibrillation, hypertension and hypercholesterolaemia (PHE, 2019d). Therefore, the CVD ambitions
are particularly important for GPNs, and engaging people in lifestyle discussions
using motivational techniques to help them make some changes is a vital skill.

Many long-term diseases and conditions such as CVD are measured by
the Quality Outcomes Framework (QOF), which is a set of measures (indicators) and attached points that help GP practices understand how they are
doing. Much of the work of GPNs is now linked to these long-term conditions, for example, heart attack, stroke, diabetes, chronic obstructive pulmonary disease, heart failure, chronic kidney disease, peripheral arterial disease
and dementia. More information on the QOF can be found here: https://digital
.nhs.uk/data-and-information/data-tools-and-services/data-services/general
-practice-data-hub/quality-outcomes-framework-qof.

Leading with care

A further dimension of the NHS Leadership Model (NHS Leadership Academy,
2013) is leading with care, and placing more emphasis on the importance of
strong nursing leadership has been evident since the launch of the NHS ten-
point plan for GPNs (NHSE, 2016b). Many existing GPNs would not necessarily consider themselves as leaders because many associate the term 'leader'
with a position of authority rather than influence. Many GPNs support, motivate
and inspire not only their general practice teams but also the expanding group of
allied health care professionals who are working in general practice. GPNs can
lead in specific areas of responsibility to assist the running of the practice. This
is particularly so since the launch of Care Quality Commission (CQC) inspections after the Health and Social Care Act in 2008; information on the CQC can
be found at: http://www.legislation.gov.uk/ukpga/2008/14/contents.

GPNs have an opportunity to lead with supporting patients with learning
disabilities in conducting physical health checks. It is possible to build up trust
and become a familiar figure to really make a difference in this area. In general
practice, there is a unique opportunity to really get to know patients and their
families and carers, which enables personalised care planning. Knowing the
local community and what is available means that GPNs can signpost and work
with organisations to provide some much-needed support, for example, arranging

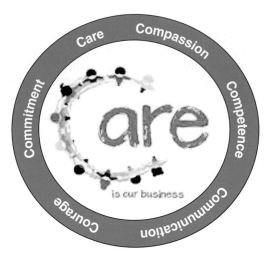

Fig. 1.3 The six fundamental values of compassionate care. (From NHS England. (2012). *Compassion in practice.* https://www.england.nhs.uk/wp-content/uploads/2012/12/compassion-in -practice.pdf.)

for someone to go swimming with a person with a learning disability, or to facilitate an exercise programme along with advising where weight management support groups meet.

Leading with compassion

The Compassion in Practice strategy (NHS England, 2012), incorporating the six Cs (care, compassion, competence, communication, courage, and commitment), which was launched in 2012 by the previous Chief Nursing Officer, Jane Cummings, set out a vision for compassionate care and can be found here: https://www.england .nhs.uk/6cs/wp-content/uploads/sites/25/2015/03/cip-6cs.pdf (Fig. 1.3).

These values embody the GPN role, which focuses on assisting people to remain independent, maximise their wellbeing and improve their health. GPNs get to know their practice population and often use their intuition or rely on their hunches about people, perhaps having a sense that something is not right. This can sometimes make it difficult to explain why there might be a problem, but working in general practice in partnership and collaboration with GPs and other health care team colleagues means that someone else in the team may also know the individual personally, so concerns may be shared. This can enable more personalised care and support to be offered to really lead the delivery of high-quality care.

Evaluating information

An essential part of a patient consultation involves evaluating information to decide the direction of care. The uniqueness of the GPN role is that it includes regular follow-up and annual review, which enables evaluation of the care provided, and this in turn enhances job satisfaction, especially when a person returns after making some changes, and health issues have improved. For those nurses new to the role, it can feel quite daunting, particularly with time-pressured appointment systems and only 10 to 15 minutes with a patient in which to evaluate all the information gathered and decide about ongoing care. Addressing the immediate priorities is crucial, but in general practice, there is always the option to offer a further appointment if necessary to discuss issues further. The opportunity of time or a 'wait and see approach' can be an advantage in general practice nursing, as GPNs can also focus on prevention, and then adopt a more proactive approach in subsequent follow-up visits.

Leading change

GPNs are in a valuable position to use information held on the general practice computer systems, which provide data that can be used to help them to innovate and lead new ways of working. For example, if a practice has a high number of people with diabetes on the QOF register, a GPN could consider how these patients might access care in a way that will both meet their needs and support the practice. One example of this could be to introduce group consultations for patients to provide health education, which in turn would also offer peer support (NHS England, 2019d). 'Group work is valuable because it provides opportunities for social inclusion, connection, creativity and care' (Gillam, 2018). An example of where GPNs have led on one such initiative can be found in the following case study.

Case study

General practice nurses in the Premiere Health Team, Leigh (Wigan CCG) and West Gorton (Manchester CCG) medical practices introduced group consultations for adults with type 2 diabetes (NHS England, 2019d). This new approach has led to better outcomes, experiences and use of resources locally.

---

https://www.england.nhs.uk/atlas_case_study/introducing-group-consultations-for-adults-with-type-2-diabetes/

Connecting our service

With the new models of care and a range of new allied health care professions joining general practice, GPNs are in a good position to connect everyone and act as team leaders. Digital resources enable health professionals to connect even though they work in isolation, and are an essential way of sharing information and resources.

Digital champions

The use of digitally enabled care is supported in the LTP, and advances in digital technology are improving clinical care. Digital nurse champion roles have been developed to lead the change in general practice (Chambers et al., 2018a).

Box 1.2   General practice nurse single point site

The General Practice Nurse (GPN) Single Point platform can be used to:

- Access national programme resources such as nursing workforce induction templates and national clinical protocols
- Share information on recruitment, retention and return-to-practice initiatives
- Obtain direct access to regional GPN workforce data
- Find good practice case studies
- Be part of the regional GPN transformation
- Access the clinical supervision model and supporting digital platform
- Contribute to discussion forums

Access to the platform can be obtained by emailing england.gpnsinglep@nhs.net. (From NHS. (2020). *Future NHS Collaboration Platform: GPN single point* [online]. Available at: https://future.nhs.uk.)

Computer tablet devices are being used in consultations, for example, to share information on health apps or to take digital clinical photographs to upload to patient records. Video technology (e.g., Skype), can be used for discussions with professional colleagues or to enable remote consultations between health care professionals and patients (Chambers et al., 2018b). This will be discussed further later in the book, and progress had been made in this area, especially during the COVID-19 pandemic.

Sharing the vision

General practice nurse single point site

As part of the NHS England GPN ten-point plan, a GPN Single Point site has been set up to share resources, news and ideas (Box 1.2).

Engaging the team

Source4Networks

Using platforms such as Source4Networks can link GPNs in a community of practice to share useful information and provide a much-needed support network of information. Source4Networks is an online platform for leaders developed by the NHS Sustainable Improvement team and London South Bank University; further information can be found at the following link: https://www.england.nhs.uk/sustainableimprovement/source4networks/.

Holding to account

The advent of the Health and Social Care Act in 2008 and the CQC inspections has ensured that general practices are held to account for the care that they provided. As a result, this has provided an opportunity for GPNs to take on additional roles, such as being the Lead for Infection Prevention and Control in their general practice. Resources including posters, workbooks, audit tools and policies, such as those available on the Infection Prevention Control website are useful for promoting good practice and procedures. GPN lead nurses and practice managers may find these resources helpful in preparations for CQC visits; they can be found at the following link: https://www.infectionpreventioncontrol .co.uk/gp-practices/.

Safeguarding

GPNs have a vital role in safeguarding children and adults. The Safeguarding Accountability and Assurance Framework (NHS England and NHS Improvement, 2019) brings together important documents and clarifies the roles and responsibilities of all involved in promoting the safety, protection and welfare of children, young people and adults. Because of the varied nature of the GPN role, there may be many occasions when safeguarding concerns may be raised, and this document provides links to guidance and legislation. The framework can be found at the following link: https://www.england.nhs.uk /wp-content/uploads/2015/07/safeguarding-children-young-people-adults-at -risk-saaf-1.pdf.

The NHS Safeguarding app is available on mobile devices. The app provides instant access to information that defines abuse and explains the statutory responsibilities. It also includes a Children and Young Persons Guide and an Adult Guide and a Staff Guide, with information on training timeframes, length and minimum hours. The link to the site can be found at: http://www.myguideapps .com/projects/safeguarding/default/.

Developing capability

It has been mentioned that one-third of GPNs are planning to retire in the next 5 to 10 years, so there is an urgent need to encourage more student nurse placements and to develop the current and future workforce (QNI, 2016). Some general practices have had preregistration student nurses on placements supported by GPNs for many years (Boast, 2015; Lane and Peake, 2015) and have been able to grow their own future workforce through employing them as newly qualified nurses. The Shape of Caring Review (HEE, 2015) highlighted the importance of training our future nurses and focused on raising the bar further in this area to make assessor and supervisor roles commonplace in general practice. The Shape of Caring Review can be found at the following link: https:// www.hee.nhs.uk/sites/default/files/documents/2348-Shape-of-caring-review -FINAL.pdf.

The General Practice Nursing Workforce Development Plan (HEE, 2017) and the GPN ten-point action plan (NHS England, 2016b) also recommended increasing the number of placements for preregistration nursing students in general practice and developing the role of the GPN educator to support this. In this role, GPNs work with CCGs and Training Hubs to improve the experience for student nurses and those new to general practice nursing. In the future, linking this role up to the PCNs will also enhance the training and support available. The NMC Standards for Student Supervision and Assessment (NMC, 2018b) highlight that all nurses have the responsibility of supervising others. The following link provides access to the standards: https://www.nmc.org.uk/standards-for -education-and-training/standards-for-student-supervision-and-assessment/.

ACPs are multiprofessional health care professionals, including nurses, educated to Master's level or equivalent, with the skills and knowledge to allow them to expand their scope of practice to better meet the needs of the people they care for. ACPs are deployed across all health care settings and work at a level of advanced clinical practice that pulls together the four ACP pillars of clinical practice, leadership and management, education and research. A definition of ACP, its underpinning standards and governance, can be found in the multiprofessional framework for advanced clinical practice: https://www.hee .nhs.uk/our-work/advanced-clinical-practice/multi-professional-framework. The framework ensures there is national consistency in the level of practice across multiprofessional roles that is clearly understood by the public, advanced clinical practitioners, their colleagues, education providers and employers.

Influencing for results

GPNs work in a unique situation, and there is a real opportunity for GPNs to develop leadership skills to influence improvement that will lead to change and add value (NHS England, 2016c). There are opportunities for GPNs to influence within the PCNs, reviewing the needs of the PCN populations and working across the network to effect change and improvement. For example, GPNs could work together with GPNs from other practices to ensure adequate skill sets are available to cover the whole area. This would work well for long-term condition expertise or wound care, for example, especially in view of the workforce issues. Some nurses in general practice have taken up clinical director roles within PCNs or have become nurse partners within a general practice (Penfold, 2019; Belton & Sears, 2017).

Addressing frailty

Frailty has been referred to as a 'syndrome' that encompasses the effects of ageing alongside multiple long-term conditions (Lyndon, 2018). A person who is frail loses the ability to maintain homeostasis, leading to complications such as dehydration, increased falls, inadequate nutrition and lowered resistance to infection, leading to adverse outcomes of hospitalisation, disability, nursing home admission or mortality (Clegg et al., 2016).

It is inevitable that GPNs will encounter patients living with frailty as the syndrome becomes more prevalent across our society because of an ageing population, and as the number of people living with long-term conditions increases. The British Geriatric Society (2019) identifies 10% of the population over 65 years of age, and a quarter of those over 85 years of age as having frailty. According to Smith and Wallington (2019), frailty is not inevitably linked to ageing, although it occurs more often as people get older. The term frailty has been used to describe the condition of patients with multiple morbidities (multiple long-term conditions) and people living with a physical disability. Although there may be an overlap in the management of these two patient populations, it is important to understand the differences. A patient with multiple long-term conditions may not have been assessed for frailty if the focus of care is on each individual disease, and there may be a cohort of patients worthy of undergoing a more focused review. Patients with a long-term physical disability may not have frailty, whereas those with frailty may have a disability (British Geriatric Society, 2019). Frailty varies in severity, and care should be taken so that patients are not labelled. Remembering that frailty is a long-term condition, but not a static state, ensures that the care of the patient is individualised.

A person living with mild frailty has twice the risk of mortality compared with an older, fit person (British Geriatric Society, 2019). The strongest risk factor for frailty is age, alongside gender, with a higher prevalence found in women (Turner, 2014). There are over 4000 admissions a day for people living with mild, moderate or severe frailty. The British Geriatric Society refers to five frailty syndromes, as shown in Fig. 1.4.

The central problem with frailty is the potential for adverse reactions to minor stressors or changes that can range, for example, from a minor episode of influenza to an unplanned admission following a fall. Thus, interaction with a health care professional in general practice can be a trigger to initiate

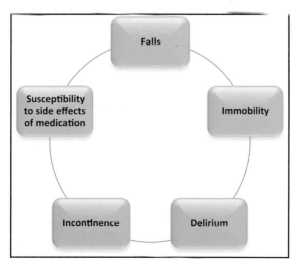

Fig. 1.4 Frailty syndromes. (From Turner, G. (2014). *Introduction to frailty, fit for frailty.* https://www.bgs.org.uk.)

an assessment for frailty. It needs to be acknowledged that the frailty state is not static, and interventions can be put in place to support the patient.

There are two broad models of frailty. The first, which has central features of physical frailty, is known as a 'Phenotype Model' (Fried et al., 2001) and encompasses a set of symptoms. The presence of three out of the five symptoms is a predictor of the presence of frailty.

- Unintentional weight loss
- Reduced physical activity
- Slow walking speed
- Weakness
- Self-reported exhaustion, low energy expenditure

The second model is described as a 'Frailty Index' that defines an accumulation of physical to psychosocial deficits over time (Davies et al., 2018). The British Geriatric Society (2014) refers to this second model as the 'Cumulative Deficit Model', which encompasses physical, cognitive and social factors that influence the condition. Through liaison with clinical pharmacists in practice, patients' medication should also be reviewed, as there is a developing area of interest linking certain medicines and polypharmacy to the development of frailty.

There is global concern that existing health care systems cannot meet the demand of the increasing number of patients with frailty. The NHS Plan (NHS England, 2019b) recognises the need to put systems in place to support this vulnerable group of patients and pledges to improve care of older people living with frailty and those with long-term conditions. To reduce unwarranted variation in services across health and social care through a collaborative approach with key stakeholders, NHS Right Care has produced the 'NHS Right Care Frailty Toolkit' (British Geriatric Society, 2019), which supports the NHS Plan in caring for older people and signposts the way in recognising older people with frailty and supporting them to live well for longer.

Promotion of healthy ageing offers the chance to avoid the onset of frailty. GPNs can play an integral role in supporting the ageing well agenda, offering advice on preventable or modifiable risk factors and signposting to available resources that support care and long-term health. GPNs would benefit from enhancing their knowledge and skills in recognising and managing frailty. RCN (2019b) offers online resources to support health professionals in the recognition and management of frailty. A partnership between NHS England and NHS Improvement along with Health Education England has supported Skills for Health to develop a framework for frailty core capabilities that supports the development of knowledge and skills across four domains. Understanding these principles will aid the GPN in undertaking a training needs analysis and producing a development plan. This framework can be found at: https://www.skillsforhealth.org.uk/services /item/607-frailty-core-capabilities-framework.

It is imperative that GPNs recognise people living with frailty so that appropriate care plans can be put in place to support the patient; validated screening tools are available to aid risk stratification. Introduced into the GP Contract 2017/18 and becoming a contractual requirement, the electronic frailty index uses information stored within the electronic patient record to aid in identifying the degree of frailty, prompting the clinician to review the patients care in those over 65 years of age, which can aid in the planning and delivery of appropriate services (British Medical Association, 2018). The tool uses the Cumulative Deficit Model that measures frailty based on a range of deficits, and then generates a score indicating a frailty category of fit, mild, moderate or severe. Using correct read coding during consultations helps identify patients for frailty registers; it is therefore important that any new general practice staffs are offered information technology (IT) systems training to become familiar with IT infrastructure and systems.

End-of-life care

You matter because you are you, and you matter to the end of your life. We will do all we can not only to help you die peacefully, but also to live until you die.
Dame Cicely Saunders, nurse, physician, writer, and founder of
hospice movement (1918–2005)

End of life is a term used by professionals to signify the final stages of life. Every year over half a million people die in the United Kingdom, mainly within the hospital setting (RCN, 2019c). It is now acknowledged that, as people are living longer, they may not always get the right care they need in the right setting at the right time or at a particularly vulnerable time; people at the end of life need these structures in place (National Institute for Health Research, 2015). The NHS LTP (NHS England, 2019b) is investing in care closer to home, developing teams that can support care out of hospital and pledging to introduce personalised care and proactive care planning for individuals in the last year of life. In England, it is estimated that each general practice will have approximately 20 deaths per year. Nevertheless, with the changing demographics of an ageing population, it is projected that there will be an increase in the number of individuals approaching end of life in the next few years. By the time people reach the end of their lives, they often have multiple conditions with complex needs (NHS Improving Quality, 2014); it is therefore important that roles and skills are refined to equip primary care staff to support these patients.

End-of-life care has often been seen as the role of a specialist nurse. However, this is no longer the case: the RCN (2019c) states that it is the role of every nurse working in any setting that is involved with an individual who is dying. The individual and his or her family must be assured that all staff members involved in their care are competent, compassionate and confident. A systematic review undertaken by Mitchell et al. (2018) reviewed key journal articles dating from 2000 to 2017 regarding end-of-life care in general practice and identified a lack of evidence that GPNs play a key role in these pathways of care, therefore recommending further research in this area. Nonetheless, as the role of GPNs expands, their key skills and attributes can be valuable to support patients at the end of life. Key skills needed to deliver this care identified by RCN (2019c) are cited in Table 3.0. A study by Matthews (2019) suggests training of health care professionals can often be challenging because of lack of access and staff shortages. Health Education resource e-learning for Health offers valuable online training and education for end-of-life care, which covers a wide range of interactive sessions that are suitable for the GPN to access. Other suitable learning resources are available from Macmillan Learn Zone (2020), which offers a foundation online course in palliative and end-of-life care and can be accessed here: https://learnzone .org.uk/macprofs/238.

Improving care for patients nearing the end of their lives is a highly valued aspect of the work within general practice and one that requires a whole-team approach. Although there remains a stigma attached to dying, which results in avoidance of discussing issues surrounding death and dying, a key aspect of end-of-life care is identifying the patient's wishes. The GPN can be proactive in this area by starting these discussions, allowing patients to express how and where they wish to be cared for and starting the conversations for care planning (Table 1.1).

End-of-life policy

A report by the Primary Care Workforce Commission (2015) called for each patient to have a named clinician who leads on his or her care. The LTP (NHS England, 2019b) encourages GPs over the next 5 years GPs to further improve

Table 1.1 **Key skills for end-of-life care.**

Communication	The ability to initiate and take part in conversations about death and dying
Assessment	The ability to assess people's needs in partnership with the individual, family and carers. Discuss with everyone involved, ensuring this is written down and shared
Coordination	All care, treatment needs and wishes of individuals are shared with everyone who has contact with them. This is coordinated by one named lead, ensuring he or she is available for the dying person, their family and other health professionals involved in the care
Competence	All nurses are competent to deliver compassionate and sensitive end-of-life care with support from the wider multidisciplinary team

From RCN (2019c).

the services they provide for patients in the last year of life and support their families. Using a collaborative approach to care across primary and secondary care, the MDT can offer a structured supportive pathway for those who are nearing the end of life, alongside their families and carers. The GP contract QOF (NHS England, 2019) sets out a quality improvement domain for end-of-life care. These standards encourage more patients to be identified and placed on a register and offered advanced care plans to live well and die well in a place of their choosing.

The Gold Standards Framework (GSF) has a huge impact on the quality of care at the end of patients' lives. Originally developed as a national strategy in 1998 to support frontline health care professionals in optimising care for patients approaching end of life, the prognostic indicator tool GSF is now truly embedded within primary care.

Communication in end-of-life care

Death, dying and bereavement are important parts of everyone's life, and, although inevitable, they are also unpredictable. Effective communication is central to caring for patients and their families when approaching the end of life (King, 2018 in Chiltern & Bain, 2018). The support not only provides information, but also acts as a comfort that someone is listening, making them feel valued and respected. Therefore, offering choice and control in things that are important to them at this time is vital. A review of the 'choice in end of life care' report (Choice in End of Life Programme Board, 2015) suggested asking those approaching end of life one simple question, 'What is important to you?' can open the gateway to conversations focused on the wishes of the patient. At the centre of good-quality end-of-life care is sensitive and effective communication with the patient and his or her family/carer. This will require a variety of knowledge and skills for the GPN to be able to demonstrate the highest standards of care.

Advanced care planning

Advanced care planning follows a person-centred approach, allowing the patient to maintain some control over decisions of how to be cared for in the future. Advanced care planning has been defined as a process that supports adults at any age and stage of health to convey their wishes (RCN, 2019c). Advanced care planning can be undertaken at any point, from being well to the end stage of dying, allowing a patient's choices to be formally recorded (RCN, 2019c). These wishes may take the form of withholding certain treatments, making advanced decisions on how the patient wishes to be cared for or appointing people under a lasting power of attorney to make decisions on their behalf when they lose capacity.

End-of-life care is discussed more openly within general practice. Because GPNs are key members of the MDT, they hold some responsibility to advocate on behalf of the patient to ensure a coordinated plan of care is followed. It is imperative that GPNs are therefore educated in the policies and procedures to follow for end-of-life care so they can effectively collaborate with the MDT to manage this life stage.

Because the population is ageing and more people are living longer with complex health care needs and long-term conditions, this will inevitably mean that GPNs will encounter patients who are approaching end of life. These patients will need good palliative care that will often involve the input from a MDT. GPNs may encounter patients who have malignancies and other life-limiting conditions who are well enough to continue to visit the GP practice. Depending on their experience, GPNs may be involved in having conversations with patients about the issue of dying. In the United Kingdom, it has been suggested that 56% to 70% of people would prefer to die at home, yet of the 500,000 people who die each year in England, 58% die in hospital (Dying Matters Coalition, 2018). Information like this is available at: www.dyingmatters.org/overview/why-talk-about-it. In recent years, end-of-life care has gained recognition, and as a result, the End of Life Care Strategy was published in 2008. The strategy set out clear guidance for the development of care pathways for patients near the end of their life.

A King's Fund report from Marie Curie Cancer Care entitled 'Improving choice at the end of life' (King's Fund, 2008) demonstrated that a pilot project helped to double the number of terminally ill people able to die at home. However, the reality is that most people die in hospital, even though around 40% have no medical need to be there. Additional research by the charity also showed that patients who were already in hospital expressed a preference to return home to die, even if they required complex care. The research proved that many patients wish to die at home, and they must be given every possible opportunity to do so, to ensure that their dignity is maintained.

Charter for end-of-life care

Health professionals including general practitioners and nurses in primary care now have a charter, developed by the Royal College of General Practitioners (RCGP, 2011), to assist with better care for patients at the end of their lives. The charter features seven key pledges to help patients live as well and as long as they can, including:

- That the primary care team will do all they can to help patients preserve their independence, dignity and sense of personal control throughout the course of their illness.
- That the primary care team will support those close to the patient, both as patients approach the end of life and through bereavement.
  Additional resources can be found at:
  https://rcni.com/hosted-content/rcn/fundamentals-of-end-of-life-care/rcn-principles
     -of-nursing-practice
  https://www.rcgp.org.uk/endoflifecare
  https://www.nhs.uk/conditions/end-of-life-care/

Conclusion

General practice nursing has evolved from being a task-orientated role in which GPNs act as an assistant to the GP, to an autonomous and proactive career. It clearly offers many varied opportunities, and many report the joy of working in such a diverse role. People in the care of GPNs benefit from the continuity of care provided in general practice, and there are reported improvements in clinical outcomes, uptake of preventative services, medication concordance and overall care experience among patients who receive care from a GPN (Palmer et al., 2018). GPNs are in the unique position of being able to provide care and follow families throughout their lives. GPNs are generalists, but are also specialists within their roles, particularly in long-term condition management. Many take the lead in some clinical areas and motivate and coach patients to reflect on their own health to make positive changes. Enthusiasm and self-motivation are needed especially, as the role may also involve lone working, so building supportive networks and reaching out to colleagues will be important to control stress and get the balance right. A calm, steady, flexible and resilient approach will help GPNs manage the autonomy of the role.

References

Baker, P. (2016). Men's health: An overlooked inequality. *British Journal of Nursing, 25*(19), 1054–1057.

Belton, J. & Sears, C. (2017). How to become a nurse partner. *Nursing in Practice.* https://www.nursinginpractice.com/how-become%E2%80%A6-nurse-partner.

Boast, G. (2015). Highlighting the value of mentoring students in general practice. *Practice Nursing, 26*(11), 560–563.

British Geriatric Society. (2014). *Introduction to frailty good practice guide.* https://www.bgs.org.uk/resources/introduction-to-frailty.

British Geriatric Society. (2019). *NHS right care, Frailty Toolkit.* https://www.bgs.org.uk/resources/nhs-rightcare-frailty-toolkit.

British Medical Association. (2018). *Focus on identification and management of patients with frailty.* https://www.bma.org.uk/advice/employment/contracts/general-practice-funding/focus-on-identification-and-management-of-patients-with-frailty.

Brown, S. L. (2010). Foreword. In G. Plester & C. Montgomery (Eds.), *A to Z handbook for nurses in General Practice: Reference Guide and Practical Tool.* Montgomery Plester.

Centers for Disease Control and Prevention. (2019). *Fetal alcohol spectrum disorders.* https://www.cdc.gov/ncbddd/fasd/facts.html.

Chambers, R., McKinney, R., Schmid, M., & Beaney, P. (2018a). Digital by choice: Becoming part of a digitally ready general practice team. *Primary Health Care, 28*(7), 22–27.

Chambers, R., Schmid, M., Jabbouri, A. A., & Beaney, P. (2018b). *Making digital healthcare happen in practice: A practical handbook.* Otmoor Publishing Ltd.

Chiltern, S. & Bain, H. (2018). *A textbook of community nursing.* Routledge.

Choice in End of Life Programme Board. (2015). *What's important to me. A review of choice in end of life.* https://assets.publishing.service.gov.uk/government/uploads/system/uploads/attachment_data/file/407244/CHOICE_REVIEW_FINAL_for_web.pdf.

Clegg, A., Bates, C., Young, J., et al. (2016). Development and validation of an electronic frailty index using primary care electronic health record. *Age and Ageing, 45*(3), 353–360.

Coventry University. (2016). *General Practice Nursing – leadership for quality. Programme evaluation May 2015 to March 2016*. GPNLQ report. Coventry University.

Davies, B., Baxter, H., Rooney, J., et al. (2018). Frailty assessment in primary health care and its association with unplanned secondary care use, a rapid review. *BJGP Open Journal, 2*(1), bjgpopen18X101325.

Department of Health. (2019). *Abortion statistics, England and Wales*. https://assets.publishing .service.gov.uk/government/uploads/system/uploads/attachment_data/file/808556/Abortion _Statistics__England_and_Wales_2018__1_.pdf.

Dying Matters Coalition. (2018). *Why talk about it?* www.dyingmatters.sorg/overview/why-talk -about-it.

Fried, L. P., Tangen, C. M., & Walston, J. (2001). Frailty in older adults: Evidence for a phenotype. *The Journals of Gerontology. Series A, Biological Sciences and Medical Sciences, 56*(3), M146–M156.

Gillam, T. (2018). *Creativity, wellbeing and mental health practice*. Palgrave Pivot.

Harding, M. (2016). *Planning to become pregnant*. https://patient.info/pregnancy/planning-to -become-pregnant.

Health Education England, NHS England/Improvement and Skills for Health. (2020). *Core capabilities framework for advanced clinical practice (nurses) working in general practice/ primary care in England*. https://www.skillsforhealth.org.uk/images/services/cstf/ACP%20 Primary%20Care%20Nurse%20Fwk%202020.pdf.

Health Education England. (2019). *The GP training programme*. https://gprecruitment.hee.nhs.uk /recruitment/training.

Health Education England. (2017). *The General Practice Nursing workforce development plan*. https://www.hee.nhs.uk/sites/default/files/documents/The%20general%20practice%20nursing%20workforce%20development%20plan.pdf.

Health Education England. (2017b). *Multi-professional framework for advanced clinical practice in England*. https://www.hee.nhs.uk/our-work/advanced-clinical-practice/multi-professional -framework.

Health Education England. (2015). *Shape of Caring Review. Raising the bar: A review of the future education and training of registered nurses and care assistants*. https://www.hee.nhs.uk/sites /default/files/documents/2348-Shape-of-caring-review-FINAL.pdf.

King's Fund. (2008). *Improving choice at the end of life*. https://www.kingsfund.org.uk/publications /improving-choice-end-life.

Lane, P. & Peake, C. (2015). A scheme to increase practice nurse numbers*111*(13), 22–25.

Legislation.gov.uk. (2020). *Human Fertilisation and Embryology Act (1990)*. http://www .legislation.gov.uk/ukpga/1990/37/contents.

Lyndon, H. (2018). How GPNs can meet the challenges of frailty in primary care. *Journal of General Practice Nursing, 4*(4), 47–52.

Macmillan Cancer Support. (2020). *Learn zone*. https://learnzone.org.uk/macprofs/238.

Matthews, E. (2019). Surprise questions that can improve end of life care. *Nursing Older People, 31*(6), 15.

Men's Health Forum. (2019). https://www.menshealthforum.org.uk/.

Mitchell, G., Senior, H., Johnson, C., et al. (2018). Systematic review of general practice end-of-life symptom control. *BMJ Supportive & Palliative Care, 8*(4), 411–420.

National Institute for Health and Care Excellence. (2017). *Vitamin D: Supplement use in specific population groups*. https://www.nice.org.uk/guidance/ph56.

National Institute for Health and Care Excellence. (2019a). Pre-conception – advice and management. *Clinical Knowledge Summary.* https://cks.nice.org.uk/pre-conception-advice-and-mana gement#!scenario:1.

National Institute for Health and Care Excellence. (2019b). Antenatal Care for uncomplicated pregnancies. *Clinical Guideline CG62.* https://www.nice.org.uk/guidance/cg62/chapter/1 -Guidance#lifestyle-considerations.

National Institute for Health Research. (2015). *Better Endings Right care right place right time.* https://content.nihr.ac.uk/nihrdc/themedreview-000826-BE/Better-endings-FINAL -WEB.pdf.

National Office of Statistics. (2019). *Conceptions in England and Wales: 2017.* https://www.ons .gov.uk/peoplepopulationandcommunity/birthsdeathsandmarriages/conceptionandfertilityrates /bulletins/conceptionstatistics/2017.

National Voices. (2017). *Person-centred care evidence from service users.* https://www .nationalvoices.org.uk/sites/default/files/public/publications/person-centred_care_in_2017 _-_national_voices.pdf.

NHS Employers. (2019). *Agenda for change. NHS Terms and Conditions.* https://www .nhsemployers.org/pay-pensions-and-reward/agenda-for-change.

NHS England. (2012). *Compassion in practice.* https://www.england.nhs.uk/wp-content/uploads /2012/12/compassion-in-practice.pdf.

NHS England. (2014). *Five year forward view.* https://www.england.nhs.uk/wp-content/uploads /2014/10/5yfv-web.pdf.

NHS England. (2016a). *General practice five year forward view.* https://www.england.nhs.uk /wp-content/uploads/2016/04/gpfv.pdf.

NHS England. (2016b). *General practice – developing confidence, capability and capacity: A ten point action plan for general practice nursing.* https://www.england.nhs.uk/wp-content /uploads/2018/01/general-practice-nursing-ten-point-plan-v17.pdf.

NHS England. (2016c). *Leading change adding value. A framework for nursing, midwifery and care staff.* https://www.england.nhs.uk/wp-content/uploads/2016/05/nursing-framework .pdf.

NHS England. (2019a). *General practice nursing induction template.* https://www.qni.org.uk /wp-content/uploads/2019/05/General-Practice-Nursing-Induction-Template.pdf.

NHS England. (2019b). *Long term plan.* https://www.longtermplan.nhs.uk/.

NHS England. (2019c). *Universal personalised care: Implementing the Comprehensive Model.* https://www.england.nhs.uk/publication/universal-personalised-care-implementing the -comprehensive-model/.

NHS England. (2019d). *Atlas of shared learning: Introducing group consultations for adults with Type 2 diabetes.* https://www.england.nhs.uk/atlas_case_study/introducing-group-consultations -for-adults-with-type-2-diabetes/.

NHS England. (2020a). *Making every contact count.* https://www.makingeverycontactcount.co.uk/.

NHS England. (2019). *GP Contract.* www.england.nhs.uk.

NHS England. (2020b). *Personalised care and support planning.* https://www.england.nhs.uk.

NHS England and NHS Improvement. (2019). *Safeguarding children, young people and adults at risk in the NHS: Safeguarding accountability and assurance framework.* https://www .england.nhs.uk/wp-content/uploads/2015/07/safeguarding-children-young-people-adults-at -risk-saaf-1.pdf.

NHS Improving Quality. (2014). *Capacity, care planning and advanced care planning in life limiting illness.* https://www.england.nhs.uk/improvement-hub/publication/capacity-care-planning -and-advance-care-planning-in-life-limiting-illness-a-guide-for-health-and-social-care-staff/.

NHS Leadership Academy. (2013). *Healthcare Leadership Model: The nine dimensions of leadership behaviour.* http://www.leadershipacademy.nhs.uk/wp-content/uploads/2014/10/NHSLeadership -LeadershipModel-colour.pdf.

NHS Smokefree. (2020). *Smoke free support.* https://www.nhs.uk/smokefree/why-quit/smoking -in-pregnancy.

Nursing and Midwifery Council. (2001). *Standards for Specialist Practice education and practice.* https://www.nmc.org.uk/standards/standards-for-post-registration/standards-for-specialist -education-and-practice/.

Nursing and Midwifery Council. (2018a). *The Code: Professional standards of behaviour for nurses, midwives and nurse associates.* https://www.nmc.org.uk/standards/code/.

Nursing and Midwifery Council. (2018b). *Realising professionalism: Standards for education and training. Part 2: Standards for student supervision and assessment.* https://www.nmc.org.uk /standards-for-education-and-training/standards-for-student-supervision-and-assessment/.

Palmer, W., Hemmings, N., Rosen, R., Keeble, E., Williams, S., Padison, C., Imison, C. (2018). *Improving access and continuity on general practice: Practical and policy lessons.* Nuffield Trust. Available at: https://www.nuffieldtrust.org.uk/files/2019-01/continuing-care-summary -final-.pdf.

Penfold, J. (2019). General Practice Nurses are stepping up to the challenge of leadership. *Primary Health Care, 29*(5), 14–16.

Primary Care Workforce Commission. (2015). *The Future of Primary Care creating teams for tomorrow.* https://www.hee.nhs.uk/sites/default/files/documents/The%20Future%20of%20 Primary%20Care%20report.pdf.

Public Health England. (2019a). *All Our Health: About the framework.* https://www.gov.uk /government/publications/all-our-health-about-the-framework/all-our-health-about-the-framework.

Public Health England. (2019b). *All Our Health: Personalised care and population health.* https:// www.gov.uk/government/collections/all-our-health-personalised-care-and-population-health.

Public Health England. (2019c). *Cardiovascular disease prevention: Applying All Our Health.* https://www.gov.uk/government/publications/cardiovascular-disease-prevention-applying-all -our-health.

Public Health England. (2019d). *Health matters: Preventing cardiovascular disease.* https://www .gov.uk/government/publications/health-matters-preventing-cardiovascular-disease/health -matters-preventing-cardiovascular-disease.

Queen's Nursing Institute. (2015). *General Practice Nursing in the 21st Century: A time of opportunity.* The Queen's Nursing Institute. https://www.qni.org.uk/wp-content/uploads/2016/09 /gpn_c21_report.pdf.

Queen's Nursing Institute. (2016). *Transition to General Practice Nursing Toolkit.* https://www.qni .org.uk/wp-content/uploads/2017/01/Transition-to-General-Practice-Nursing.pdf.

Queen's Nursing Institute. (2019). *The Ellen Mary Memorial Prize.* https://www.qni.org.uk /explore-qni/qni-awards/the-ellen-mary-memorial-prize/.

Queen's Nursing Institute. (2020). *The QNI Standards of Education and Practice for Nurses New to General Practice Nursing.* https://www.qni.org.uk/nursing-in-the-community/practice -standards-models/general-practice-nurse-standards/.

Royal College of General Practitioners. (2011). *Charter for end of life care.* RCGP.

Royal College of General Practitioners. (2015). *General Practice Nurse competencies.* RCGP.

Royal College of Nursing. (2017). *Termination of pregnancy; An RCN Nursing Framework.* https://www.rcn.org.uk/professional-development/publications/pub-005957.

Royal College of Nursing. (2018). *RCN Credentialing for Advanced Level Nursing Practice: Handbook for applicants.*

Royal College of Nursing. (2019a). *Cardiovascular disease prevention.* https://www.rcn.org.uk /clinical-topics/public-health/cardiovascular-disease-prevention.

Royal College of Nursing. (2019b). *Frailty in older people.* https://www.rcn.org.uk/clinical-topics /older-people/frailty.

Royal College of Nursing. (2019c). *End of Life Care; The nursing role* [online.] Available at: https:// www.rcn.org.uk/clinical-topics/end-of-life-care/the-nursing-role.

Smith, K. & Wallington, S. (2019). Assessment of frailty in Alzheimer's: A literature review. *Practice Nursing, 30*(7), 327–329.

The Health Foundation. (2016). *Person-Centred Care made simple.* https://www.health.org.uk /sites/default/files/PersonCentredCareMadeSimple.pdf.

The King's Fund. (2017). *What is social prescribing?* https://www.kingsfund.org.uk/publications /social-prescribing.

Turner, G. (2014). *Introduction to frailty, Fit for Frailty.* https://www.bgs.org.uk.

World Health Organisation. (2012). *Preconception care; maximizing the gains of maternal and child health: Policy brief.* https://www.who.int/maternal_child_adolescent/documents /preconception_care_policy_brief.pdf.

Chapter 2

General practice and system working

Sheinaz Stansfield

Learning outcomes

After reading this chapter, you should be able to:

1. Understand the business element of General Practice
2. Understand income streams for individual practices
3. Understand operational functions in General Practice at the administrative, operational and strategic levels

Introduction

Many practices function as small businesses, albeit some may have remodelled to have the operation functions provided by a federation or may have integrated the administrative workings known as 'back office functions' provided through a scaled-up model. For this reason, it will be important for nurses new to general practice to spend some time with the Practice Manager (PM) as part of their early induction. Understanding the nonclinical systems and processes in place that provide a foundation to clinical service delivery will be essential knowledge for General Practice Nurses (GPNs) to help understand how the rest of the team functions and will contribute to helping new GPNs embed well into the team.

PMs deal with the day-to-day management of the practice and with the business elements and the processes of the practice. Processes are concerned with planning, budgeting, organising, staffing, controlling and problem solving (Kotter, 1996). Over the past four decades management of general practice has changed with different iterations of national health policy designed to expand primary health care services.

Management functions in general practice have evolved as new models of care have emerged, with the general practice model evolving from a simple 'cottage industry model' to a 'corner shop model', and now a scaled-up 'supermarket model' of super practices, and most recently scaling up and working together in Primary Care Networks (PCNs). There is, however, variation in the extent to which individual practices engage in these new models of care.

In this context, there is no standardised model for practice management, but management functions are organised at three levels within individual practices and the emergent new models of care delivery:

1. Administrative
2. Operational
3. Strategic

This chapter provides a brief overview of the development of general practices and the increasingly complex National Health Service (NHS) organisational architecture within which individual practices exist. At the time of writing this chapter, the majority of practices are owned by General Practitioners (GPs); however, with the introduction of the recent review of the GP Contract in 2019 the partnership model is starting to change, with the inclusion of nurses, allied health professionals and other non-clinical partners. Responsibility for the delivery of management functions varies across practices, dependent on the structure, culture and leadership style of the organisation. Predominantly, practice management functions are determined by senior partners who are usually the business owners, and functions are delivered by PMs. The introduction of a more diverse leadership team will have a positive impact on both the leadership style and culture of the organisation.

Background

General practice constitutes the range of services provided traditionally by GPs. The terms 'family practice' or 'primary care' are also used to describe general practice. However, primary care in England has now extended to also include services provided by community pharmacy, dental surgery, optometry and community services providers. For the purposes of this chapter, the term 'general practice' is used specifically to denote services provided in general practice surgeries.

In the United Kingdom general practice has emerged from a pattern of services which were largely established by the National Insurance Act in 1911. The 'list system' which came from the 'friendly societies' across the country was established. Initially this 'list' included only those that were able to make national insurance contributions. In 1948 it was extended to the whole population when the NHS was established. GPs retained their lists as part of their independent contractor status. Every patient is entitled to be on the list, or panel, of a GP, which now provides the basis of payment currency to general practice.

The unique skills and education of GPs enabled them to become the first independent contractors in the NHS. They became self-employed individuals who paid their own tax and national insurance. As independent contractors, GPs and the staff they employ deliver services on behalf of the NHS but are not NHS employees, which means they are not subject to the same pay and terms and conditions of employment as NHS staff. Evolving from a simple corner shop model, practice management was predominantly an administrative function. With services often provided from the GP's front room, the management 'administrative' function was usually undertaken by the GP's spouse. GPs were family practitioners who had a gatekeeper role to other services, mainly in secondary care.

The General Medical Services (GMS) contract brought the first GP contracting charter, with the introduction of accountability and governance into general practice. A three-part payment system and incentive schemes were introduced. The work of Barbara Starfield started to highlight that general practice was an essential ingredient of a cost-effective health service, managing up to 80% of the health care needs (Caley, 2013).

Early intervention and prevention were introduced to the practices, and they started to become more complex organisations, with the introduction of ancillary staff receptionists and GPNs, forming the early 'Primary Health Care Team'. The profile of general practice as the jewel in the crown of the NHS began.

The purchaser and provider split of the 1990s brought competition into the NHS, as well as the introduction of the internal market. Larger partnerships were emerging with formal practice management roles to manage more complex funding arrangements and increased system complexity. With this evolving infrastructure, fundholding, community fundholding and Personal Medical Services (PMS) contracts were introduced to complement the existing GMS contract. The supermarket model started to emerge, with a focus on quality, effectiveness, efficiency and experience.

The profile of GPs was raised further in the political arena with a realisation that general practice could deliver good outcomes for patients and maintain the gatekeeper role with only a fraction of NHS expenditure. General practice received 11% of gross domestic product (GDP) in the late 1990s. By 2019 this had reduced to 8% GDP, amidst increasing demand and complexity of population need.

External organisations

Clinical Commissioning Groups

Clinical Commissioning Groups (CCGs) were created following the Health and Social Care Act in 2012 and replaced Primary Care Trusts. Since April 2013 these changes required all general practices to be a member of a CCG. CCGs are clinically led statutory NHS bodies responsible for the planning and commissioning of health care services for their local area. These changes required GPs and nurses to be involved in activities related to planning and service design and provided the opportunity to work outside of the practice setting. They became involved in developing local health care policy and became clinical leaders for external and NHS organisations such as NHS England and NHS Improvement, as well as CCGs. GPs and nurses became involved in redesigning secondary care services or were involved in system-wide educational activities and developments. Nursing roles started to change, and opportunities emerged for nurses to be involved in quality assurance and patient safety roles within a CCG.

The NHS Five Year Forward View (NHSE, 2016) introduced primary care co-commissioning, giving CCGs an opportunity to take greater responsibility for general practice commissioning at three levels:

- Level 1: Greater involvement: CCGs work more closely with their local National Health Service England (NHSE) teams in making decisions about primary care services.
- Level 2: Joint commissioning: CCGs jointly commission general practice with NHSE regional teams through a joint committee.
- Level 3: Delegated commissioning: CCGs take on full responsibility for commissioning of general practice services.

Case study

Sandra is Macmillan Primary Care Lead Nurse for the Southwest (SW) London Health and Care Partnership. This is a novel role developing the role of primary care nurses in relation to cancer as a long-term condition through leadership, education and influencing of key stakeholders. Working within a Sustainability and Transformation Partnership (STP) provides the opportunity to influence and lead change at scale. Having a senior nursing role in the STP ensures that the unique and invaluable role of primary care nursing is both recognised and supported in development. Sandra previously worked with the Transforming Cancer Services Team for London to develop a model for primary care follow-up of patients with stable prostate cancer that has now been adopted across London.

Sandra Dyer, Macmillan Primary Care Lead Nurse, SW London Health and Care partnership.

Integrated care systems

At the time of writing this chapter, strategic planning and reorganisation are happening through Sustainability and Transformation Partnerships, which were introduced in 2016. They bring together NHS organisations, local councils and the voluntary sector to work together to improve health care for patients. In some areas these have evolved to form integrated care systems (ICSs). ICSs provide strategic collaboration of these organisations with a collective responsibility for managing resources, delivering NHS standards and working together to improve the health of the population across regional areas. ICSs nationally have tested this model of integrated working. The aim is to expand to 42 ICSs across the country to help people live longer, healthier lives in their communities with care provided closer to home, with shorter stays in hospital. During 2021 CCGs are being replaced by ICSs, meaning there will be fewer commissioners who will become responsible for larger geographical areas.

Integrated care partnerships

Integrated Care Partnerships (ICPs) are collaborative networks of care providers, health care professionals, community providers, voluntary organisations, patients, carers and service users. The role of ICPs is to design and coordinate delivery of local health and social care services. This 'place-based' integrated style of working covers populations of circa 150,000 to 500,000 people and will be the focus for partnership working between the NHS and local authorities across cities, boroughs and neighbourhoods. As general practice scales up through federations and PCNs, they will also have an active role for the first time in planning and designing care at population level.

Provider landscape

Individual practices

The business structure of General Practice has not changed much since the inception of the NHS in 1948. Essentially, practices are run by clinical partners in a vertical structure. Changes in the GP contract have sought to stimulate working within a broader primary health care team; however, in many practices Senior Partners control and maintain decision-making power. General practice is still delivered mainly through a 'cottage industry' model in which practices of varying sizes provide a limited range of first contact services (Kings Fund, 2014).

Increasingly, these practices must function in a more complex commissioning and provider landscape. Practices need to understand the benefit of working within each element of the system, prioritising how much time and energy they give to each to maximise the potential both for practices and their patients.

Federations

The British Medical Association (BMA) describes a federation as a group of practices working together within their local area, in a locally agreed collective legal or organisational entity. As a provider organisation, federations provide economies of scale to help sustain individual practices by managing workload and coordinating services across a geographical area. There are several different organisational forms that a federation can take. Two of these are:

1. A very loose arrangement based, for example, on a memorandum of understanding.
2. A legal entity, such as a company limited by shares or guarantee, a community interest company or a limited liability partnership.

Governance of federations has emerged to suit local arrangements. There are different ownership and management structures dependent on local arrangements and needs. Operational and administrative processes can be standardised to reduce workload and save money, through joint provision or commissioning of back office functions such as human resources (HR) and payroll, which may be centralised. Staff, whether clinical or operational, can also be employed and support practices through the provision of services, and at times facilitation of sharing good practice.

In all models, individual practices remain independent organisations, but profit, contractual and pension arrangements will vary according to the model chosen. This includes whether practices or the federation holds GMS/PMS/ alternative provider medical services (APMS) contracts.

Primary care networks

Although general practices have been finding different ways of working together for many years (e.g., in super-partnerships, federations, clusters and networks) the NHS long-term plan (NHSE, 2019) and the new Five Year Framework for the GP contract, published in January 2019, put a more formal structure around this way of working through PCNs, but without creating new statutory bodies. PCNs were introduced in 2019 and are being developed within the context of 'Place-Based Care'. Within these areas, PCNs are an effort to scale up general practice through collaboration, managing a population of between 30,000 and 50,000 people. There is more detail on PCNs in Chapter 12 – (Primary Care Networks and Multi Disciplinary Team-Based Working).

Testimonial

Ben Scott is a nurse who was one of the first Clinical Directors (CDs) and based in South Primary Care Network in Doncaster. Ben has now become a partner in general practice. 'My experience as a CD has been one of enthralling challenge; there has been ups downs, ins outs and roundabouts. But I have loved every minute. Primary has enabled me to reach a position whereby I can have a positive influence large scale on patients and workforce. I have evolved as an individual and embraced more than I could have ever imagined.'

Organisational culture

Corporate culture as a subject of interest to managers first appeared in the management literature in the early 1980s. Observation of Far Eastern companies and the writing of Peters and Waterman, particularly their book 'In Search of Excellence' (Peters & Waterman, 1982), highlighted the importance of culture within organisations. Indeed, they indicated that culture had to be a central part of organisational strategy for successful or excellent organisations. Every organisation has a culture, whether it is designed or evolves through neglect, accident or omission.

In some practices a command and control culture has been perpetuated in alignment with the vertical organisational structure and senior partner model of leadership. These command and control cultures are associated with:

- Incompatible vision, mission and goals, and a lack of understanding about the future direction of the organisation, which may lead to failure.

- Lack of leadership, poor direction from senior managers, competition between managers and poor role models within the senior management team, which may lead to failure.
- Lack of quality of service provision, poor running of the organisation and priorities externally perceived as being incorrect, which will lead to either failure or demise.

With introduction of PCNs, a different, more collaborative, culture and leadership style will be key to success. While shared values, beliefs and a collective interest in building an organisation are key elements of culture, the behaviour of senior managers and leaders is a key factor in developing culture. It is both the implicit and explicit understanding of culture and the organisation's core values that provide the unifying power to develop excellent organisations (Covey, 1994).

A strong culture is evident in practices where all members have a shared understanding of the core beliefs and values of the organisation. These beliefs and values infiltrate all aspects of the organisation and are a key element of the strategy. Internally, culture has other functions, providing the 'glue' that binds the organisation together. It is practices with this culture and collaborative leadership style that are forging the way forward towards successful new models of care and scaled-up General Practice.

Reflection
___
Consider the organisational culture of your practice, how this is influenced and what role you can play in influencing the nursing contribution.

Quality management

Over the past two decades, there has been an increasing focus on quality in the NHS, including in general practice. The Health and Social Care Act and the NHS Constitution strengthened the commitment to quality, and the infrastructure needed to confer quality on every aspect of the organisation's business has been embedded.

In 1998, Lord Darzi's report 'High Quality Care for All' set out a vision in which high-quality care was central to the NHS, and quality was defined in terms of safety, effectiveness and patient experience. This definition has now been enshrined in legislation, and the NHS quality agenda built around this simple, yet effective, definition encompasses three components:

- Patient safety: Reducing adverse impact on patients and preventing medical and systems errors that may lead to unsafe care or harm to patients.
- Clinical effectiveness: The extent to which specific clinical interventions do what they are intended to do (i.e., maintain and improve the health of patients and secure the greatest possible health gain from the available resources), providing evidence-based care and robust clinical and information governance arrangements.

- Patient experience: Different from patient involvement, this is about treating patients with dignity, respect and compassion, ensuring that the patient receives the best possible experience of care and recovery.

This definition has been adopted throughout the NHS in England and was used as the basis of the NHS Outcomes Framework and incorporated into the regulatory framework developed by the Care Quality Commission (CQC) in 2013 (Ross & Naylor, 2017).

In October 2014, the Five Year Forward View made a commitment to 're-energise' the National Quality Board (NQB), providing system alignment and leadership, ensuring that quality becomes integral to the core business of every NHS organisation. The role of the NQB to date has focused on delivery of the quality agenda, predominantly in secondary care. Implementation of a range of quality standards and quality accounts in secondary care and other provider organisations has resulted in these providers having board-level responsibility for a systematic approach to quality assurance.

CCGs use a range of quality improvement measures, including the National Institute for Health and Care Excellence (NICE), quality dashboards, clinical commissioning information systems (locally developed) and audit activity, to measure quality in general practice. CCGs have the flexibility to develop locally relevant reward and incentive schemes in delivery of the Commissioning Outcomes Framework. In addition, practices have become financially accountable for their clinical decision-making through the introduction of quality outcome indicators. These incentives are structured to enable general practices to work differently, shifting their focus from individuals to population health and achievement of health improvement outcomes. It is the role of CCGs to ensure all measures of quality at every level of the system are transparently available to support accountability, patient choice and prioritisation.

Incentives support reductions in health inequalities, for example, by focusing on those members of the local population who have the greatest need for specific interventions, and agreed-upon indicators to measure quality are outcomes-focused rather than quantity-focused:

- meaningful clinical audit
- involvement in development of quality measures and agreeing baselines
- freedom to identify locally relevant indicators for quality impartment
- organised learning and sharing and feedback loops for continued engagement
- identification of a local tool for total quality improvement and a commissioning process that enables access to general practices

To date there has been no legal requirement and certainly no compelling reason for general practices to engage in continuous quality improvement. Commissioning and contracting have been at arm's length, with no real power to address poor practice. A monopoly in care provision and the existing contracting system have guaranteed a regular income. This has been possible because of patient loyalty and a compliant workforce, which has resulted in little change. However, service regulation, more rigorous performance management and an increasingly demanding customer and workforce base are providing a compelling mix that challenges organisational culture and structure to enable delivery of high-quality care.

Quality assurance

General practitioners performers list

All GPs are required to be on a performers list, which is administered by Primary Care Support Services on behalf of NHSE. This list provides an extra layer of assurance that the clinician is suitably qualified, has up-to-date training and has the appropriate English language skills. In addition, relevant checks such as Disclosure and Barring have been completed. No such measure exists currently for nurses working in general practice.

Care quality commission

Quality assurance is the provision of services that meet an appropriate standard, through transactional processes. It is the role of the CQC to drive improvement, through assurance, in quality of health and social care standards. From April 2013 general practice was 'legally' required to meet these 'essential standards of quality and safety'. Compliance with the CQC standards is intended to enable general practice to function effectively in an environment within which patient expectations and performance management have become more challenging than ever before. For general practice this has been resource-intensive and onerous. However, as it evolves, this should prove to be the most comprehensive tool for systematic quality assurance, encompassing all three components of quality (effectiveness, efficiency and experience).

In addition, the CQC has the power to address poor practice. Where providers are found not to be meeting these minimum quality standards, the CQC has the power to issue warning notices, penalties, suspensions or restriction of activities. In extreme cases, this has resulted in closure of some services.

To date, performance management of general practice has been limited, with commissioning organisations having limited power or influence over poor performance, or ability to hold failing organisations to account. Therefore, the concept of regulation has caused significant anxiety amongst the general practice community. This level of scrutiny and regulation has provided a compelling rationale for change. This strong organisational infrastructure, along with nurse involvement, will enable practices to strengthen quality assurance. A key role for nurses will be to ensure that policies and procedures relating to clinical systems such as infection control are in place and implemented in preparation for CQC inspection.

Quality improvement

Quality improvement is a continuous process involving all levels of the organisation working together to produce better services and care, through transformational processes and action. Quality improvement relies on the use of methods and tools to continuously improve quality of care and outcomes for patients. This works best when it is at the heart of organisations and local plans for redesigning NHS services.

Exposure to quality improvement to general practices came through the General Practice Forward View (GPFV), published on 21st April 2016. It set out national investment and commitments to strengthen general practice in the short term and support sustainable transformation of primary care for the future. It included specific, practical and funded investment in five areas:

- investment
- workforce
- workload
- practice infrastructure
- care redesign

The NHSE GPFV Time for Care programme introduced the concept of quality improvement into general practice, with a fully funded suite of quality improvement programmes designed to increase capacity and capability in general practice. Programmes are provided at the individual, practice and across-practice level. At the heart of this development programme are the 10 High Impact Actions that aim to help practice teams manage their workload. These actions help adopt, adapt and spread innovations that speed up clinical and non-clinical tasks. This programme also left a legacy of new skills and confidence for practice teams to lead local improvement work. The 'Time For Care' programme was further extended by NHS England and NHS Improvement in 2019 and provided development support for PCNs.

Case study

Have a look at the 'Time For Care' case studies at: https://www.england.nhs.uk/gp/case-studies/

Quality outcomes framework

The Quality Outcomes Framework (QOF) was introduced as part of the 2004 general practice contract review as an initial attempt to align rewards and incentives in the pursuit of quality improvement, and included both clinical and managerial indicators. The QOF provided the first opportunity to gather data on primary care quality nationally. This set critical foundations of embedding evidence-based care and an organised (not systematic) approach to addressing health inequalities and chronic disease management.

However, despite the introduction of prevalence weighting in 2009/2010, case finding remains challenging. Attendance and admission through Accident and Emergency (A&E) continue to increase for chronic conditions that should be managed upstream in primary and community care services, adding pressure to a system that is already financially constrained. As people live longer with two or more long-term conditions and increased complexity, a different model of care delivery is becoming necessary. Nurses with personalised care planning and case management skills will have a key role to play in this proactive approach to care provision (Last, 2019).

The Quality and Productivity (QP) indicators introduced by NICE in 2010/2011 were aimed at securing a more effective use of NHS resources through improvements in the quality of primary care. Six QP indicators covering outpatient referrals and emergency admissions were agreed on in 2010/2011 and extended to 2011/2012. Introduction of this new process of monitoring and review of evidence-based clinical and cost-effectiveness indicators will ensure that the activities being measured become standardised in clinical practice, and no longer need to be incentivised, allowing new indicators to evolve through the modification of thresholds or to be replaced when they become standard practice. Increasingly, GPNs are taking a leading role in delivering care to improve clinical outcomes for patients. Examples of this can be seen nationally where GPNs lead management of people with two or more long-term conditions through a 'Year of Care' approach to care management, as well as group consultations for management of long-term conditions.

Contracting and finance

The GP partnership model has underpinned general practice since before the establishment of the NHS and is thought to be a major component of the success of general practice in England (Watson, 2019). GPs remain the first point of contact for between 80% and 90% of patients.

Increasingly, nurses and nonclinical partners have a key role to play in implementation of general practice contracts that outline obligations and provide details of funding. NHS England and NHS Improvement have three main contract options that they use to commission primary medical services. These are:

- GMS contracts: These deliver core medical services and are agreed nationally. The funding for these types of contract is calculated based on the practice's registered list size, with a fixed, nationally agreed price per patient, and the actual amount paid is calculated on a practice-by-practice basis.
- PMS contracts: PMS contracts provide similar core medical services to GMS contracts but can also include extra health services that are considered to be 'over and above' the usual core services – for example, special clinics for homeless people in areas of high need. PMS contracts make it possible to address specific local health needs. The funding for PMS contracts is worked out locally.

- APMS contracts: APMS contracts enable Primary Care Organisations (PCOs) to commission/provide primary medical services within their area to the extent that they are necessary. APMS contracts provide the opportunity for locally negotiated contracts and allow PCOs to contract non-NHS bodies, such as voluntary or commercial sector providers or GMS/PMS practices, to provide enhanced and additional primary medical services.

In addition to these three core contracting mechanisms, additional services are contracted through Directed Enhanced Services (DESs) or Locally Enhanced Services (LESs):

- DES: A DES is a nationally negotiated service, over and above that provided under usual contracts. These are commissioned by an NHSE regional team and are voluntary contracts for GP practices.
- LES: An LES is locally negotiated and commissioned by CCGs, or in some cases, public health LESs through local authorities. These schemes are also voluntary and designed to meet local needs, such as those commissioned by the local authority to address population health needs. Nurses working in primary care have a key role to play in the provision of these services, as they are often related to health promotion and prevention, including services such as family planning, smoking cessation and heart health checks.

Core practice income

Statement of financial elements

Core general practice contract payments are outlined in the 'Statement of Financial Elements' (SFE). SFEs outline the general groupings under which funding is allocated to general practice. These are revised by NHSE regularly, and may have a retrospective effect and amendments, which are published periodically with delivery dates and associated payment changes.

How the practice receives funding

Global sum

The global sum is an annual sum that covers payment for delivery of essential and additional services. Funding is calculated quarterly and paid monthly. The global sum is determined by the practice list size and adjusted for practice demographics. Costs for staff employment are also included. This is a regular monthly payment that enables practices to plan income and expenditure.

Private income

About one-third of practice income comes from private sources, although there will be significant variation across practices. It will be important for GPNs to identify what role they will have in delivering private services, as not all practices provide these. Some of these include:

- Some travel vaccinations
- Prescribing of drugs for foreign travel
- Provision of some services excluded from the core GP contract
- Heavy goods vehicle and taxi driver medicals

Clinical quality

The QOF was introduced as part of the 2004 contract negotiations. Participation in the QOF rewards general practices for implementing 'good practice' in their surgeries and is voluntary for each partnership. For most under the present contract, the QOF is almost the only area where practices can make a difference to their income, and requires all to participate. Most practices get a significant proportion of their income through the QOF. In many practices GPNs have a lead role in managing long-term conditions and other clinical requirements for the QOF. They, therefore, have an important role to play in planning, delivering and also ensuring appropriate claiming for services delivered.

QOF points and indicators are revised and negotiated by the BMA on an annual basis. The criteria are designed around best practice and have several points allocated for achievement. At the end of the financial year the total number of points achieved by a practice is collated by the Calculating Quality Reporting Services, an approval, reporting and payments calculation system for GP practices. It helps practices to track, monitor and declare achievement for the QOF, DES and Vaccination and Immunisation programmes.

To move away from process-driven QOF indicators, outcome-based indicators have been tested as part of the QOF. Many of these have included indicators on population health and reduction in secondary care activity, particularly unplanned activity.

The QOF criteria are grouped into four domains:

Clinical. The clinical element awards points for achieving specified clinical 'indicators'. The formula includes the number of patients and the numbers diagnosed with certain common chronic illnesses. In the clinical domain the value of points includes the prevalence of a condition in the practice; increased case finding attracts additional funding. Indicators change every year (NHSE, 2019). Those that nurses contribute to may change every year and cover:

- management of some of the most common chronic conditions, e.g., asthma, diabetes, cardiovascular disease
- management of major public health concerns such as smoking and obesity
- provision of preventative services such as screening and blood pressure checks

Organisational. Organisational indicators include such things as the availability of practice leaflets and practice staff education. In the organisational domain the value of points is proportional to the number of patients registered with the practice.

Patient Involvement/Experience. The process for patient involvement in general practice decision-making has, to date, been transactional, incentivised through the GP contract, QOF and enhanced services.

Patient Participation Groups (PPGs). PPGs were introduced to general practice following the April 2016 contract negotiations (BMA, 2016). PPGs are defined by the NHS as the 'active participation of citizens, users and carers and their representatives in the development of healthcare services and as partners in their own healthcare'. There is no requirement, nor description in statute, of what constitutes a PPG, what it can do, how it should be organised or whether it should be a face-to-face group or a virtual group, or both, making it difficult for some practices to successfully embed this approach to achieve their purposes. Therefore, there is significant variation in the adoption of PPGs and their level of engagement or influence in general practice.

The family and friends test

The friends and family test, a national scheme first introduced into hospital settings, was introduced to general practice in 2015. It is a single-question survey which asks patients whether they would recommend the practice to their friends or family. Practices use a variety of methods to collect this information, predominantly a card in reception.

Patient survey

The general practice patient survey is undertaken annually at a national level by NHS England and NHS Improvement. It is used to assess patients' experiences of health care services provided by general practices, including experience of access and making appointments, as well as the quality of care received from all health care professionals, including nurses. A requirement assessed as part of CQC is that practices review results, develop action plans and upload these onto the practice website for the public to review.

Additional services

Additional services are part of the public health and prevention aspects of the QOF, predominantly delivered by GPNs. Practices have the flexibility to opt in or temporarily opt out of the provision of additional services, some of which include:

- Child health surveillance
- Contraceptive services
- Cervical screening
- Vaccinations and immunisations

A test bed programme is being set up to test quality improvement approaches to some QOF indicators. On an annual basis individual PCNs will be identified to test network-wide indicators. These will see a shift of QOF indicators from practices to across the networks. Some of these include medicine management, early cancer diagnosis and cardiovascular case finding.

Primary care networks

PCNs will have the responsibility of delivering seven national service specifications set out in the contract. Although it is anticipated that new roles will contribute to PCN-wide achievement, GPNs will also have a role in achieving practice-specific targets, as achievement at practice level will impact PCN-wide funding (Table 2.1).

A multidisciplinary approach will be required to maximise income through these indicators, and GPNs will have a key role, moving from reactive, process-based management of patients through QOF to a proactive case management approach with early intervention, prevention and proactive management of patients. Different skills and multidisciplinary working will be essential to achieving these indicators.

Reflection

Take some time to find out what contract your practice delivers.

Are there any services that your practice has opted out of or delivers as extra?

How can you find out about your practice's involvement in a primary care network (PCN)?

How are other general practice nurses involved in PCNs in your area?

Table 2.1   **Primary care network advanced services.**

2019/2021	Structured medicines review and optimization	• Directly tackling overmedication, including inappropriate use of antibiotics • Medication reviews for priority groups, including frail elderly patients
2020/2020	Enhanced health in care homes	• Improving case management and care planning in care homes
2021/2022	Anticipatory care	• Primary care networks to work with community services to collaborate in proactive case management/care planning
2021/2022	Personalised care	• Personalised care planning
2020/2021	Supporting early cancer diagnosis	• Early intervention and prevention
2020/2022	Early intervention and prevention of cardiovascular disease	• Quality improvement tools used to test existing Quality Outcomes Framework indicators to find the best approaches to case finding and prevention

From Network-Contract-DES-Specification-PCN-Requirements-and-Entitlements-2020-21-October-NHSE.

Workforce

Faced with changing demographics, people living longer with long-term conditions and with increasingly complex health needs, alongside a shortage of GPs and GPNs primary care, is resulting in unprecedented pressures. To date, the workforce in general practice has remained simple, with GPs, GPNs, Health Care Assistants and administrative staff. However, as general practice evolves and the average size of practices increases, more GPs are choosing to work in a salaried (employed) role (GOV.UK, 2019). There is a trend towards more part-time and flexible working, with an increase in portfolio careers. Therefore, 'partnerships' have become less popular with GPs in recent years, and there is a risk that the model of traditional general practice could be lost (GOV.UK, 2019). Interestingly, there are nurses who have become partners in general practice. At the time of writing, NHS England/NHS Improvement are developing a formal pathway which will increase the opportunity for more nurses to become partners in general practice.

The workforce in general practice is being transformed through new models of care introduced to manage these changes. To expand the workforce to become a more multiprofessional model with a greater mix of skills, 5000 new 'non-medical' roles are being introduced to work alongside general practice staff and are seen as complementary to nursing roles. These new roles intend to extend the skill mix of professionals to include Pharmacists, Paramedics, Physician's Associates and First Contact Physiotherapists. This will bring a different dynamic to the traditional general practice team, ensuring that patients and populations can receive care at the right time and by the right professional appropriate to their health care requirements.

Reflection

What different professionals work in your practice or primary care network?
What range of conditions and patients do they see?
How may you work as an integrated team with these other team members?

Testimonial

Zuzana Khan was one of the first Primary Care Network Clinical Directors working as an Advanced Nurse Practitioner in General Practice. 'This was not something I'd ever imagine I would be.' Nominated by her practice, she led a network of five practices with a population of just under 49,000 patients in a busy, deprived inner city area (Newham, East London). This allowed her to develop connections with people of influence to work together to meet the needs of the population of Newham.

Managing human resources

PMs manage resources in the practice. The 1991 NHS reforms and the new GP Contract of 2004 brought new funding arrangements, functions and services, which have required a different infrastructure for organisational and staff management in general practice. This, coupled with the introduction of CQC 'Well Led' and 'Safe key lines of enquires,' has resulted in an increased focus on the management of resources in the practice.

HR management is concerned with management of employees in the practice and focuses on development of organisational policies and procedures. Employee recruitment, retention, training, development, remuneration, conditions and development, are key components of HR management.

Pay, terms and conditions of employment

It is important for new GPNs to be aware that general practices, as independent organisations, have no formal mechanism for agreeing pay and conditions for nursing and administrative staff. Many practices have taken some aspects of the NHS Agenda for Change and adapted them for their staff, but this will differ from practice to practice. Most GPNs will negotiate their own pay and terms and conditions of employment, which has led to a wide variance across general practices in England.

Remuneration of partners is governed through partnership agreements for those practices that have them. A partnership agreement (deed) is a formal document that defines the partnership and the relationship between partners. HR arrangements will be covered in the partnership agreement, as will arrangements for drawings (pay) of partners. Nurses wishing to become partners in general practice will need to consider impact on terms and conditions and pension.

In 2004, the BMA developed a model contract for salaried GPs which covers all the expected terms and conditions for salaried GPs. The model contact is in line with terms and conditions of other doctors employed in the NHS. The Doctors and Dentists Review Body makes annual recommendations as to the pay and remuneration of salaried GPs. Currently no such measures exist for nurses employed in general practice.

Through CQC inspections and increasing complexity of the general practice workforce, many practices either individually or through their federations are starting to develop more robust arrangements for HR management. Many are choosing to outsource this function, with others commissioning jointly across practices. Introduction of information technology (IT) platforms such as 'Clarity intranet' will enable the standardisation of policies and procedures across practices.

Health and safety

As for all small businesses, there has always been a responsibility for general practices to abide by health and safety legislation (HSE, 1974). However, until 2016, many practices did not support the requirements of health and safety legislation. The introduction of CQC resulted in the development of policies and procedures in practice to support evidence that practices were meeting health

---

Box 2.1   Health and safety requirements impacting nursing standards

- Building maintenance, risk assessments and monitoring
- Equipment maintenance and monitoring
- Portable appliance testing and collaboration regarding medical equipment
- *Legionella* testing
- Recycling all waste and medication
- Calibration of medical equipment
- Safe handling and storage of medications
- Control of substances hazardous to health
- Infection control/cleaning schedule
- Trained first aiders
- Disaster recovery plan/business continuity plan
- Fire safety training
- Ensuring personal protective equipment and clothing are available
- Ensuring spill kits are available and in-date
- Reporting of Injuries, Diseases and Dangerous Occurrences Regulations/accident book

---

From Oxford Terrace and Rawling Road Medical Group: Policies and Procedures.

and safety standards; these are required as evidence for CQC assessments. Some requirements that impact on nursing functions are listed in Box 2.1.

PMs have a responsibility for operational management of health and safety policies and procedures. However, as scrutiny increases and requirements become more complex, some practices outsource support to external organisations. Federated working has enabled standardisation and joint commissioning of health and safety support in some areas. Development of PCNs may enable standardisation and cost-sharing across practices; this will be particularly important for the safety of PCN staff working across practices and in the community.

Information and digital technology

NHS Digital IT programmes are being developed to enable a paperless NHS by 2020. Many practices are already paperless and use EMIS or System One as their preferred clinical systems, although other clinical systems are also available. Some 73% of clinical systems are procured via the NHS Digital Framework (NHS Digital, 2020).

NHS Digital is supporting the use and design of technology to:

- enable self-care and self-management for patients
- help to reduce workload in practices
- enable practices to work together through data and document sharing to operate at scale
- support greater efficiency across the whole system
- improve access through the use of online services

Priorities to expedite the use of digital technology in practices and across PNCs include the following:

- Practices are expected to make 25% of appointments bookable online
- Practices provide online and video consultations
- Practices should not have or use fax machines for NHS work or patient correspondence
- Data relating to activity, capacity and waiting times will be published alongside secondary care data
- A new measurement of patient-reported satisfaction with access and data will be implemented

Clinical coding

Clinical coding is the translation of medical terminology to describe problems, diagnosis, treatment, and clinical symptoms. SNOMED Clinical Terms (NHS.UK, 2018) are used in general practice. Coding systematically organises computer-processable collections of medical terms, synonyms and definitions used in clinical documentation and reporting.

It is important that clinical data are coded accurately and consistently, because this information not only helps decision-making processes in general practices, but it is also essential for claiming and payment, and so is vital for the practice's financial viability.

GP2GP

GP2GP is used to transfer patient records securely between general practices and is only available in England. New patients are registered into the clinical system, and a search is undertaken to find out if personal demographics already exist on the system. Once received, the file is integrated into the clinical system automatically.

Electronic Prescription Service

The Electronic Prescription Service (EPS) allows prescribers to send prescriptions electronically to the pharmacy of the patient's choice. This makes the prescribing and dispensing process more efficient and convenient for patients and staff. Some 93% of practices have successfully adopted EPS, a process that makes paper prescriptions redundant. From April 2019 it became a priority for all patients to be able to access prescriptions through EPS.

Summary care record

Since April 2019, all new patients have had access to their own digital record, known as the Summary Care Record (SCR). SCRs are an electronic record of patient information created from the general practice medical records. To support safer care, they can be seen and used by authorised staff across the health system, including in hospital settings if a patient attends A&E or is admitted to a hospital or care home. SCRs include information on current medication, details of allergies and previous bad reactions to prescribed medication and personal details. The SCR is created automatically through the clinical system in general practices and uploaded automatically onto the NHS system. Patients are asked to give consent for others to access their records electronically and to include additional information into the SCR. In 2019, 98% of practices were using this system.

In April 2020 all patients will have online access to their full record, including the ability to add their own information and access online correspondence. Therefore, contemporaneous record keeping and robust recording will be essential. The introduction of the NHS App in 2019 allows patients to securely access their own health records, order repeat prescriptions and make appointments using their mobile phones, allowing even greater accessibility.

National Health Service 111

NHS 111 is a free 24/7 telephone triage service designed to help patients who are experiencing an urgent health care need. They can speak to a call handler who uses decision support software to assess the patient and signpost to the most appropriate health care professional. This avoids overburdening general practices and provides timely, appropriate and accessible care to the public. The service is commissioned locally, but within an NHS standard of care, and is provided by a range of different organisations nationally. As part of the new GP contract, from April 2019 there will be a requirement for one appointment per 3000 patients to be available for direct booking into the practice appointment system through NHS 111.

Conclusion

Nurses new to general practice will be mainly concerned with the clinical elements of their work in the general practice setting. Understanding the business elements and workings of the practice helps GPNs develop an appreciation of the organisation that they work in and contribute to the business.

The general practice model has evolved from a corner shop model to a supermarket model over a period of four decades. However, individual practices continue to function on a continuum between the two models. Management functions have also evolved to meet the business needs of organisations that are growing in a variety of formal and informal structures. As the NHS environment within which general practices exist becomes more complex and challenging to navigate, management functions too must evolve from administrative to operational and increasingly strategic to function across a wider system.

A workforce crisis has arisen amidst the NHS system because of changing demographics, increasing complexity of illnesses and people living longer with two or more long-term conditions. This, along with the changing NHS architecture, has resulted in increased pressure on general practice and is making the GP partnership model less favourable, with many GPs now choosing portfolio careers. This crisis has been the catalyst for new models of care and integrated working, with an increased focus on practices collaborating and working together to manage a reduction in resources.

GPNs have, to date, worked in isolation, managing the condition and not the patient. This catalyst for change will require GPNs to develop new skills, particularly focused on case management and personalised care planning to function as members of a broader, primary health care team, taking multidisciplinary approaches to manage changing demographics and patient needs.

Changing population needs and the aforementioned workforce crisis have also brought recognition that patients' needs cannot be managed by GPs alone in a 10-minute appointment. The valuable role of GPNs is required more than ever and complements the new roles that are being introduced to implement new ways of working. This constitutes a move away from managing the condition through reactive processes to managing the person through proactive, person-centred and personalised care, an area in which nursing has much to offer (Last, 2019).

Nurses have worked in general practice since the 1990s in extended roles, although their development needs have not had national exposure until now. The NHS England and NHS Improvement GPN Ten Point Plan (NHS, 2017) recognises the ability of general practice nurses to transform care and address the workforce challenges to deliver an NHS fit for the future.

Through exposure to quality improvement and new models of care, general practice is going through transformation in structure, culture and leadership style. This, coupled with multidisciplinary working and training, will make general practice a more desirable first destination career choice for nurses.

References

BMA 2016. (2016). *Involving patients and communities checklist.* https://www.google.com /search?client=safari&rls=en&q=BMA+2016:+Involving+Patients+and+Communities+Che cklist&spell=1&sa=X&ved=2ahUKEwj4yp6KnpDpAhVPTxUIHW5tBEcQBSgAegQIDB An&biw=1388&bih=1282.

Caley, M. (2013). Remember Barbara Starfield: Primary care is the health system's bedrock. *BMJ, 347*(3), f4627.

Covey, S. (2004). The 7 Habits of Highly Effective People: Powerful Lessons in Personal Change. New York: Free Press.

Datadictionary.nhs.uk. (2018). *Supporting information: SNOMED CT.* https://www.datadictionary .nhs.uk/web_site_content/supporting_information/clinical_coding/snomed_ct.asp?shownav=1.

GOV.UK. (2019). *GP partnership review.* https://www.gov.uk/government/collections/gp-partnership -review.

Hse.gov.uk. (1974). *Health and Safety at Work Etc Act 1974 – Legislation Explained.* https://www.hse.gov.uk/legislation/hswa.htm.

Kingsfund.org.uk. (2014). *Commissioning and funding general practice: Making the case for family care networks.* https://www.kingsfund.org.uk/sites/default/files/field/field_publication_file/commissioning-and-funding-general-practice-kingsfund-feb14.pdf.

Kotter, J. P. (1996). *Leading change.* Harvard Business School Press.

Last, R. (2019). Making personalised care happen: Implementing the 'Comprehensive Model' in general practice. *Practice Nurse, 49*(9), 33–37.

NHS Digital. (2020). *Home – NHS Digital.* https://www.digital.nhs.uk.

NHS Digital. (2019). *Quality Outcomes Framework (QOF) – NHS Digital.* https://www.digital.nhs.uk/data-and-information/data-tools-and-services/data-services/general-practice-data-hub/quality-outcomes-framework-qof.

NHS England. (2016). *NHS England 2016 General Practice forward view.* https://www.england.nhs.uk/gp/gpfv/.

NHS England. (2019) *NHS long term plan.* https://www.longtermplan.nhs.uk/wp-content/uploads/2019/01/nhs-long-term-plan.pdf.

NHS England. (2019). *A five-year framework for GP contract reform to implement the NHS long term plan.* https://www.england.nhs.uk/publication/gp-contract-five-year-framework/.

NHS England. (2019). *Releasing time for care.* https://www.england.nhs.uk/gp/gpfv/redesign/gpdp/releasing-time/.

NHS England. (2019). *General Practice Nursing ten point plan.* https://www.england.nhs.uk/wp-content/uploads/2018/01/general-practice-nursing-ten-point-plan-v17.pdf.

NHS England. (2020/21). *Network Contract Directed Enhanced Service (DES) Contract Specification: Primary Care Network Entitlements and Requirements.* https://www.england.nhs.uk/publication/des-contract-specification-2020-21-pcn-entitlements-and-requirements/.

Peters, T. J. & Waterman, R. H. (1982). *Search of excellence: Lessons from America's best-run Companies.* Harper & Row.

Ross, S. & Naylor, C. (2017). *Quality improvement in mental health. London: the king's fund.* https://www.kingsfund.org.uk/publications/quality-improvement-mental-health.

Chapter 3

Styles of communication

Janet Procter-King, Heather Henry, Georgina Craig

Learning outcomes

After reading this chapter you should be able to:

1. Discuss effective verbal and nonverbal communication in general practice
2. Describe the three parts of a group consultation
3. Explain how patients can become the main change resource in motivational interviewing

Introduction

Being able to effectively listen to, communicate with and motivate your patients is an essential skill for any General Practice Nurse (GPN) delivering person- and community-centred care. Some components of good communication include good verbal and nonverbal communication, active listening, showing compassion, developing trust in the nurse–patient relationship and exhibiting cultural awareness.

Traditional consultations in primary care have involved the nurse and the patient interacting within short, 10- to 20-minute appointments, with the nurse there to assess, plan, implement and evaluate care.

Over the last few years, however, different ways of communicating and consulting with patients in general practice have been successfully introduced. Two of these approaches are presented in this chapter: motivational interviewing and group consultations.

Firstly, this chapter will cover the principles and approach behind motivational interviewing: how nurses in primary care can help their patients address their lifestyle issues by tapping into their own internal values and motivations. Secondly, the chapter will address how people with the same condition can come together as a group to learn how to self-manage their conditions and offer each other support.

What both approaches have in common is that they work from the assumption that patients are resourceful people who know how they might need to heal themselves. The nurse becomes the enabler and lets patients lead the clinical conversation. In this way, patients gain confidence and become more capable of self-care and less reliant on the nurse. Over time individuals and communities may demand less of primary care teams. This chapter offers insight into new ways of working that offer a satisfying way to support patients in resolving their own problems, and over the longer term may reduce demand overall.

Why motivational interviewing?

A nurse wanting to survive in general practice will be keen to know the best way to encourage behaviour change to support primary, secondary or even tertiary health promotion interventions. But the experience can be tricky both for patients, who may feel the need to defend themselves, and for health professionals, who may feel that their well-meaning advice falls on deaf ears, affecting their job satisfaction.

This chapter gives a brief overview of how to be more successful in supporting patients using a technique called motivational interviewing. The chapter aims to enthuse the reader to learn more rather than provide comprehensive information. It is written from the experience of a nurse who realised that she had to change.

Reflection

I climbed higher and higher up the general practice career ladder, driven by my desire to make a difference, but at each level I became frustrated as no matter how much I learned about causes, therapies, risk reduction, lifestyle changes, nothing seemed to be very effective at helping people change their behaviour. As a national nurse helping to develop national policy, I heard from other nurses 'It's all very well, but whatever we say they just don't listen.'

Ticking those boxes and developing a patter which just rolled of the tongue, such as, you must not drink more than x number of units, you should really do exercise x minutes y times per week, avoid eating too much and so on, was often heard in general practice nurse rooms up and down the land, including my own.

But despite all my effort of enthusing about the health benefits, explaining the process and extolling the virtues of various behaviour changes to patients or health care students for them to share, it felt increasingly pointless.

I wish I had appreciated as a newer nurse, the potential positive impact of motivational interviewing for my patients, colleagues and myself, rather than believing that my knowledge and enthusiasm would make that difference.

Jan Proctor-King (2019)

Without exception, the behaviour of the people you interact with as a GPN will be the cornerstone to their current and future health. They may blow into a spirometer, receive test results, complete forms, answer questions, be prescribed to or be referred during a health care interaction. And ultimately, it will be what they choose to do, not what you tell them that they should do, that will make the major difference.

This chapter describes how motivational interviewing techniques enable patients to talk and manage themselves towards a change in their lifestyle behaviours based on their own values and beliefs. The positive changes they make may improve outcomes for long-term conditions, relieve pressure on health services by reducing repeat visits and ease frustration for GPNs who may feel that their engagement with the patient has been unsuccessful.

Current practice

How many times have you heard someone say, 'I don't understand it, because I hardly eat a thing!' Are these patients being resistant? Or are they simply defending themselves from the nurse's advice, judgement and patter?

Behaviour change is an important part of any health promotion or disease management interaction. Nurses are encouraged to 'Ask, Advise, Action' (National Centre for Smoking Cessation and Training) and 'Make Every Contact Count' (Public Health England, 2016). But seeking out every opportunity to advise, for example, 'Breast is Best,' or 'People should stop smoking' may lead to burnout unless an effective approach is adopted.

What do we mean by motivational interviewing?

Motivational interviewing is about arranging conversations so that people talk themselves into change based on their own values and interests.

Miller and Rollnick (2012)

William Miller, a clinical psychologist from the University of New Mexico, and Stephen Rollnick, a professor of clinical psychology at Cardiff University, are the cofounders of motivational interviewing.

In 1980, Miller noticed, during a clinical trial of behaviour therapy for problem drinkers, that those counsellors who displayed a client-centred, empathic approach were more successful than those trained in traditional behaviour-change techniques. Those clients who had received support from a therapist with a more empathic style had 66% better outcomes 6 months later (Miller et al., 1980). This was an unanticipated outcome that set Miller thinking. He went on sabbatical to Bergen, Norway, where he was invited to role-play and discuss his approach with a group of young psychologists, causing him to verbalise his intuitive approach. Miller then wrote a conceptual model and clinical guidelines for motivational interviewing. The difference seemed to be around empathic listening and giving clients space to talk themselves into a way to change that they themselves discover, rather than a more confrontational and directive style.

Several clinical trials followed, after which Miller met Rollnick in Australia, and together they wrote the first book on motivational interviewing in 1991 called 'Motivational interviewing: preparing people to change addictive behaviour'. Rollnick went on to test motivational interviewing in health care.

Evidence

In 2005 Rubak et al. conducted a meta-analysis of 72 trials and discovered that, in 80 cases, motivational interviewing outperformed simple advice-giving. By 2009 over 200 studies had been undertaken in health fields as diverse as diet, problem gambling and cardiovascular rehabilitation (Miller & Rose, 2009).

The importance of verbal and nonverbal communication

Motivational interviewing is a way of being with a client, not just a set of techniques for doing counselling.

Miller and Rollnick (1991)

GPNs are fully conversant with the importance of communication with patients, both verbal and nonverbal.

Verbal communication between the patient and the nurse may take the form of welcoming reassurances to try to put the patient more at ease, direct and open questions to establish a history, and comforting conversation and supporting language during any treatment or diagnostic procedure. An appointment may end with a series of directives from the nurse to the patient detailing the next appointment, treatment intervention, prescribed medicines and dosages, procedures or discharge.

Nonverbal communication is very powerful and exceedingly important, as observations made by the nurse as the patient enters the surgery or assessment room regarding signals such as mobility, vulnerability, dependency, oppression, repression or malnourishment can be important to note to aid diagnosis and nursing care. But they can also be important triggers to be used during motivational interviewing.

Throughout a consultation, there is often no clear feedback from patients that they have understood all or part of the process, or that they feel that they have ownership of their own health and outcomes of any treatment. This may be particularly true of those with long-term conditions, who may experience many different emotions when attending a consultation, including: accepting that this is their fate, fearing being judged by the clinician, viewing their appointment and practice visit as a social opportunity, or being unable or unwilling to fully understand the advice and instructions given to them. The result may be that the consultation and prescription may be considered unsuccessful.

Motivational interviewing is about shifting power towards the patient and avoiding the creation of resistance. Through respectful observation and two-way communication, the clinician is no longer offering advice. Instead, he or she is offering information, and consequently people do not feel the need to defend themselves.

Below are two scenarios for behaviour-related communication. Ask yourself which is more likely to lead to long-lasting change and which would be the most satisfying and effective for everyone concerned. Also note who did most of the talking.

Case study

Scenario A

How many cigarettes are you smoking?

Only about 10 a day now; I've cut down.

So you are still smoking. It is good that you have cut down, but often people don't realise how the amount creeps up again. Can I just say that of all the things you could do for your health, stopping smoking would be the best?

Yes I know, but it is my only pleasure these days.

You could get pleasure from other things in life. Cigarettes are costing you a fortune. You are probably spending more than enough for a couple of good holidays a year. That has got to be more pleasurable than smoking? It is also increasingly affecting your lungs, as we can see today by the spirometer results. There's no time like the present. It's never too late. Let's get this sorted while you are here.

Yes, I realise that, but I've smoked for years now and it's just too hard to stop.

The smoking cessation service are great, they have all sorts of patches, etc., to help you succeed, and it's all free. Just think of all the cash you would save and the holidays you could go on. The other thing is your chest is getting worse each time, and there is only so much these inhalers can do. I don't want you ending up on oxygen all the time.

Well, no I don't, but as I say, it's not that easy. I'll think about it.

Listen, how about I refer you today? They are really good; honestly, just give it a go. You won't regret it. Here you are. I'll pop the date and time on this card so you won't forget.

Thanks, bye.

Don't you forget, you know it's best for you.

Scenario B

So how is it going with the smoking?

It's hard, you know; I've smoked for years and it is just a habit, a bad habit, but you know how it is.

 (Silence but obviously listening)

I'm not daft; I realise it's the worst thing I can do for my health, but at this stage in life it can feel like your only pleasure.

 (Silence but obviously listening)

Everyone goes on and on about, you must stop, you shouldn't be smoking, and they speak to you like you never heard it before. Good grief, I have seen the adverts on the packs and the telly. If I could give up, I would love to. I have cut down, but it's really hard. To be honest, I always say 10 a day, but it's more like 20 really.

You understand the health effects of smoking. You try to keep the amount down and would really love to stop if you could?

I would, yes.

 (Silence but obviously listening)

I did stop before, a few years ago. I just went cold turkey. Then a couple of years later after my wife died, one thing led to another and I started again. You get lonely and it's a bit like an old friend, I suppose.

Continued

You started again after your wife died but had managed to stop for 2 years before that.

Yes, it's daft really; she would be ever so cross with me. It was her banging on that made me stop that time.

Your wife really cared about your health.

She did, yes.

What was she banging on about that made you stop last time?

Well, my chest was getting bad then. We both noticed that I got out of breath when I wouldn't normally. That's when we came to you and I blew in that thing and you gave me my first inhaler… ooh, she was so cross with me, so I stopped, just like that. It wasn't actually as hard as you would imagine. I kept really busy and spent time with friends who didn't smoke, mostly the bowls crew. Yes, that was the tricky bit, avoiding smokers. Only for the first couple of months then funnily enough, I couldn't even bear the smell of cigarettes. Yes, playing bowls helped.

I can see you are single-minded. When you decided to stop, you did it, and found that being with people who didn't smoke and playing bowls with that group of nonsmokers really helped you.

I did; my wife called it something else, but yes, I am a determined sort of person.

So when you put your mind to it, kept busy and away from people who smoked, you stopped and found it easier than you thought.

I did, yes, you're right.

What are you thinking?

I'm thinking, you're right, it's silly, I should stop. Most of my friends have stopped, those that aren't dead already anyway. We were talking about it the other week and some friends used the patches from somewhere, you know, the service that does all that for free. To be honest I have been thinking about it, not only because of my health but the cost is absolutely ridiculous, and it's not going to get any cheaper is it?

So you have been thinking about this for a while and doing a bit of asking around.

Yes, I have, I suppose. Can I ask you then, are you able to get me in with the free patches service?

Yes of course; while we find an appointment which suits you, may I ask, apart from being free, which you told me before, what else, if anything, do you know about our local smoking cessation service?

Nothing. Oh, my friend said they were very friendly.

Oh, super, would it be OK if I tell you a little bit more about them?

Yes, that would be really helpful ……………

Change talk: desire, ability, reason, need

Note that in Scenario A the power in the conversation lay with the nurse, who gave the patient no opportunity to talk about what might have happened before and what might be in the patient's mind. It was all about advice-giving and telling the patient what was best for him and making decisions for him. Note also

> **Box 3.1 DARN**
>
> D Desire to change: 'How would you feel if you managed to make this change?'
>   *'I would feel so much better; just doing everyday things would be easier.'*
> A Ability to change: 'How might you be able to do it?'
>   *'I could go to Zumba with my friend on Wednesday.'*
> R Reason to change: 'What is your main reason for wanting to make this change?'
>   *'If I stop smoking, then I'll have enough puff to play with the grandkids.'*
> N Need to change: 'If you managed to make this change, what would you be able
>   to do?'
>   *'I would be able to walk farther and become more independent.'*

the resistance back from the patient, who says: '*..but I've smoked for years now, and it's just too hard to stop'*.

In the second scenario, the nurse actively listens and encourages the patient to speak by remaining silent, enabling the patient to collect his thoughts and to realise that the problem is his, not the nurse's. The nurse picks out what is called 'change talk' – signs that he is thinking about changing – and encourages him to speak more about it. The patient starts with recalling his previous successful attempt to stop smoking because his wife was upset: '*... ooh, she was so cross with me, so I stopped, just like that. It wasn't actually as hard as you would imagine.'* Then, as the nurse encourages him to talk more about his previous success, he says: *'I'm thinking, you're right, it's silly, I should stop. Most of my friends have stopped, those that aren't dead already anyway.'*

So, in motivational interviewing, it is about being alert to change talk. The mnemonic DARN (desire, ability, reason, need) is often used to elicit preparatory change talk (Box 3.1).

Listening to understand

In motivational interviewing, it is very important to distinguish between 'listening to join in' and 'listening to understand'. In social situations, it is human nature to listen out for things in common, to swap stories and to join in, for example: 'Ooh, I've been to Majorca too! Did you go to that pearl factory?' In a clinical context this could manifest as using the patient's words to lead back to whatever the nurse wants to talk about.

In scenario A we get: '*so you are still smoking; it is good that you have cut down, but often people don't realise how the amount creeps up again.'*

In scenario B the nurse refrains from this. All the focus is on the patient and on listening to understand. Listening to understand helps express empathy and builds the therapeutic relationship. As patients talk, they are listening to themselves and noticing discrepancies between their current behaviours and where they want to be, and becoming more aware of the consequences.

Open questions, affirmations, and reflections

Open questions

Open questions are questions the patient cannot answer with a yes or no or a fact, such as an address. There is nothing wrong with closed questions when facts are required, such as: 'Are you allergic to penicillin?' For motivational interviewing, however, open questions are a key feature, to encourage patients to open up and reveal what they are thinking, for example:

Tell me	Tell me about your...?
Explain	Explain to me how you feel about...?
Describe	Describe what your...?
What	What are the things that you...?
Where	Where might you find that...?
When	When could you use that...?
Why	Why do you think this keeps happening...?

A really useful open question that the nurse asks in Scenario B is: 'What are you thinking?'.

It elicits the reply: *'I'm thinking, you're right, it's silly, I should stop'.*

Affirmations

Affirmations are a type of reflection that bolsters hope and confidence by acknowledging a positive action that builds self-efficacy. They are a genuine reflection rather than just a compliment. They identify the patient's skills, strengths and characteristics. In Scenario B, the nurse remarks that the patient is very strong-minded, for example. Other examples might be: determined, knowledgeable, kind, thoughtful, focused, strong, independent, a survivor, enthusiastic, practical, resourceful, skilful, principled or experienced.

Reflections

Reflections enable people to hear their change talk again, reinforcing their reasons, their needs, their desires and their abilities. When reflecting on what the person has said, it is important to keep the inflection in the voice down at the end of the sentence and avoid starting sentences with who, why, what and so on. The nurse then repeats or paraphrases what patients are thinking in the form of a statement rather than a question and includes their reasons, needs, desires and abilities which they have mentioned as a result of the open question approach. *'Of course, I'd like to be slimmer, but it's not that easy. I've tried every diet there is and nothing ever seems to work for long; it all goes back on!'*

Reflection – 'If you could, you would really like to lose some weight and keep it off.'

'I know everyone wants me to stop smoking, but it is my only pleasure.'

Reflection – 'though you really enjoy smoking, you are fully aware that everyone worries about you and would prefer you to stop.'

'I realise that the inhalers only work if I take them, but when I'm well, I just forget them.'

Reflection – 'You forget them when you feel well but recognise that to stay well it is important to remember to use them regularly.'

Delivering motivational interviewing remotely

The COVID-19 pandemic has taught GPNs much about switching from face-to-face consultations to video- or telephone-based consultations. The motivational interviewing technique used remains the same, with the addition of skills in telephone- or video-based consultations. A brief summary of these techniques is given later. Because the patient is likely to be at home or at work, it is important to encourage privacy so that the patient feels free to speak.

Telephone consultations

Conducting motivational interviewing on the telephone means that we need to listen even harder, as the nonverbal aspects of communication are missing. Tone of voice is very important. Nurses must convey that they want to help and are interested in the person by actively showing that they are nodding and listening via gentle verbal demonstrations. These are best described as facilitative murmurs – sounds such as umm, yes, or ah ha – so the patient is sure that you are listening. Active listening to understand should be continued throughout, which can be tricky in busy and noisy environments. This means the nurse should try to find a quiet place and not be afraid to ask the patient to repeat things if necessary to check understanding.

The nurse should ensure adequate documentation of the call, which could include a telephone interview proforma, as well as a handwritten, electronic or voice recording.

Conducting telephone consultations is a skill, and nurses are encouraged to seek specific training.

Video-based consultations

With video-based consultations, the advantage is that the nurse and patient can see one another's nonverbal cues. Do, however, check that:

- The nurse and patient both have appropriate skill in managing the technology or have been supplied with relevant guidance to use the platform.

- The patient feels comfortable with video; some people do not like looking at themselves. Some platforms allow people to avoid looking at themselves.
- Patients knows when to expect the call, so that they feel 'ready' to show themselves.
- Standards of dress remain professional, and the background is not distracting or unprofessional.
- Privacy is maintained.
- Lighting is such that the patient can see the nurse's face.
- The gaze is directed into the camera rather than at the patient's image to indicate eye contact.
- Nonverbal cues such as nodding and smiling are used, unlike in telephone consultations, to indicate that you are listening.

Video group clinics (VGCs) that apply the same principles and techniques as motivational interviewing techniques are also an option. You will learn more about face-to-face group consultations and VGCs in the second part of this chapter.

Summary

Motivational interviewing is a powerful way of supporting patients in making change. After the open questions and the listening for change talk, the nurse supports self-reflection through feedback to the patient, thus allowing patients to hear their change talk again. One way to see this is that it is like picking out all the positive things that the patient has said as if they were flowers and then presenting them back together, as if they were a big bouquet. This is called summarising. Taking Scenario B as an example, this might sound like:

> 'You understand the health effects of smoking; you try to keep the amount down and would really love to stop if you could. Your wife really cared about your health, and you took notice of what she said. When you decided to stop, you did it, and found that being with people who didn't smoke and playing bowls with that group of nonsmokers really helped you. So, when you put your mind to it, kept busy and away from people who smoked, you stopped and found it easier than you thought. You've now been thinking about quitting for a while and doing a bit of asking around. I can see that you're very single-minded.'

This would then be followed by a question such as:

> 'What, if anything, will you do when you leave here today?'

Ask, share, ask

This stage is about avoiding confrontation that could arise when telling the patient what to do by instead finding out what they already know, asking permission to give further information and then finding out what they are thinking after having received the information (Box 3.2).

Box 3.2 Ask, share, ask

Ask: Find out what they already know: 'What do you know, if anything, about the stop smoking support available?'

'Not a lot really; I just went cold turkey last time. I think my mate used some tablets.'

Permission: 'Would it be ok if I told you something about it?'

'Yes, go on then.'

Share: Offer information, not advice: 'The services available in this area are...'

Ask: 'What (if anything) did you think about that?'

Goal-setting and making plans

Goal-setting is the responsibility of the patient, not the nurse, based on the patient's priorities. The nurse needs to help the patient make the goals realistic and achievable. For example, if you set a goal of walking four times a week and only walked twice, how would you feel? But if you set a goal of walking twice a week and walked three times, how would you feel then? Success breeds confidence and then further success.

Summary

Actively listen, to understand, not to advise. Make the conversation about the patient; do not join in with your own stories.

Preparatory change talk (DARN)

D Desire to change: 'Why do you want to make this change?'
A Ability to change: 'What might you be able to do?'
R Reason to change: 'What is one good reason for making the change?'
N Need to change: 'On a scale of 0 to 10, how important is it and why?'

Getting moving (OARS)

O Open questions: who, why, what, where, how, when...
A Affirmations: statements that notice and appreciate a positive action
R Reflections: repetition or rephrasing of what the client says
S Summarising: drawing together what the patient has said and presenting it as a bouquet

Implementing change talk (ask, share, ask)

Ask: 'What do you know, if anything, about the stop smoking support available?'
Permission: 'Would it be ok if I told you something about it?'
Share: Offer information, not advice: 'The services available in this area are...'
Ask: 'What (if anything) did you think about that?'

Goal setting and making plans

The patient's plans, not the nurse's
Realistic
Achievable

The skills required to develop a motivational interviewing technique are not hard to learn. With practice, perhaps initially with colleagues, in developing an ease with using silence as a positive form of communication and becoming more comfortable with using open questions, free-flowing communication with the patient will become normal. Guided learning can be found in *The Nursing Times*.

Getting started with group consultations

The clinical consultation has changed very little since the inception of the NHS. Yet, the nature of the health conditions that primary care is supporting patients in living with has shifted fundamentally.

Where once clinics were populated with people needing their clinician to 'see and treat' them, increasingly general practice teams are supporting those who are living with one or several long-term conditions over many years.

Historically, the NHS's response to this challenge has been to change the system, 'redesign the pathway,' introduce new roles and up-skill clinical people. But what if the secret to success lay in transforming how we consult with our patients?

Living and coping with a long-term condition presents patients and their loved ones with a range of complex life challenges. Long-term conditions such as diabetes or chronic obstructive pulmonary disease (COPD) impact every aspect of a person's life, from mealtimes to mobility and physical exercise, sleep, family relationships, community connection and social life. Having a long-term condition also impacts on mental health. There is an independent relationship between physical health conditions and emotional distress (Delahanty et al., 2007), and the prevalence of depression amongst those with common long-term conditions such as diabetes, cardiovascular disease, COPD and musculoskeletal disorders is two to three times higher than that seen in the general population (Kings Fund, 2012).

Recognising and working with this level of complexity is challenging in a 10-minute one-to-one appointment. Often both patients and clinicians are left feeling as though they only scratched the surface and covered the basic necessities – usually the 'clinical agenda' – and did not get to what really matters to the patient.

What is more, although clinicians understand the mechanics of a clinical condition and its medical management, they rarely have experience of living with it, and so have limited understanding of the practical day-to-day challenges that people with long-term conditions face. This means that, when it comes to advising about the practicalities of everyday living and making change, clinicians may have limited credibility.

The value of peer learning and support has been well documented in over 1000 studies (NESTA and National Voices, 2015). Gaining support and advice from others in the same boat helps people feel less alone, boosts confidence and provides empathy and inspiration that ignites hope and the motivation to take control and keep going with lifestyle changes. Peer support groups – for instance the 'Breath Easy' groups organised by the British Lung Foundation for people with respiratory conditions – are undoubtedly powerful, and yet peer support is often separate from planned clinical care and reviews, which means patients have to be motivated to seek out peer support. Not everyone has time to do this or is aware of the benefits peer connection can bring.

So, what if we combined the benefits of peer and clinician support in routine, and planned reviews so that peer support was an integral part of the planned care experience? How would that change primary care's impact?

Curiosity about this question has driven the development of a new approach to consulting for patients called 'group consultation'.

What are group consultations?

Group consultations are an alternative way to deliver one-to-one care in which the clinician consults with a group of 10 to 12 patients at the same time. Each person gets one-to-one attention in the group setting, as well as the chance to listen to what the clinician says to his or her peers. Group consultations can be run face-to-face or remotely via a video platform that facilitates group meetings. The only significant difference is that it is recommended that VGCs include a maximum of eight people to ensure a positive and interactive experience for all participants in a virtual environment.

As every GPN knows, routine reviews include a lot of repetition. Group clinics cut that repetition out completely. Each participant identifies his or her questions for the clinician before the clinician comes into the room, and once common questions are dealt with as a whole group, the clinician takes around 5 minutes to talk to each individual about his or her biometrics, medication and steps he or she can take to improve his or her health whilst the other patients in the group listen in and contribute with their experiences, thoughts and advice.

One of the things GPNs like best about group consultations is that there is more time to educate patients. The evidence shows that after one-to-one consultations people forget 40% to 80% of medical information immediately, and that almost half of the information they remember is incorrect (Kessels, 2003), so when it comes to education, our current consultation model has lots of room for improvement.

Are group consultations the same as group education?

Sometimes group consultations get confused with group education initiatives such as Daphne and Desmond, which are well-established group education programmes for people with type one and type two diabetes, respectively. Of course, the desired outcome of all consultations is that people learn new things and are educated, and so in that way group education and group consultations are similar.

What makes group education different is that, like peer support, group education is often offered separately and is an adjunct to clinical care and reviews. Secondly, group education usually has a set agenda or curriculum determined by the educator or lead clinician. Furthermore, group education is often didactic, with an educator standing up front who talks to people about their condition.

In contrast, group consultations are proactive, planned clinical reviews of patients' progress that enable patients to come together and discuss how each person can improve their health, drawing on the wisdom of their peers and the clinical expert supporting the group consultation. With the clinician's role shifted to facilitating the group, patients set the agenda and start to advise each other and generate solutions to their personal challenges, thus mirroring the principles that underpin motivational interviewing.

How group consultations flow

To watch a video of group consultation flow, go to: https://youtu.be/uZKVbKUvTfs.

The group consultation has three parts:

- Set-up and preparation
- The clinical session
- Reflection and goal setting

The flow is summarised in Fig. 3.1.

The flow is identical for both face-to-face group clinics and VGCs.

The clinician is only present for the clinical session. The other two parts are led by a facilitator, who may be a health care assistant, care navigator, social prescribing link worker or member of the practice administration team, such as a receptionist.

How group consultations flow

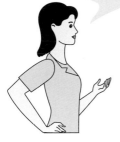

Facilitator sets up the group clinic, welcoming people, running through the flow, and agreeing group understandings. After reviewing the Results Board, people decide their question for the clinician

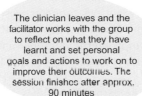

There is a quick break (5 minutes). The clinician joins after approx 15 minutes. He or she reviews the group's questions and decides with the facilitator how they will structure the clinical session. The clinician works with the group to answer their questions and do 1:1 reviews, which everyone listens to

The clinician leaves and the facilitator works with the group to reflect on what they have learnt and set personal goals and actions to work on to improve their outcomes. The session finishes after approx. 90 minutes

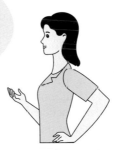

Fig. 3.1   How group consultations flow. (Copyright © 2020 Georgina Craig Associates Limited. All Rights Reserved.)

Set-up and preparation

The face-to-face group clinic or VGC begins with a blank sheet of paper. Patients consent that they will respect confidentiality, agreeing that what they hear in the room will stay in the room. This is done slightly differently depending on whether it is a face-to-face group clinic or VGC. The group is then introduced to the Results Board. An example Results Board, which includes the clinicians' notes (which patients would not see) is given in Fig 3.2.

Results Board: 20 February 2020 (Diabetes)

Consulter: Catherine Smith   **Facilitator:** Shirley Brown

Name	Hba1c	Cholesterol	BP	BMI	Urine acr	EGFR	CVD risk	Eyes	Feet	Concern/to do
Cortney	81	To do	120/70	21	To do	73	Has had CVA	Mar 2019 (abn)	Feb 2020	Chol/urine acr
Charlotte	54	4	128/80	46	n/a	73	13% (not on statin)	May 2019 (N)	Jan 2020	? consider statin?
Norman	81	3.3	148/74	46	124.6	90	35%	DNA	Jan 2020	? DRSS
Paul	74	4	129/66	24.5	2.2	90	Has had CVA	DNA	Jan 2020	? DRSS
Wendy	91	3.3	157/89	30	To do	90	32%	Mar 2019 Abn	Sept 2019	Acr, repeat Hba1c
Annette	59	5.2	122/67	25	0.7	68	8.4%	Jan 2019 (N)	Jan 2020	
Shirley	42	3.9	127/79	30	n/a	88	19.8 %	Apr 2019 (Abn)	Jan 2020	Weight?
Peter	81	3.5	128/78	31	0.3	101	10.3%	Oct 2019 (N)	Jan 2020	Hba1c control?
NORMAL	48-58	<4	<130/80	<25	<3	>90		Annual	Annual	

Fig. 3.2   Sample results board.

Pre-prepared by the group consultation facilitator or practice administration team, the Results Board summarises participants' key biometrics. Having seen their results with the benefit of comparison with their peers and the normal range, patients decide their questions for the clinician. The facilitator supports this process, collects the questions and identifies common questions that essentially become the agenda for the clinical session. Having a Results Board is critical. It leads to patients asking more insightful questions and helps them to understand their progress compared with other people, which is often enlightening and motivating.

The clinician will have reviewed the participants' notes before joining and will have proactively identified issues they want to raise with each person, for example, a note to change or adjust medication or to remind the person that he or she needs a flu vaccination. In the early days, most clinicians have a one-page printout for each patient that they can refer to and add personalised notes for recording later.

The clinician joins the group. The patients have a short comfort break and a chat; perhaps with a drink of water or cup of tea. Meanwhile, the facilitator runs through the group's questions.

The clinical session

When the clinical session begins, the clinician discusses any common questions with the whole group, making use of people's knowledge by asking, '*Does anyone know the answer?*' or '*Has anyone got any thoughts on that?*' – rather than answering the questions himself or herself.

By involving the group and letting them answer their own questions, the clinician taps into collective group wisdom and boosts participants' confidence by demonstrating that the group already knows most of the answers to their questions.

The clinician then moves into more personalised one-to-one discussions with each person in turn, referring to the Results Board as appropriate and asking how each person is getting on with managing his or her condition. All participants listen in to the one-to-ones of each other person in the circle and have the opportunity to share their experiences and thoughts, alongside any advice the clinician has to offer. The clinician encourages the group to answer any further questions that come up, offer advice and share their experiences. For instance, if someone is struggling to make a change such as losing weight, the clinician may ask, *'Has anyone lost weight? What advice would you give?'* This means that, even during the clinical session, patients are doing most of the talking. Experienced clinicians have timed how much of the group clinical session they talk for. It is often as little as 20% of the time. As a measure of quality, asking an observer to time how much you talk during the clinical session can help you assess and improve your group consultation practice. Clinicians' facilitation of group discussion is critical, because research shows that the more interactive group clinics are, the better the health outcomes for participants (Novick et al., 2013).

Setting goals and reflecting on learnings

Once the clinician has spoken to everyone on a one-to-one basis, he or she leaves the group clinic. This provides the opportunity for the clinician to generate prescriptions and update records with individual actions. Often clinicians leave a couple of appointments free directly after the group consultation in case anyone needs to speak to them individually. If these are not needed, this provides extra time for documenting.

In the meantime, the facilitator works with the group to explore what they have learnt from the clinical session and to encourage them to set a personal goal to work towards before their next review, which may be in a year's time or sooner, depending on how well controlled their health condition is.

When do group consultations work best?

Face-to-face group clinics and VGCs have been trialled in England and work well with people at all stages of life, including maternity, early years (health visiting), primary, community, outpatient and specialist care for both adults and children.

From a clinician's perspective, switching to group consultations works especially well where there is:

- A lot of repetition within the clinical review
- A heavy caseload, with regular follow-up required
- Limited capacity or access to clinical expertise

Group consultations work for most long-term health conditions, even if some of the issues to be discussed are personal. Group clinics have also been used to manage conditions characterised by flare-ups. They have been used to support urgent care. For instance, in the United States, Doctor Interactive Group Medical Appointments have supported people with chronic asthma and allergies who are frequent service users. These appointments were provided as weekly drop-in clinics with up to 10 patients per session, and patients were followed up for 4 years. Hospital presentations fell from five a year at baseline to two in the final year of follow-up (Liebhaber et al., 2009).

Once up and running and scheduled on a regular basis, a group clinic model facilitates such a 'drop-in' arrangement. This increases access, clinic flexibility and responsiveness. Knowing they can drop in and see someone if they need support urgently is also reassuring for patients who may be experiencing anxiety; this is especially important for people whose symptoms include breathlessness because anxiety may sometimes exacerbate breathlessness, and the reassurance of knowing they can access support if needed may reduce anxiety.

Because they connect people in the same boat, group consultations also complement initiatives such as social prescribing and care navigation, which have come to the fore as a result of the General Practice Forward View (NHS England, 2016) and aim to support patients who are struggling with psychosocial aspects of living with health issues by helping them become connected and gain peer support – similarly, building community and reducing social isolation – outcomes that primary care networks are tasked with supporting and improving.

What are the benefits for clinicians?

Group consultations have many positive impacts for clinicians.

They are more energising than one-to-one care and help clinicians build more meaningful relationships and get to the bottom of the story quicker with their patients; for instance, patients are more truthful about whether they are taking medication in a group setting (Gandhi & Craig, 2019).

They reduce repetition and lone working, which can be draining. They offer very significant time efficiency gains, with clinicians often seeing the same number of patients in a quarter or a half of the time it would take to see them one-to-one, which frees up time that can be spent with patients who need more support and used to develop access to new services.

Furthermore, compared with one-to-one care, people turn up more often for their group clinics, and 'do not attend' (DNA) rates are lower. Group clinics also eradicate the clinician time wasted when patients DNA because there is no waiting around between patients, and group clinics more often finish on time, helping to reduce stress and improve clinicians' work–life balance.

Finally, and key to development in primary care right now, group consultations support personal, professional and workforce development. They build primary care team cohesion and support integrated working across specialities, practice networks and organisations. Plus, group clinics are a great setting to support skills acceleration in new and returning team members and to enable more experienced clinicians to pass on their knowledge and delegate routine reviews and follow-up care to others in the team.

To hear clinicians talking about group consultations, go to: https://youtu.be /8EoN05SS164.

What are the benefits for patients?

In addition to the psychosocial benefits group care provides, this model has been shown to improve important biometrics compared with one-to-one care. In diabetes, evidence suggests that HbA1c and blood pressure improve (Edelman et al., 2015). In chronic neuromuscular disease, quality of life improves (Seesing et al., 2014). Patients' knowledge of their condition increases (Yehle et al., 2009), and patient satisfaction is high (Heyworth et al., 2014).

What are the benefits for the practice?

In the course of the clinical session and with the help of a well-designed Results Board that ticks all the Quality Outcomes Framework (QOF) boxes, clinical reviews get done that would otherwise have been completed in a one-to-one appointment.

Evaluation suggests that the Results Board may boost QOF compliance and help ensure quality of care, as well as generating additional income for the practice (Gandhi & Craig, 2019).

As highlighted, group clinics also make the most of limited clinician time and capacity, which means the practice is achieving better-quality outcomes in less time.

To hear patients talking about group consultations, go to: https://youtu.be /ZhXgOdT2FZQ.

How do I get started?

Use this chapter to discuss the benefits of group consultations with your practice team. You need a General Practitioner and your practice manager on board. Talk to your health care assistant colleagues about being your facilitator. Once you have some interest and feel your team would like to get started, go to the Group Consultation Hub on the NHS Futures website, where you will find lots of resources and discussion groups. Register for NHS Futures and follow this link: https://bit.ly/nhsvgc or go to www.elcworks .co.uk.

Case study

The challenge

In 2018, the Lancaster Medical Practice introduced group consultations for people living with cancer. Currently this group is not systematically followed up in primary care. Yet, statistics show that following cancer treatment, and when living with and beyond cancer, people have a lot of ongoing needs and concerns, including physical and mental health issues and lifestyle and information needs.

What the team did

The group consultation was built around the Macmillan Holistic Needs Assessment, which is designed to elicit peoples' concerns related to physical, emotional, lifestyle and information needs.

The practice undertook an EMIS search to generate a list of patients eligible for a cancer review. The general practice nurse invited patients to attend. Before the session, the practice sent out information packs and rang to remind people about their appointment.

Six patients were seen and then followed up at 3 and 6 months.

Findings

Clinician efficiency
- Doing the group consultation saved 30 minutes of clinician time compared with six one-to-one reviews
- Usually the General Practitioner did all the cancer reviews for patients in the surgery. The group model facilitated General Practice Nurses' skills development and delegation of the review
- The team plans to combine cancer reviews with reviews for concomitant long-term conditions (e.g., hypertension), to make the reviews even more person-centred

Wellbeing
- At baseline, 66% of patients reported at least one area of concern. At follow up, 66% had no concerns, representing a 100% increase in the number of people with no concerns
- At baseline, amongst those reporting concerns, people had, on average, 4.0 physical, 2.5 emotional and 1.8 lifestyle and information concerns ($n = 8.3$). At follow-up, those reporting concerns had, on average, 4 physical, 1 lifestyle and information and 2 emotional concerns ($n = 7$), a 15% reduction
- The total number of concerns amongst the patients at baseline was 33. At follow-up, the total number of concerns was 14, a reduction of 60%
- At baseline, the average self-assessed 'overall level of concern' was 3. At follow-up, it was 2.2, a reduction of 36%

Experience of care
Patients felt group consultation worked well and that it could also have worked for their initial primary care review following diagnosis. Patients were happy to talk and learnt from each other. The Lancaster Medical Practice team also reported that they enjoyed delivering the group consultation.

Conclusion

This chapter has explored two of the most exciting emergent consultation practices that GPNs are using to improve communication and outcomes from consulting with patients.

What both approaches have in common is that the nurse enables patients to build on their strengths and sees them as resourceful people who know how to heal themselves.

Both practices build confidence and patients' motivation and capacity for self-care. Over time, both aim to help individuals to take control. Furthermore, group consultations support patients in building social networks and community so that patients grow and need primary care teams less.

To master both practices, like any skill, takes practice. The framework presented here gives you an overview of the two techniques and some tips on getting started. Use what you have learnt to reflect on how you currently run your consultations and what you might do differently to deliver more satisfying interactions that leave patients even more motivated to change.

References

Delahanty, L. M., Grant, R. W., Wittenberg, E., et al. (2007). Association of diabetes-related emotional distress with diabetes treatment in primary care patients with Type 2 diabetes. *Diabetic Medicine, 24*(1), 48–54.

Edelman, D., Gierisch, J. M., McDuffie, J. R., Oddone, E., & Williams, J. W., Jr. (2015). Shared medical appointments for patients with Diabetes Mellitus: A systematic review. *Journal of General Internal Medicine, 30*(1), 99–106.

Gandhi, D. & Craig, G. (2019). An evaluation of the suitability, feasibility and acceptability of diabetes group consultations in Brigstock Medical Practice. *Journal of Medicines Optimisation, 5*(1), 39–46.

Heyworth, L., Rozenblum, R., Burgess, J. F., Jr., et al. (2014). Influence of shared medical appointments on patient satisfaction: A retrospective three year study. *Annals of Family Medicine, 12*(4), 324–330.

Kessels, R. P. C. (2003). Patients' memory for medical information. *Journal of the Royal Society of Medicine, 96*(5), 219–222.

Kings Fund. (2012). *Long Term Conditions and mental health: The cost of co-morbidities.* https://www.kingsfund.org.uk/publications/long-term-conditions-and-mental-health.

Liebhaber, M. I., Banister, R. B., Raffetto, W., Dyer, Z. A., & Gershenhorn, G. (2009). Doctor interactive group. Medical appointments (DIGMA) for patients with asthma: A four year outcome study. *Journal of Allergy and Clinical Immunology, 123*(2), S42.

Miller, W. R. & Rollnick, S. (1991). *Motivational interviewing: Preparing people to change addictive behavior.* Guilford Press.

Miller, W. R. & Rollnick, S. (2012). *Motivational interviewing: Helping people change.* Guilford Press.

Miller, W. R. & Rose, G. S. (2009). Toward a theory of motivational interviewing. *The American Psychologist, 64*(6), 527–537.

Miller, W. R., Taylor, C. A., & West, J. C. (1980). Focused versus broad-spectrum behavior therapy for problem drinkers. *Journal of Consulting and Clinical Psychology, 48*(5), 590–601.

National Centre for Smoking Cessation and Training. https://elearning.ncsct.co.uk/vba-launch.

NESTA and National Voices. (2015). *Peer support: What is it and why does it work?*

NHS England. (2016). *General Practice Forward View (GPFV).* https://www.england.nhs.uk/gp/gpfv/.

Novick, G., Reid, A. E., Lewis, J., Kershaw, T. S., Rising, S., & Ickovics, J. R. (2013). Group Prenatal care: Model fidelity and outcomes. *American Journal of Obstetrics and Gynecology, 209*(2), 112.e1–112.e6.

Nursing Times. (2010). *Motivational interviewing 1: Background, principles and application in health care.* https://www.nursingtimes.net/clinical-archive/motivational-interviewing-1-background-principles-and-application-in-healthcare-28-08-2010/.

Public Health England. (2016). *Making every contact count.* https://www.gov.uk/government/publications/making-every-contact-count-mecc-practical-resources.

Royal College of Nursing. *How motivational interviewing works.* https://www.rcn.org.uk/clinical-topics/supporting-behaviour-change/motivational-interviewing.

Rubak, S., Sandbaek, A., Lauritzen, T., & Christensen, B. (2005). Motivational interviewing: A systematic review and meta-analysis. *The British Journal of General Practice, 55*(513), 305–312.

Seesing, F. M., Drost, G., Groenewoud, J., van der Wilt, G. J., & van Engelen, B. G. (2014). Shared medical appointments improve QOL in neuromuscular patients: A randomized controlled trial. *Neurology, 83*(3), 240–246.

Yehle, K. S., Sands, L. P., Rhynders, P. A., & Newton, N. D. (2009). The effect of shared medical visits on knowledge and self-care in patients with heart failure: A pilot study. *Heart Lung, 38*(1), 25–33.

Chapter 4

Treatment room skills

Helen Donovan, Jane Chiodini, Helen Crowther, Paula Spooner,
Gill Boast

Vaccination in primary care by Helen Donovan

Learning outcomes

After reading this chapter you should be able to:

1. Understand the fundamentals of core treatment room skills to nurses new to general practice (General Practice Nurses)
2. Appreciate the principles and rationale for vaccination, travel health, cervical cytology and wound care
3. Identify where to access appropriate and evidence-based information to facilitate best practice

Introduction

Vaccination is a fundamental part of primary care, and in the United Kingdom it is primarily a role for general practice nurses (GPNs). Vaccines are highly effective at reducing infectious disease and are recognised by the World Health Organization (WHO) as second only to clean water at effectively controlling disease (Andre et al., 2008). In the United Kingdom, a number of different vaccines have been successfully introduced over the last 50 years, and, as such, many once-common infections are now rarely seen.

The success of any vaccine programme relies on enough people being vaccinated to control or stop the spread of infections. To ensure continued disease control, it is essential to maintain a high vaccine uptake and to make sure that vaccines are given safely and effectively. To achieve this, those who advise on and/or administer vaccines need to be knowledgeable and skilled. They also need to be able to answer patients'/parents' questions confidently and accurately and to be able to explain why vaccines are needed, while dispelling any myths that may be believed or any concerns that may arise.

This chapter discusses the various elements required to successfully and safely provide vaccines in general practice. It provides this information alongside key resources to support best practice and to help GPNs stay well informed and up to date as vaccinators. The importance of vaccination has become even more apparent in the management of the COVID-19 pandemic.

Immunisation is the process where a person is made immune or resistant to an infectious disease. This may be by the administration of a vaccine, which stimulates the body's own immune system to protect the individual against subsequent infection or disease. It may also occur after exposure to the infection and recovery from the disease. The terms immunisation and vaccination are often used interchangeably, but for the purpose of this chapter, which is about the principles of giving vaccines, the term vaccination will be used.

This chapter is intended to provide an overview for GPNs to support best practice and to give vaccinators the necessary knowledge, skills and competence to undertake this essential role. It provides a background to the principles of and rationale for vaccination and the routine vaccination schedule for the United Kingdom to support vaccine administration, and addresses how to discuss vaccination with individuals and carers. It is beyond the scope of this chapter to detail every aspect of vaccination, but the chapter will direct readers to the most appropriate and evidence-based sources to find out more. Each section is supported with key resources to support more in-depth understanding.

The programme is broadly similar across the United Kingdom, but there are some differences to schedules and guidance. Vaccinators should familiarise themselves with the relevant public health information on immunisation and vaccination, and also any local information.

The UK vaccination policy, including the recommended schedule, the rationale for each vaccine and the principles of best practice in vaccination, is set out in 'Immunisation against infectious disease,' also known as the 'Green Book' (Public Health England [PHE], 2020). This resource is applicable across the United Kingdom, is constantly being updated and should always be accessed online. Throughout this chapter individual chapters from this resource are referred to for vaccinators to look at for further detail.

Background to vaccination

The use of vaccines to protect individuals from the risk of dying or experiencing serious consequences from having an infectious disease has had a significant impact on our health. The WHO states that 2 to 3 million deaths a year are averted through successful vaccine programmes; and yet there are still 1.5 million deaths attributed to vaccine-preventable disease per year, and one in five children remain unvaccinated (Okwo-Bele, 2015), which shows the need to continually improve on vaccination services.

In the United Kingdom most children receive the vaccines they need, and globally the programme is highly respected. It is constantly being evaluated, and vaccines are now recommended for individuals across their life to protect them from a wide range of infections. The effectiveness of the programme is evident in the significant reductions seen in the number of cases of disease after

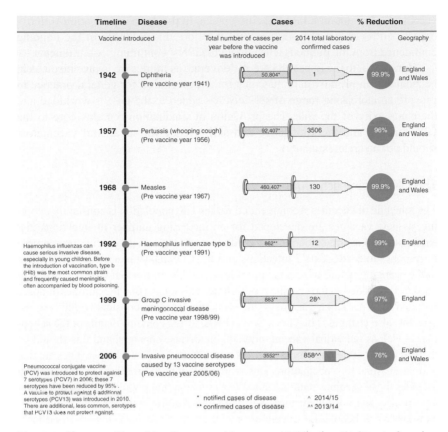

Timeline	Disease	Cases		% Reduction
Vaccine introduced		Total number of cases per year before the vaccine was introduced	2014 total laboratory confirmed cases	Geography
1942	Diphtheria (Pre vaccine year 1941)	50,804*	1	99.9% England and Wales
1957	Pertussis (whooping cough) (Pre vaccine year 1956)	92,407*	3506	96% England and Wales
1968	Measles (Pre vaccine year 1967)	460,407*	130	99.9% England and Wales
1992	Haemophilus influenzae type b (Pre vaccine year 1991)	862**	12	99% England
1999	Group C invasive meningococcal disease (Pre vaccine year 1998/99)	883**	28^	97% England
2006	Invasive pneumococcal disease caused by 13 vaccine serotypes (Pre vaccine year 2005/06)	3552**	858^^	76% England and Wales

Haemophilus influenzas can cause serious invasive disease, especially in young children. Before the introduction of vaccination, type b (Hib) was the most common strain and frequently caused meningitis, often accompanied by blood poisoning.

Pneumococcal conjugate vaccine (PCV) was introduced to protect against 7 serotypes (PCV7) in 2006; these 7 serotypes have been reduced by 95% . A vaccine to protect against 6 additional serotypes (PCV13) was introduced in 2010. There are additional, less common, serotypes that PCV13 does not protect against.

* notified cases of disease   ^ 2014/15
** confirmed cases of disease   ^^ 2013/14

Fig. 4.1   Vaccines. (From https://www.gov.uk/government/publications/the-impact-of-vaccines-infographic.)

vaccines against them were introduced (PHE, 2016; Fig. 4.1) and consequently the substantial effects on mortality and morbidity.

As the incidence of vaccine-preventable diseases declines, because of the success of vaccine programmes, GPNs need to be able to explain why vaccinations are still so important and dispel any misconceptions about vaccines that may arise. As the infections become uncommon, the public increasingly worries about the rare risks of the vaccines (Cooper et al., 2008), or even has unfounded safety concerns which amount to no more than myth. A key factor critical to the ongoing success of the programme is the knowledge, skills and expertise of those who provide information and advice on immunisation and give the vaccines. It is evident from recent surveys that the public recognises and trusts this expertise and values being able to get advice from professionals who are both skilled and knowledgeable about the vaccines they need (Campbell et al., 2015; Campbell et al., 2017; Edwards et al., 2017; PHE, 2019c). It is therefore vital that vaccinators are confident, well-informed and up to date to ensure public confidence in vaccines and maintain a high vaccine uptake. In the main, vaccination is delivered by GPNs in general practice, and therefore this evidence of the ongoing confidence from the public is a testament to GPNs' continuing commitment.

The shift in the way health care is delivered, as more care is provided out of hospital and in primary care, has meant the expectation for general practice to provide an increasing range of services has added to the GPN's workload and the complexity of the role. The provision of vaccination remains core to the GPN's remit, and the knowledge and skill needed for successful vaccinators should not be underestimated.

The UK vaccine schedule

The schedule of vaccines recommended for the UK population is constantly evolving, as new vaccines are developed for an increasing number of infectious diseases, but also as the epidemiology of diseases changes. The vaccine programme in response to SARS-CoV2 infections and the COVID-19 pandemic is testament to the changing nature of vaccine programmes. This means that new and different vaccines are added to the vaccine programme. This means that the number of doses required for a particular vaccine or the schedule for when boosters would be most effective also changes. The Green Book (PHE, 2013) contains details of the schedule, as well as individual vaccine-preventable disease chapters, and this should be the first point of reference for any GPN looking for advice on what vaccines are due and the reasons for vaccination. This is in relation to the routine schedule, which includes those vaccines recommended for anyone in the population based on their age. It also sets out where there are particular requirements for vaccination, for example when people are travelling or if they or others in their household have conditions which mean that additional or further vaccines would be recommended.

Resources

Useful tools for general practice nurses regarding the routine vaccination schedule; these are updated regularly. Check the country-specific pages for any variations.

● The 'complete immunisation schedule' part of the Public Health England immunisation collection: https://www.gov.uk/government/publications/the-complete-routine-immunisation-schedule

● 'A visual guide for vaccines to the routine programme' – poster with images of all the vaccines in the current schedule: https://www.gov.uk/government/publications/a-visual-guide-to-vaccines-poster

---

The routine schedule details the vaccines required for anyone in the population, the number of doses required and the gaps required between doses of the same vaccine to maximise the effect. Certain vaccines are only recommended for individuals at a specific age, depending on how old people are likely to be when they catch the disease, when the disease is most likely to be of significance or when the maximum impact of offering routine vaccination would be

Box 4.1 Three steps to establishing vaccine requirements

1. Identify what the person has had already. If possible, use his or her vaccine record, online translation tools and the relevant county vaccination schedule:
   - European Centre for Disease Control vaccine scheduler: https://vaccine-schedule.ecdc.europa.eu/
   - World Health Organization vaccine-preventable diseases: monitoring system, global summary: http://apps.who.int/immunization_monitoring/globalsummary/schedules
   - Unless there is a reliable vaccine history, individuals should be assumed to be unimmunised, and a full course of immunisations planned
2. Determine what they now need. This will depend on their age and previous vaccinations:
   - The Public Health England (PHE) algorithm 'Vaccination of individuals with uncertain or incomplete immunisation status': https://www.gov.uk/government/publications/vaccination-of-individuals-with-uncertain-or-incomplete-immunisation-status
   - The PHE 'UK and International Immunisation Schedules Comparison tool' looks at the UK schedule and compares it to that of the 20 most common immigrant countries: https://www.gov.uk/government/publications/uk-and-international-immunisation-schedules-comparison-tool
3. Plan the schedule for the individual. Use the minimum number of visits and the shortest timescale to provide protection as soon as possible.
   - Where individuals come into the United Kingdom partway through their immunisation schedule, aim to get them onto the UK schedule and immunised as appropriate for age
   - If a vaccine schedule has been started, there is no need to repeat doses, however long the gap; just resume the course

seen. For example, *Haemophilus influenzae* type B is very uncommon in children over 10 years. Shingles infection can occur at any age, but the maximum impact of routine vaccination is seen when it is given to people between 70 and 80 years of age. Pertussis infection in neonates is life-threatening, and vaccination of the mother in pregnancy helps provide passive immunity to protect infants until they are old enough to have the vaccine themselves (Box 4.1).

Determining what vaccines people need is complex and can be time-consuming, particularly where people have missed out on vaccines at the recommended time or when people come from other countries.

The reality is that this probably cannot all be done in one appointment. If possible, arrange for an appointment with enough time or bring people back to go over the steps and plan their future appointments.

Administration of vaccines

For anyone unused to injecting infants and children, this can be daunting, and the best advice is to arrange to spend time with one or preferably a few experienced vaccinators to pick up tips, such as how to position wriggling babies or reluctant children and getting parents or carers to hold small children and keep them still and secure.

It may seem a minor consideration for many nurses, but the thought of having an injection and experiencing the associated pain, however slight, can put many people off. A significant proportion of the population will have a needle phobia, and Taddio et al. (2012) warned that these fears need to be taken seriously to support vaccine uptake and manage vaccine clinics. The WHO position paper on minimising pain at the time of vaccination (WHO, 2015) suggests that between 24% and 40% of people are concerned about the pain associated with injections. The paper provides some strategies to help with minimising the pain, including keeping calm, being organised and collaborative, providing distraction for children, making sure children are held securely and making the process as quick and efficient as possible.

The best practice for vaccine administration is set out in Chapter 4 of the Green Book; these recommendations are based on the currently available evidence and experience. On occasion they may differ from the information in the vaccine manufacturers' summaries of product characteristics; in these cases, the Green Book advice should be followed. Vaccinators need to familiarise themselves with the information and guidance in the Green Book for the vaccine being given.

The vaccine needs to be prepared according to the guidance and just before administration because the efficacy may be compromised if the vaccine is prepared too far in advance.

Route of vaccine delivery

Most vaccines are given via the intramuscular (IM) route. The needle length needs to be appropriate, and the vaccine efficacy depends on the vaccine being delivered in the correct way and at the correct site. This will normally be the deltoid muscle in adults and children over 1 year. In infants and babies under 1 year the anteriolateral aspect of the thigh provides a larger muscle mass. Where more than one vaccine is needed in any one limb, there needs to be a gap of approximately 2.5 cm between each injection. For most IM injections in infants, children and adults a 25 mm 23G (blue) or 25 mm 25G (orange) needle should be used. Only in preterm or very small infants is a 16 mm needle suitable for IM injection. In larger adults, a longer length (e.g., 38 mm (green)) may be required, and an individual assessment should be made.

IM injections for vaccines should be given with the skin held tight, not bunched. There is no need to cleanse the skin before injection unless it is visibly dirty, in which case it should be cleaned with soap and water, not alcohol wipes (PHE, 2017). There is no need to aspirate the syringe before administration, and it is best to administer the vaccine as quickly as possible to minimise the time the needle is in the skin (Taddio et al., 2015). Gloves are not necessary when administering a vaccine by injection, providing the health worker's skin is intact (WHO, 2010), as gloves may exacerbate skin problems in health care workers;

see the Royal College of Nursing (RCN) guidance on the appropriate use of gloves (RCN, 2018a).

Vaccinators need to be familiar with the route of delivery for any other vaccines they give, such as Bacille Calmette–Guérin, which is given intradermally, and occasional vaccines that may need to be given by subcutaneous injection. The live attenuated influenza vaccine given to children is administered via the intranasal route, and some other vaccines, such as the rotavirus vaccine, are given orally.

Consent

Consent is described by the National Health Service (NHS) as the permission given by a person before they receive any type of medical treatment, test or examination (NHS, 2019a). This must be done based on an explanation by a clinician.

Consent needs to be given voluntarily by someone who has enough information to make the decision, as well as the capacity to make the decision. The individual or the parent or guardian needs to be informed of what vaccine is being given and give their consent.

This is an area which often causes GPNs concern. Chapter 2 of the Green Book describes the principles and process of consent in greater detail, and vaccinators should familiarise themselves with this information. It is important, however, that vaccinators do not put in place unnecessary barriers to vaccination.

Legally, consent can be given verbally. There is no requirement for consent to immunisation to be in writing, and, although it does provide a record of the decision, this consent can also be made verbally.

Children aged 16 and 17 years can give consent on their own behalf. Although it is usual to seek parental consent for younger children, a child under 16 can give valid consent, provided that the child is sufficiently mature to understand the benefits and risks of vaccination and the risks of not vaccinating.

Where consent is sought from parents, it is not necessary to insist on a letter from parents or a signed consent form. Indeed, it should be noted that a signature alone on a form is not conclusive proof that consent has been given.

Vaccinators need to work closely with families and know who has attended for vaccines with the child. Legally it is acceptable for the person with parental responsibility to give permission to another person, such as a child minder or grandparent, to bring in the child to be vaccinated and to give consent on behalf of the parent (Children Act, 1989). However, vaccinators need to be clear that this permission is in place, and, where consent is given by a person other than the individual, the person who has given consent should be clearly documented in the medical record.

The consent of one person with parental responsibility is all that is necessary. If, for example, one parent brings the infant for vaccination, it is not necessary to check if the other parent consents. If, however, the nurse becomes aware that the other parent objects to the vaccination, it should not be given until the dispute has been resolved.

If an adult lacks capacity to consent, for example, because of a severe learning disability, there may be a lasting power of attorney giving consent. If not, the vaccinator may lawfully administer the vaccine, if it is in the best interests of the adult. The consent of relatives is not necessary. It is, however, good practice to involve the relatives and to answer all their questions.

Vaccine safety and adverse reactions

Vaccines stimulate an immune response in the body, and as a result, adverse reactions can occur. Most of these are predictable and resolve spontaneously without specific treatment. Chapter 8 of the Green Book details the common side effects which vaccinators can expect. Very occasionally more serious adverse reactions can occur, and all vaccinators need to be trained and up to date with what to do in the event of anaphylaxis. Although the risk of anaphylaxis associated with vaccines is rare (1:1,000,000), the resuscitation council recommends that vaccinators should have a regular update. There are e-learning resources to support this: https://www.resus.org.uk/anaphylaxis/emergency-treatment-of-anaphylactic-reactions/.

The individual receiving the vaccine, or his or her parent or carer, also needs to be made aware of possible side effects, as well as more serious adverse reactions and advice on what to do; fever is a common side effect and can be easily treated with an appropriate dose of paracetamol or ibuprofen. Leaflets are available to give people at the time of having a vaccine. There is no evidence to support keeping people for a period of time post vaccination, but obviously, any immediate adverse reactions should be noted. Any adverse reaction needs to be recorded on the Yellow Card notification system, whether by the individual or the parent or by the vaccinator; this is detailed in Chapter 9 of the Green Book.

Record keeping

The vaccine details need to be recorded in the patient record. This needs to include the name of the vaccine, the batch number and the expiry date. The dose and the site at which the vaccine has been given need to be recorded. Where more than one vaccine is given, the record needs to clearly indicate where each vaccine has been given; and where more than one vaccine is given in a limb, then the position of each needs to be recorded clearly. It is imperative that this is done accurately and using the correct codes so that there is an exact reporting on vaccine uptake for the practice and the wider population. The information also needs to be recorded in the individual's personal vaccination record.

Appointment times

Vaccine administration errors contribute to the overall rate of adverse events following vaccination, as indicated in Chapter 8 of the Green Book. It is therefore essential for clinic management to consider how to avoid errors and make the process as easy as possible for the vaccinator and the person receiving the vaccine. The RCN publication 'Managing immunisation clinics' (2018) provides a practical tool to support GPNs in managing a childhood vaccine clinic and making sure that the right vaccines are used in the right way. One of the key factors is having enough time. As we have already seen in this chapter, the schedule itself is complex, and the process needed to make sure vaccines are given correctly and safely requires detailed attention, as well as having time to determine which vaccines are needed and to answer queries or concerns. The average GPN appointment is 10 to 15 minutes, and in practice this often is not enough time. For most childhood vaccine appointments 20 minutes is the minimum, and more time may be needed where there are multiple vaccines to give or a complex history (RCN, 2018b). Similarly, the RCN travel competencies (Boyne et al., 2018) also suggest that, at minimum, a 20-minute appointment is required for a travel consultation. Influenza vaccines can often be given safely in a much shorter time, depending on how the clinic is arranged and what administration support is available.

Resources

Alongside the Green Book there are other useful resources to ensure best practice:
- The World Health Organization 'Best practice for injections and related procedures':   https://www.who.int/infection-prevention/publications/best-practices_toolkit/en/
- The Royal College of Nursing 'Practical and clinical guidance for vaccine administration': https://www.rcn.org.uk/clinical-topics/public-health/immunisation/practical-and-clinical-guidance-for-vaccine-administration

---

Maximising uptake and addressing barriers to vaccination

Although individual protection acquired from vaccines is important, successful control of many vaccine-preventable diseases requires that significant numbers of people are vaccinated. This means that every effort needs to be made to vaccinate as many people as possible and to maintain a high uptake of the recommended vaccines.

In general, the United Kingdom has relatively high vaccination uptake; however, the rates fall short of the 95% coverage generally agreed to be needed for most vaccines to stop disease spreading. Although there is a lot of speculation that there is an increasing antivaccine movement and that social media messaging may be undermining peoples' trust and confidence in vaccines, the evidence does not support this. The public trusts the information it gets on vaccination from health care professionals over and above other sources of information (PHE, 2019c). The reasons for lower than ideal uptake are multiple. The evidence suggests that organisation of services and the way in which people can access services contribute, and that various strategies are needed to improve uptake and remove barriers (Crocker-Buque et al., 2016). A report from the

Royal Society for Public Health (2019) showed that the key barriers to vacci-nation were the timing and availability of appointments and getting child care. Health care workers who took part in the survey acknowledged that parents, especially those who work, struggle to fit in vaccine appointments with busy schedules.

Key elements for improving uptake

- Call and recall: Sending reminders when vaccines are due, and then further reminders, is crucial. It is unreasonable to expect people to remember from a previous appointment or a conversation they may have had that their vac-cine is due. Appointments and reminders for these appointments need to be built into the delivery of the service.
- Checking and reminding individuals: This should occur when people con-tact the surgery receptionists to check if their vaccines are up to date, par-ticularly for children and young people up to 25 years, and appointments for them to have the vaccines they need should be arranged. The patient records and information technology system can be used to support this and post alerts when vaccines are due.
- Keeping accurate records: This should include accurate codes so that data is reported properly. It is important that practice staff know who is due for vaccines. Use the practice patient record system to run searches to identify those missing vaccines within the practice population and plan strategies accordingly.
- Scheduling appointments: Make sure that there are enough appointments, and that these are flexible to allow people to come at different times. It is also useful to have options for people to call in to discuss vaccines.
- Providing information: It is imperative that vaccinators speak about vaccines with confidence and answer people's questions. Have resources, leaflets and posters available, signpost people to reputable sources of information online and educate patients on how to look for these information sources. Being able to talk to people about vaccines is crucial. Based on the evidence, the sort of questions people ask can often be predicted (Kennedy et al., 2011), and therefore nurses can be prepared to answer their questions and tailor their response based on what people are asking and the level of understand-ing (Donovan & Bedford, 2013).

Reflection

Consider how the vaccination clinic is organised in your practice, taking into con-sideration all that has been mentioned above regarding timings.

What is the uptake within your population for vaccines given at 1 year, 2 years and 5 years of age?

What could be done to improve the service and increase coverage?

Education and training in vaccination

The national minimum standards and core curriculum for immunisation training were first developed in 2005 by the then Health Protection Agency, with the overall aim being to describe the minimum training that should be given to all practitioners engaging in any aspect of immunisation so that they are able to confidently, competently, safely and effectively promote and administer vaccinations. The original standards have subsequently been revised and updated, and there are now two sets of training standards and core curricula: one for registered health care professionals (PHE, 2018a) and one for health care support workers (PHE, 2015), who are becoming increasingly involved in advising and/or administering certain vaccines.

The standards define the responsibilities of vaccinators and employers in relation to immunisation training. They describe the need for foundation training encompassing twelve core areas of knowledge for those new to immunisation and discuss the importance of regular updates, what should be covered in update training and ways to stay up to date in immunisation.

One of the consequences of a successful vaccination programme is that the public and many health care workers themselves have limited knowledge or experience of the diseases they are vaccinating against and the burden the diseases have on individuals. The ongoing development of new and improved vaccines, and the prevalence and trends of infectious diseases frequently changing, mean that many new programmes have been introduced and existing programmes modified. Alongside this, media messages and social media can rapidly spread concerns and myths about vaccine safety and about the necessity of some vaccines, all of which impacts on public confidence.

Given that trust in the information and advice provided by health care practitioners appears to be pivotal in influencing patient and parental decisions about immunisation (Campbell et al., 2015; Campbell et al., 2017; Edwards et al., 2017; Leask et al., 2014), and consequently in achieving and maintaining high vaccine uptake, high levels of knowledge and confidence and a positive attitude to vaccination in health care practitioners are crucial. This can only be achieved through receiving comprehensive foundation training and ongoing updates.

It is also essential in preventing vaccination errors. With the increasing complexity of and frequent changes made to the programme, and progressively more complex conditions and medication regimes which may affect whether some patients can receive certain vaccines, comprehensive education is vital. Mistakes not only put patients at risk of adverse reactions and of being inadequately protected, they also decrease public confidence in immunisation. This could ultimately mean fewer people choosing to be vaccinated, which will lead to more cases and outbreaks of vaccine preventable disease and a loss of herd immunity.

Box 4.2 Core areas of immunisation knowledge

1. The aims of immunisation, national vaccine policy and schedules
2. The immune response to vaccines and how vaccines work
3. Vaccine-preventable diseases
4. The different types of vaccines, their composition and the indications and contraindications
5. Current issues in immunisation
6. Communicating with patients, parents and carers about vaccines
7. Legal issues in immunisation
8. Storage and handling of vaccines
9. Correct administration of vaccines
10. Anaphylaxis and adverse reactions
11. Documentation, record-keeping and reporting
12. Strategies for optimising immunisation uptake

From the Public Health England National Minimum Standards and core curriculum for registered health care practitioners: https://www.gov.uk/government/publications/national-minimum-standards-and -core-curriculum-for-immunisation-training-for-registered-healthcare-practitioners.

The national minimum standards are designed to support any health care practitioner with a role in immunisation to request and gain access to comprehensive training. The standards provide best practice guidelines, and, whereas they are not mandatory, given the wider need for professional and practice standards they should be seen as a useful tool to support safe, effective and quality immunisation services, rather than as a barrier to practice.

The core curriculum describes the 12 core topics that should be included in all foundation immunisation training and provides detail as to the key areas each topic should cover (Box 4.2).

The curriculum is designed so that it can be adapted to meet the needs of the particular workforce. The level of detail within the topics covered can be adapted based on the particular nature of the work, the role of the practitioners and the vaccine(s) they advise on and/or administer.

It is also recommended that there is flexibility in the way that immunisers gain their knowledge, for example through a blended approach using e-learning alongside face-to-face taught courses and gaining practical experience with the support of a mentor. The comprehensive interactive e-learning programme found at https://www.e-lfh.org.uk/programmes/immunisation/ covers all aspects of the curriculum and can be used as a foundation for those new to vaccination or as a refresher for people to update their knowledge. Practitioners should also keep up to date through a combination of e-learning, webcasts, subscribing to the monthly Vaccine Update publication from PHE (https://www .gov.uk/government/collections/vaccine-update), reading journal articles, performing self-assessment against a knowledge and competency framework and attending study days and courses. Clinical supervision is an important tool that can help people stay up to date. It can also be helpful to have a colleague available to discuss complex cases, review the information in Vaccine Update and go through the competency tool, such as the RCN Immunisation Knowledge and Skills Competence assessment tool (https://www.rcn.org.uk/professional -development/publications/pdf-006943). There are specific disease and vaccine sections within the e-lfh platform for those only involved in certain programmes such as the influenza or COVID-19 programmes.

Assessment of knowledge and competence

Following training, a period of supervised practice to allow acquisition and observation of clinical skills and application of knowledge to practice for practitioners new to immunisation is recommended, as is the completion of an immunisation competency checklist (PHE, 2018a). A knowledge and competency assessment tool is available for both registered health care professionals and health care support staff to use; it is included in an appendix in the training standards (PHE, 2015; PHE, 2018a) and as an RCN publication (RCN, 2015). The tool has been designed to assess a practitioner's knowledge, core clinical skills and vaccine administration process. It can be used by those who are new to immunisation or by experienced practitioners to check their knowledge and as part of their update. It can be adapted depending on the individual service area and the specific range of vaccines the individual gives or advises on, and can be used as a self-assessment tool, as an assessment tool for use with a supervisor, or both.

Vaccine ordering and storage

Vaccines recommended for the routine schedule are ordered in to general practice from a central stock; the practice does not pay for them directly. Influenza vaccines and travel vaccines will be purchased directly from the manufacturer. It is an essential part of the vaccine clinic process to have enough vaccines, but also store them in the correct way so that they are effective. They are sensitive biological substances and can become ineffective if stored outside of the correct environment. Vaccines are also a significant cost to the NHS. Chapter 3 of the Green Book covers the ordering, storage and disposal of vaccines.

Ordering and management

- Have named people within the team who are responsible for the ordering and management of vaccines; however, all members of the team need to be aware of how important it is to ensure vaccines are kept in the optimum conditions.
- Vaccines need to be maintained in what is referred to as the 'cold chain': this means that they need to be kept according to the manufacturer licence

or authorisation. This is normally between 2° C and 8° C from the point of manufacture through to administration to the patient.

- The vaccines need to be kept refrigerated, and the stock should be rotated so that new vaccine stock is placed at the back to make sure vaccines are used within their expiry date.
- Only enough vaccines should be ordered for the needs of the practice, every 2 to 4 weeks.

Vaccine fridge

- Vaccines need to be stored in an approved and validated fridge designed for pharmaceutical products. Do not be tempted to use an ordinary domestic fridge.
- The fridge should only be used to store pharmaceutical products. Do not store food and clinical specimens alongside vaccines.
- The temperature of the fridge needs to be kept between 2° C and 8° C. Keep the vaccine fridge secure and accessible only to authorised practice staff.
- Have the fridge installed with a switchless socket or clearly label the plug 'Do not unplug/switch off'.
- Use a large enough fridge to allow enough space around the vaccine packages for air to circulate. Do not overfill the fridge.
- Keep the fridge clean, with no build-up of ice. Follow the manufacturer's servicing recommendations and ensure the fridge is calibrated to check the temperature gauge.
- Keep vaccines in their original packaging and prevent them from being exposed to light. Keep the fridge organised so it is easy to see where vaccines are.

Fridge temperature recording

- The temperature of the fridge should ideally be recorded twice a day during the working week.
- Use the four Rs: Read, Record, Reset, React
  - Read: the current, maximum and minimum temperature
  - Record: on a chart to show the temperature
  - Reset: the fridge temperature
  - React: if the temperature falls outside 2° C to 8° C
- Ideally, have a second thermometer independent to the integral thermometer in the vaccine fridge. This is so you can crosscheck the accuracy of the temperature and monitor the temperature should the electricity supply fail.
- A data logger is useful to help show detailed information about the fridge temperature if there is a cold chain failure.
- If a data logger is used, however, you still need to read and record temperatures on the fridge (minimum, maximum and current) and reset the min/max

thermometer. This will assure you the fridge contents have been stored correctly and are safe to use.

Resources
- Public Health England vaccine handling protocols: https://www.gov.uk /government/collections/immunisation#vaccine-handling-and-protocols
- Care and Quality Commission Nigel's Surgery 17: Vaccine storage and fridges in GP practices: https://www.cqc.org.uk/guidance-providers/gps/nigels-surgery -17-vaccine-storage-fridges-gp-practices

---

Medicines administration

Vaccines are prescription-only medicines (POMs), which means they need to have the appropriate authorisation to supply and/or administer to a patient. The regulation of medicines is clearly defined under the Human Medicines Regulations 2012 (HMR, 2012) and is applicable across the United Kingdom. Chapter 5 in the Green Book (PHE, 2017) provides greater detail. All vaccines are POMs, and under the legislation medicines cannot be sold or supplied unless there is a valid prescription or a patient-specific direction (PSD) from an appropriate practitioner.

The prescriber is responsible for the assessment of the patient(s) named, and the prescription or PSD provides directions in writing detailing the medicines to be supplied or administered.

There are some specific exemptions in the legislation which are relevant to those providing vaccines:

- A Patient Group Direction (PGD) provides a legal framework for some health care professionals, including registered nurses, to administer a POM.
- In the case of an occupational health scheme, a 'Written Instruction' signed by a medical practitioner can allow for certain listed health care professionals to administer medicines.
- Certain medicines such as adrenaline can be administered in an emergency without the directions of a prescriber.
- In addition to these under the Coronavirus and Influenza Amendment to the HMR (2020) the use of a national protocol was introduced to authorise administration of specific vaccines in an emergency situation.

However, best practice is for any medicine or treatment to be provided on a named patient basis. Vaccination clinics should be set up so that vaccines can be provided to anyone who is eligible either in booked clinics or at other times, in an opportunistic way. In practice, unless the nurse administering the vaccine is an independent prescriber the usual mechanism for supply and or administration of vaccines is with a PGD which provides a legal framework for some health care professionals, including registered nurses, to administer a POM. Although many people get confused with the legal requirements, the reality is that PGDs have allowed a great deal of flexibility in the way services are delivered. It is important to note that, for unregistered staff, such as health care assistants, or for registered nursing associates, the legislation does not allow for the use of a PGD, and if these staff are supporting vaccination clinics, they will need a prescription or PSD to administer the vaccine (RCN, 2019a; RCN, 2019b).

Immunisation training is a key requirement for the use of PGDs. The Medicines and Healthcare products Regulatory Agency (MHRA, 2017) states that only competent, qualified and trained professionals can use PGDs for the supply and/or administration of vaccines, and National Institute for Health and Care Excellence (NICE) guidance on PGDs (NICE, 2013) recommends that a comprehensive and appropriate training programme be provided for all people involved in using PGDs, with competency assessed post-training. Additionally, the Nursing and Midwifery Council (NMC) Code states that nurses must be up to date with skills and knowledge and use the best available evidence (NMC, 2015), and the NMC standards for medicines management state that PGDs should only be used once the registrant has been assessed as competent (NMC, 2007).

Resources

- Royal College of Nursing Clinical Topic 'Medicines Management': https://www .rcn.org.uk/clinical-topics/medicines-management/medicine-supply-and -administration
- Care and Quality Commission Nigel's surgery 19; Patient Group Directions/ Patient-Specific Directions: https://www.cqc.org.uk/guidance-providers/gps/nigels -surgery-19-patient-group-directions-pgds-patient-specific-directions
- Specialist Pharmacy Service, the first stop for professional medicines advice: https://www.sps.nhs.uk/

Challenges for childhood vaccination during COVID-19

A novel coronavirus SARS-CoV-2 and resulting coronavirus disease (COVID-19) was declared a pandemic by the WHO on 12th March 2020. Across the world this meant that all countries including the United Kingdom had to implement strategies to minimise the spread of infection to mitigate the impact of the disease on the population as well as on the health and care system.

There is always a need to balance within any business continuity planning, those services which can be reduced or limited and those which need to continue as essential (NHS, 2020).

Vaccination is a prime example of something that needs to continue given the overall impact that vaccines have on preventing disease saving and lives (WHO, 2008). Experience demonstrates that even small declines in vaccine uptake leads to increases in cases of vaccine preventable diseases and deaths. In March 2020, the European region of the WHO warned that even a short disruption to immunisation programmes during a pandemic could result in an increase in vaccine preventable diseases, further adding to the burden on health care (WHO, 2020a).

The Joint Committee for Vaccination and Immunisation (JCVI) clearly recommended that the childhood programme should continue (JCVI, 2020). Many parents will need additional reassurance and support as they will be understandably concerned about the risk of infection if they attended their GP surgery.

The RCN guidance to support the practicalities of maintaining vaccination services (RCN, 2020) supports how to manage the services themselves as well as the importance of promoting vaccination to parents. The need for this and constant vigilance to maintain vaccine services has been seen with a reduction in vaccine uptake since the start of the pandemic from the PHE analysis (PHE, 2021).

Vaccination programme for SARS-CoV2/COVID-19

The vaccine programme for the novel virus SARS-COV2 with the aim of helping control COVID-19 disease commenced in the UK on the 8th December 2020. The programme is driven primarily through primary care with general practice nurses being at the forefront of the programme. The programme is certainly the largest ever involving partners from across the health and social care system and wider to manage the specific vaccine requirements, workforce needs and logistics. The clear aim of the programme is to protect those at greatest risk from disease first but with an eventual aim to vaccinate the adult population and hopefully help control transmission of infection. As with all other UK programmes it has been led and advised by the JCVI to inform government and policy (JCVI, 2021) which is set out in the Green Book chapter for COVID-19 disease, Chapter 14b.

The UK programme has a variety of vaccines and the details are included in the Green Book. There is also separate education resources relevant to the overall vaccine programme and the individual vaccines available.

Conclusion

It is a routine and core element of general practice to provide vaccination, and this is nearly always a role played by GPNs. Although vaccine administration is routine, the complexity should not be underestimated, right through from the management of the clinic and being able to talk to people confidently and with the most up-to-date evidence and advice for ordering and storing vaccines and administering them safely, all of which rightly takes considerable time. Given the vital importance to both individual protection against disease and the huge public health benefits gained through immunisation, this is time well spent. The impact of COVID-19 will be far reaching. The role of educated and skilled health care professionals to deliver vaccination programmes is acknowledged, and nurses need to make sure they can access the appropriate education and continue their professional development to maintain their role and make sure they can help maintain public confidence improve accessibility to vaccines across the population and a high vaccine uptake.

Reflection

- Read the national minimum training standards and complete the competency assessment tool (PHE, 2018; RCN, 2015), taking action for any competencies you do not feel confident or competent in.
- Those new to vaccination will need to complete a core immunisation and vaccination course covering all the core elements outlined above. Best practice would be to also have a mentor in the workplace to help learn the vaccination skills and work through the competency assessment tool. Where this is not possible, work with other skilled vaccinators in other areas to develop skills.
- Register to undertake the immunisation e-learning programme and try the knowledge assessments: https://www.e-lfh.org.uk/programmes/immunisation/
- Find out what education and training is available in your local area, from your manager or local health protection/screening and immunisation team.
- Familiarise yourself with the many different resources available on national or local immunisation web pages. It is worthwhile spending a little time looking through country and local information every few months, including the Green Book (Immunisation against infectious disease) (PHE, 2020), vaccine schedules, the uncertain/incomplete immunisation status algorithm, parent/patient information and vaccine incident guidance.
- Sign up to 'Vaccine Update'. This newsletter from Public Health England provides updates on vaccine schedules, policies and procedures: https://www.gov.uk/government/collections/vaccine-update
- Familiarise yourself with the resources and various links available on the Royal College of Nursing Clinical Topic 'Immunisation': https://www.rcn.org.uk/clinical-topics/public-health/specialist-areas/immunisation
- Look at the Oxford Vaccine Knowledge Project website and read the frequently asked questions and the section on vaccine ingredients: http://vk.ovg.ox.ac.uk/

Travel health by Jane Chiodini

Introduction

In 2018 there were 71.7 million visits overseas by UK residents, with the most common reason being holiday travel. Within that number were 16.7 million visits overseas to visit friends and family (ONS, 2018), and this group represents the highest risk group of travellers returning to the United Kingdom with malaria (PHE, 2019c). Travel health has been a role of the GPN for many years.

This field of practice is complex and challenging, with no two travel consultations ever being the same, but once the GPN has acquired skills and competence, the subject and care can be exciting and enjoyable.

The provision of travel health care in a primary care setting

What must a general practice provide?

Protecting the traveller's health in terms of disease protection is not only important for patients, but also in preventing the spread of infectious disease on their return home to the United Kingdom, and thus is of great public health importance. General Practice is funded in a number of ways, including the Global Sum, which is a distribution of core funding to cover the cost of providing routine primary care services to its registered list of patients. Historically travel health has not been part of this funding, but was provided as an 'Additional Service'. However, the new general practitioner (GP) contract for England, negotiated with the government for 2020/2021 to 2023/2024, was announced in February 2020 (NHS England, 2020). It stated that vaccinations and immunisations will become an essential contractual service amid a payment model overhaul. All practices will be expected to offer all routine, pre-exposure and post-exposure vaccinations and NHS travel vaccinations to the eligible practice population. A named lead for vaccination services who is responsible for meeting the core standards and requirements of the contract and 'maximising' vaccination opportunities will be introduced in all practices. In recent years many GP practices had unofficially stopped providing a travel service, but this new information clarifies that travel health care must continue to be provided. Although the announcement focussed on vaccines, travellers can also be at personal risk from other threats such as road traffic accidents, solar damage, personal safety and security and need to be advised appropriately, based on an individual pre-travel risk assessment. Travel health is frequently misunderstood by some working in general practice. The viewpoint that travel health care is 'just about giving the injections' is not only incorrect but can be detrimental to the care of the traveller and the professional integrity of the health care practitioner delivering this care (Box 4.3).

Box 4.3 Travel-related vaccines which must be provided to national health service patients as a national health service provision

Hepatitis A (and all vaccines which have a hepatitis A component)
Typhoid (both injectable and oral presentations)
Cholera
Polio (administered for a traveller as Revaxis, which is a combination vaccine of tetanus, polio and diphtheria, therefore all three components are provided on the NHS because none are available as single-antigen vaccines)

The following factors also need to be provided as part of the travel health service:

- An initial travel risk assessment
- Advice on the travel health risks (which would include risk of diseases that could be prevented by private travel vaccines which may not be administered within the individual surgery)
- Signposting to a selection of centres where the private travel vaccines may be provided if the GP surgery opts not to provide them
- Malaria prevention advice if required by the itinerary
- Signposting towards additional reading and advice for individual health risks
- Documentary evidence of vaccine history

What can a general practice additionally provide?

The majority of general practices only provide the NHS vaccines; however, they can also provide a private service if they choose. This results in a more holistic provision of care to the traveller and can also be a substantial income generator if undertaken effectively.

In addition to the list of vaccines in Box 4.4, malaria tablets and travel equipment, for example, mosquito nets, repellents and first aid kits, may be charged for privately. There are other administrative duties such as provision of fitness-to-fly certificates and the international certificate of vaccination or prophylaxis that can be charged for as well.

Training and knowledge to provide travel health care

Although this information aims to provide an overview of travel health, training is required for further knowledge and to become competent as a practitioner. The RCN guidance suggests a minimum of 15 hours of training initially, which would include some mentorship (RCN, 2018c). Courses are available;

Box 4.4 Travel-related vaccines which must be charged for if provided in a national health service setting

Rabies
Yellow fever
Japanese encephalitis
Tick-borne encephalitis
Meningitis ACWY (for travel purposes)
Hepatitis B[a]

---

[a]Guidance for hepatitis B indicates this vaccine may be charged for (BMA, 2018). It is the decision of the individual surgery as to whether or not they charge their patient if given for the purpose of travel; however, the Medicine Management Committees within Clinical Commissioning Groups often stipulate it must be charged for.

however, there is no official requirement to undertake one, either for the practice of travel medicine or for those training in the subject. However, a nurse must of course always abide by the Nursing and Midwifery Council code of practice (NMC, 2018). Yellow fever vaccine can only be administered in registered yellow fever centres, and practitioners doing so need to undertake training every 2 years (NaTHNaC, 2016). All those undertaking travel health training should be competent in immunisation and have undertaken a 2-day course on this subject before administering travel guidance or travel immunisation (PHE, 2018a). The author recommends the Royal College of Physicians and Surgeons of Glasgow, which has a Faculty of Travel Medicine (FTM) that focusses on education and standards in the field (Chiodini et al., 2012). The FTM has published a new document entitled 'Good Practice Guidance for Providing a Travel Health Service' (Chiodini et al., 2020), which includes a competency tool and is essential reading.

Travel health care is more effectively delivered in a dedicated travel clinic as opposed to opportunistic appointments. Late afternoon and evening appointments are more popular for travellers. A minimum of 20 minutes per traveller appointment is advised (RCN, 2018), with more complex scenarios requiring even longer. Details and suggestions on how to manage the travel consultation can be found on page 18 of the RCN document 'Competencies: Travel health nursing: career and competence development'.

Travel risk assessment

No travel health consultation should take place without undertaking a travel risk assessment (RCN, 2018). This process will determine the level of risk for the individual traveller with regard to his or her travel itinerary and personal health history. A number of travel risk assessment forms have been developed, and many of them have been transformed into templates used within computer systems in a general practice. Examples are listed in the resources section. Table 4.1 identifies the information required to perform a travel risk assessment.

The impact of a travel risk assessment

Travellers generally do not appreciate the rationale for requesting this information, but the detail could impact the outcome. Many resources have written comprehensive explanations of the importance of the questions asked, and GPNs are advised to become familiar with these texts (see Resources box), but the following information provides an initial insight.

Travel risk assessment is based on a number of factors, and the evaluation of the risk assessment will inform the management of the advice subsequently given, vaccines advised and malaria prevention advice required, if this is also a risk in their trip. The key areas to consider are shown in Fig. 4.2.

Table 4.1 Information required for a travel risk assessment.

Traveller-focussed questions	Trip-focussed questions
Age and sex	Country to be visited and exact location or region – capture all details for a multidestination trip, including time spent at all destinations
Traveller country of origin	Whether travel will be rural or urban
Current health status	Total length of stay for the trip
Previous medical history including: heart disease; diabetes; anaemia; bleeding or clotting disorders; epilepsy/seizures; gastrointestinal complaints; liver or renal problems; HIV/AIDS; immune system conditions; mental health conditions; neurological illness; respiratory disease; rheumatological conditions; previous surgical operations including thymectomy or splenectomy; splenic disorders; and, for women only, pregnancy, planning pregnancy, breast feeding, female genital mutilation previously performed	Type of travel and accommodation – examples include: holiday; business trip; visiting friends and family; expatriate travel; volunteer work; health care work; military work; cruise ship travel; safari; adventure; diving; backpacking; school trip; pilgrimage; medical tourism; staying in hotel/hostel/camping
Current medication	Budget for the trip if appropriate
Allergies to food, latex and medication	Mode of travel: air travel; by sea; overland trucking, etc.
Previous vaccine history	Future travel plans
Tendency to faint with injections	Travel insurance obtained

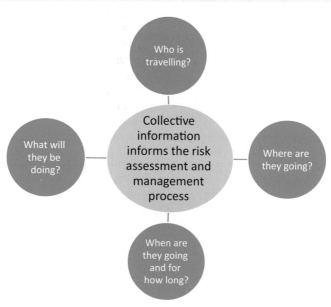

Fig. 4.2   Travel risk assessment.

Case study

A 70-year-old woman is taking a 2-week package holiday to Kenya, staying in Mombasa. She has a medical history of myocardial infarction 8 years ago but is currently fit and well, and is on a daily statin, but no other medication. She is travelling with her married daughter and two teenage children, staying in a hotel, except for 2 days on the trip when they will be in a safari lodge. She is unsure about her vaccine history, and there are no previous records on the computer system except for three doses of tetanus vaccine; the last one was given 20 years ago.

Issues to consider: an overview

Older travellers present a greater risk because their immune system is waning with increasing age (immunosenescence), and travel vaccines given may not provide optimum protection (NaTHNaC, 2017). Senses are reduced in older travellers, which can put them at increased risk of dangers such as road traffic accidents; in addition, they are more likely to have previous medical history, which may complicate aspects of their trip and put them at greater risk of requiring medical attention whilst abroad in a country where health care facilities may not be of a standard they may be used to. It is important to establish previous medical history, current health problems and any medication taken. These aspects form one of the most time-consuming aspects of the consultation, especially if further advice is required. This individual needs to be brought up to date with immunisations required for the United Kingdom. The nurse would need to administer a further dose of the tetanus, polio and diphtheria vaccines (as one combined vaccine), check on measles, mumps and rubella vaccine (MMR) status and offer two doses of vaccine a minimum of a month apart, using vaccine stock from ImmForm, and establish whether she has received influenza and pneumococcal disease protection. Although these are important vaccines in the national schedule, they are used also for travel purposes. Varicella status could also be checked. If after rechecking records, (which may involve paper notes, if still held because many surgeries sometimes do not transfer this information across onto the computer record), there is no evidence of her having received them, she should also be advised to consider having hepatitis A and typhoid vaccines. Her travel description would probably not indicate that hepatitis B or meningococcal disease are significant risks, but awareness of risk and advice on prevention remains important. Rabies would be a risk, and again comprehensive advice should be given, including management of a potential risk of exposure, which is essential whether or not she chooses to have rabies vaccine pretravel (NaTHNaC, 2019a). Yellow fever is a risk in parts of Kenya (NaTHNaC, 2019b); however, there is also a risk of serious adverse events to vaccination, which is increased in those aged 60 years and above (NaTHNaC, 2019c). If risk of disease is significant, then vaccination must still always be considered, but a very thorough risk assessment needs to undertaken by a health care professional trained in yellow fever vaccination (MHRA et al., 2019). Mombasa is in a low-risk area for yellow fever, so vaccine would not be advised for this patient; however, mosquito bite avoidance will be essential, also in view of other mosquito-borne infections present in the country, including dengue and Rift Valley fever. Malaria is the most dangerous mosquito-borne infection in Kenya, and Mombasa is a high-risk area for

Continued

the most dangerous species, *Plasmodium falciparum*. Chemoprophylaxis will be required, and the consultation will require explanation of the various antimalarial tablets available, allowing this patient to make an informed choice as to which she prefers to purchase and take (NaTHNaC, 2019b).

Other risks in Kenya include altitude if going to such areas, safety and security, road traffic accidents, sun exposure, food and water cleanliness, travellers' diarrhoea, and so on.

Resources

- Royal College of Nursing. (2018). Competencies: Travel health nursing – career and competence development. Royal College of Nursing. https://www.rcn.org .uk/professional-development/publications/pdf-006506
- For the risk assessment/management section, see pages 11–20.
- Centers for Disease Control and Prevention. (2020). The Yellow Book 2020 (Health Information for International Travel). https://wwwnc.cdc.gov/travel /page/yellowbook-home
- Chapter 2 – Pre-travel consultation can be found at: https://wwwnc.cdc.gov /travel/yellowbook/2020/preparing-international-travelers/the-pretravel -consultation
- The National Travel Health Network and Centre have an e-learning course on risk assessment: https://travelhealthpro.org.uk/news/238/e-learning-course-on -risk-assessment

Travel risk management

Advice on the many health risks travellers may be exposed to needs to be tailored to their individual travel risk assessment. It is also not feasible to cover all aspects of care within the consultation time, nor would the traveller be able to absorb all detail given, so backup written advice is useful, or direction to suitable websites to gain the knowledge and undertake further research. The author has a general travel advice leaflet available for travellers to use at https://www .janechiodini.co.uk/help/tar/, and the National Travel Health Network and Centre's website TravelHealthPro at https://travelhealthpro.org.uk/ or Health Protection Scotland's public website Fit for Travel at https://www.fitfortravel. nhs.uk/home are good sites to refer the traveller to.

See Box 4.5 for the principles of general travel advice.

Specialist advice is also sometimes required, dependent on the risk assessment in addition to the general advice. Examples could include:

- Travelling at altitude: https://www.fitfortravel.nhs.uk/advice/general-travel -health-advice/altitude-and-travel and https://travelhealthpro.org.uk/factsheet /26/altitude-illness

Box 4.5   Principles of general travel advice

Insect bite avoidance advice

Infected mosquitoes will bite day or night depending on the mosquito type, but in all situations stringent bite prevention methods are essential to minimise disease risk. For malaria prevention, the insect repellent commonly recommended is N,N-diethyl-m-toluamide (DEET), up to a 50% concentration. Alternatives are available for those who do not wish to use DEET. Repellents should be applied to any exposed skin at high-risk times and reapplied as required, remembering that in a hot and humid country the traveller may sweat off the repellent more quickly. Repellents and insecticides can be used on cotton clothing. Room protection may be by the use of air conditioning units, screening over the windows, insect vapourisers (electric or battery operated), knock-down sprays and impregnated mosquito nets. The UK Malaria Guidance document has an excellent section on insect bite prevention which should be studied for greater knowledge: https://www.gov.uk/government/publications/malaria-prevention-guidelines-for-travellers-from-the-uk

Animal bites

Because rabies is present in many countries of the world, advice regarding rabies risk is essential, as the consequence of disease is usually death (see rabies section later in this chapter). Advice would include not touching any animals, particularly dogs, cats and monkeys; if licked on broken skin, scratched or bitten by an animal in a country with rabies risk, wash the wound thoroughly with soap and running water for 15 minutes, then apply an antiseptic if possible (e.g., povidone iodine or alcohol) and seek medical advice immediately (WHO, 2019b). This is essential advice for all travellers, even if they have received pre-exposure vaccine.

Food, water and personal hygiene advice

Specific advice on appropriate food and drink is applicable even if a vaccine has been given to help protect against diseases transmitted by the faecal-oral route, as vaccines may not give the traveller 100% protection. Safe food would include hot, thoroughly grilled or boiled items, processed or packed foods, cooked vegetables and fruits (e.g., bananas), and safe drinks would include carbonated soft drinks and water, boiled water and purified water treated with iodine and chlorine. Unsafe drinks would include tap water, chipped ice and unpasteurized milk, and unsafe foods would include salads, uncooked seafood, and raw or poorly cooked meats. Handwashing with soap and clean water after going to the toilet, before eating and before handling food is advised. If handwashing is not feasible, then sanitising hand gel can also be used.

For details on prevention and management of travellers' diarrhoea, see later in this chapter under non-vaccine-preventable risks.

Blood and bodily fluid risks

Although a vaccine is available to protect against hepatitis B, other blood-borne infections such as hepatitis C and human immunodeficiency virus constitute a risk to travellers, especially if going to areas of the world where the risk is greater and

Continued

health care facilities are less optimal. Preventive advice is important, including only accepting adequately screened blood if a transfusion is required; refusing medical procedures with nonsterile equipment; not sharing needles (e.g., tattooing, body piercing, acupuncture and drug use) and always practising safe sex, including the use of condoms. Travellers could also be advised to travel with a sterile medical kit; one which is commercially purchased and will have a certificate within it to prove the traveller is carrying it for medical reasons only.

Accidents
Accidents are leading causes of death in travellers abroad, predominantly road traffic accidents and swimming/water accidents. Travellers can help prevent them by following sensible precautions such as: avoiding alcohol and food before swimming; never diving into water where the depth is uncertain; only swimming in safe water, checking for currents, sharks, jellyfish, etc.; avoiding alcohol when driving, especially at night; avoiding hiring motorcycles and mopeds and, if hiring a car, renting a large one if possible and ensuring the tyres, brakes and seat belts are in good condition; using reliable taxi firms; and knowing where emergency facilities are.

Personal safety and security
This is really important when abroad. The Foreign and Commonwealth has individual country advice on the subject at https://www.gov.uk/foreign-travel-advice that includes details of crime, sexual assault, scams, political situations, terrorism, local customs and laws.

Insurance cover should also be addressed with the traveller, particularly if there are any underlying medical conditions. The traveller would need to inform the insurance company of these and also secure cover for medical repatriation.

Air travel
Long-haul flight advice would include comfort on the journey, getting up and exercising when possible and keeping rehydrated with nonalcoholic fluids. Risk of venous thromboembolism (VTE) is low in most travellers; those at greater risk are older travellers, pregnant women, those with a previous history of VTE or recent surgery, those with certain blood clotting disorders, malignancy or certain heart conditions and those taking oestrogen-containing medicines. Correctly fitted compression socks may be advised (NaTHNaC, 2018a).

Sun and heat
Sunburn and heatstroke can cause serious problems in travellers. Precautionary guidelines include gradual sun exposure, use of sunblocks which contain UVA and UVB protection, sufficient sun protection factor (SPF) and observation of minimum SPF levels (e.g., minimum of SPF 15 in adults and SPF 25 in children). If using a repellent, apply the sun protection before the repellent; if DEET is used, a higher SPF is required, as DEET can reduce the SPF protection. Avoid the sun at its peak time of 11am to 3pm, taking special care of those with pale skin/red hair and children. Wear protective clothing and ensure adequate hydration with nonalcoholic fluids.

- Guidance on how to advise individual travellers on the duration of preventative measures against sexual transmission of Zika virus: https://www.gov.uk/government/publications/zika-virus-sexual-transmission-advice-algorithm – useful for those who are planning a pregnancy
- Travel advice for the diabetic traveller: https://travelhealthpro.org.uk/factsheet/4/diabetes and https://www.travax.nhs.uk/health-advice/special-groups/diabetes/
- Travel during pregnancy: https://travelhealthpro.org.uk/factsheet/45/pregnancy and https://www.travax.nhs.uk/health-advice/special-groups/pregnancy-and-pre-conception/
- Travelling with additional needs and/or disability: https://travelhealthpro.org.uk/factsheet/80/travelling-with-additional-needs-andor-disability and https://www.travax.nhs.uk/health-advice/special-groups/disabilities/

Vaccine-preventable diseases

There are a number of vaccine-preventable diseases from which travellers can be at risk, but the morbidity and mortality from such infections is extremely low in comparison to other risks from travel abroad, such as road traffic accidents. However, after the provision of clean water, vaccination is the most important public health measure. It is important to ensure travellers are up to date with the national immunisation schedule during the pre-travel consultation. This includes checking their vaccination history and giving any further necessary vaccines required. Influenza and pneumococcal vaccines are also important considerations for travellers, especially those travelling to the southern hemisphere in the UK summer period, when it will be the winter season in that part of the globe, and infections such as flu will be of greater intensity. The recent increase in the risk of measles infection both in the United Kingdom and abroad makes it particularly important to ensure that travellers have a record of two doses of MMR vaccine, and if not, that they are vaccinated; NHS stock of vaccine can be used for this purpose (PHE, 2017).

Tables 4.2 and 4.3 provide brief information about the diseases, what causes them, the vaccines available and additional preventive measures that should be taken. This information forms a basic overview, but further knowledge on specific diseases and vaccines should be acquired. The reader is advised to refer to 'Immunisation against infectious disease', commonly known as the Green Book, found at https://www.gov.uk/government/collections/immunisation-against-infectious-disease-the-green-book, and the Summary of Product Characteristics for the individual vaccines found on the Electronic Medicines Compendium at https://www.medicines.org.uk/emc/.

A chart developed by the author of this chapter is also available as a tool to help in practice (see item no. 3 at https://www.janechiodini.co.uk/tools/), but this should be used in conjunction with national resources previously mentioned.

Table 4.2 National health service travel vaccines.

Disease	Causative organism	Main transmission	General vaccine information. All vaccines must be stored in the cold chain at 2° C–8° C	Comments
Hepatitis A	Virus	Faecal-oral (contaminated food and water)	Five vaccine products are available in the United Kingdom in adult and paediatric formulation. General rule is that two doses in a course usually given 6–12 months apart, give 25 years protection from the date of the second dose (according to current guidance). Paediatric vaccines used from 1 year of age.	Paediatric vaccines are VAQTA paediatric and Havrix Junior Monodose. Adult vaccines are VAQTA Adult, Avaxim and Havrix Monodose. Hepatitis A vaccine can also be given to adults in the combination hepatitis A and typhoid vaccine Viatim, and in combination hepatitis A and B vaccines Twinrix Adult, Twinrix Paediatric and Ambirix. For further learning on frequently asked questions see http://bit.ly/2RYG437.
Typhoid	Bacterium: *Salmonella typhi*	Faecal-oral (contaminated food and water)	Only one injectable vaccine available in the United Kingdom – Typhim Vi. One dose gives up to 3 years' protection, from 2 years of age. One oral vaccine is available in the United Kingdom – Vivotif (live vaccine), which is given from 5 years of age, three capsules in the course (for timing intervals see Green Book, Chapter 11, page 9, Table 11.2).	Injectable product is a polysaccharide vaccine which is not as effective. Oral vaccine must be taken with a cool drink 1 hour before a meal. High-risk areas of the world for UK travellers are India, Pakistan and Bangladesh. High-risk groups are those visiting friends and relatives, long-term travellers, children and those going to areas of poor sanitation.

Table 4.2 National health service travel vaccines—cont'd.

Disease	Causative organism	Main transmission	General vaccine information. All vaccines must be stored in the cold chain at 2° C–8° C	Comments
Cholera	Bacterium: *Vibrio cholerae*	Faecal-oral (contaminated food and water)	One vaccine currently available in the United Kingdom – Dukoral, which is an oral vaccine given from 6 years of age, two doses a minimum of 1 week and a maximum of 6 weeks apart gives 2 years' protection. In a 2- to 6-year-old child, three doses are given, providing 6 months' protection.	See manufacturer's instructions for preparation and administration. Must be nil by mouth for 1 hour pre- and 1 hour post-vaccine administration. A new oral vaccine is due for launch in the United Kingdom in early 2020 which will be a one-dose schedule – VaxChora.
Tetanus	Bacterium: *Clostridium tetani*	Tetanus spores in the soil or manure enter via a penetrating wound.	Each disease protection is only available within combination vaccines in the United Kingdom. Five doses are given in the national immunisation schedule. See https://www.gov.uk/government /publications/the-complete-routine -immunisation-schedule. Travellers can then have Revaxis administered at 10-yearly intervals if travelling to high-risk areas.	At the current time, the World Health Organization has named polio as a Public Health Emergency of International Concern. Eventual global eradication is planned, but in the meantime, to prevent spread of disease, regulations are in place for travellers going to certain high-risk areas for longer than 4 weeks. Evidence of polio vaccination within the past 12 months has to be provided on exit from the country (Global Polio Eradication Initiative, 2019).
Polio	Virus serotypes 1, 2, and 3	Faecal-oral (contaminated food and water)		
Diphtheria	Bacterium: *Corynebacterium diphtheriae*	Person-to-person, respiratory droplet, e.g., coughing and sneezing		

Continued

Table 4.2 National health service travel vaccines—cont'd.

The measles, mumps and rubella (MMR) vaccine is provided as part of the national immunisation programme. All individuals should have record of two doses of MMR vaccine given, irrespective of age. However, if a traveller is going to a high-risk area and does not have such evidence, then vaccination should be offered as a National Health Service (NHS) provision with the general practitioner surgery using the ImmForm stock of vaccine.

The Bacille Camille-Guerin (BCG) vaccine is not part of the national immunisation programme and is only given to small babies in certain circumstances, e.g., those born to a parent or grandparent who originates from a country where the annual incidence of tuberculosis is 40:100,000 or greater. BCG can be given for travel purposes to unvaccinated children under 16 years of age who are going to live for more than 3 months in countries where there remains a risk. A tuberculin skin test is required before vaccination for all children from 6 years of age and may be recommended for some younger children. This would not be provided in primary care, and the traveller would often be referred to the local NHS chest clinic. The vaccine is not given to travellers outside this age range except health care workers travelling who may be at risk through their activities at the destination (PHE, 2013).

From PHE. (2013). *Immunisation against infectious disease. 'The Green Book'.* https://www.gov.uk/government/collections/immunisation-against-infectious-disease-the-green-book; Electronic medicines compendium. (2019). https://www.medicines.org.uk/emc/.

Table 4.3 Private travel vaccines.

Disease	Causative organism	Main transmission	General vaccine information All vaccines must be stored in the cold chain at 2° C–8° C	Comments
Meningococcal disease	Bacterium: *Neisseria meningitidis*	Person-to-person, respiratory droplet, e.g., kissing, coughing and sneezing	There are two different brands of a conjugate ACWY vaccine in the UK – Menveo (licensed from 2 years of age) and Nimenrix (licensed from 6 weeks of age). One dose is usually required before travel (10 days before entry for those entering the Kingdom of Saudi Arabia [KSA]) and 'for travel purposes provides 5 years' protection, after which time a booster will be required if there is ongoing risk of exposure to the disease. (Note: for children <1 year receiving Nimenrix, different dosing is required; see the Green Book.)	There are six different strains: A, B, C, E, W135 and Y. The four major meningococcal groups abroad are A, C, W135 and Y. The highest risk area is the 'meningitis belt' of sub-Saharan Africa, particularly during the dry season, but travellers to KSA attending for pilgrimage (Umrah and Hajj) also require vaccination to obtain a visa, which is required by the Saudi Arabian government for entry to the country. Pilgrims will need a certificate of vaccination completion to apply for a visa.
Hepatitis B	Virus	Blood and bodily fluids	Two products available in the United Kingdom in adult and paediatric formulation – Engerix B and HBvaxPRO. There are also different schedules of 0, 1 and 6 months; 0, 7, 21 days and 12 months; and 0 and 6 months for 11- to 15-year-olds. It is important to refer to the Green Book for the different options.	Vaccination should be considered if travellers are visiting high-risk areas for long periods or are at social or occupational risk. Hepatitis B protection is also available in combination hep A + hep B vaccines – Twinrix Adult, Twinrix Paediatric and Ambirix. If these vaccines are administered in a National Health Service (NHS) setting they must be provided on the NHS programme because they confer hepatitis A protection. The hepatitis B vaccine can be given alone as a private vaccine in an NHS setting.

Continued

Table 4.3 Private travel vaccines—cont'd.

Disease	Causative organism	Main transmission	General vaccine information All vaccines must be stored in the cold chain at 2° C–8° C	Comments
Yellow fever	Virus	Mosquito bites	One licensed product in the United Kingdom – Stamaril. One dose provides lifetime protection in most travellers. See Chapter 35 of the Green Book, Figure 35.1: https://www.gov.uk/government/publications/yellow-fever-the-green-book-chapter-35. After administration, an International Certificate of Vaccination or Prophylaxis must be completed for the traveller. The vaccine is licensed from 9 months of age but can be considered in infants aged 6–9 months off licence.	Found in parts of Africa, South America, Central America and the Caribbean. Outbreaks do occur, so the country-specific database information should be read carefully. the vaccine is given for disease protection but is sometimes needed for entry requirement in accordance with World Health Organization regulations. The yellow fever vaccine can only be administered in a yellow fever centre. aSee information below this table for further details.
Rabies	Virus	Saliva of any infected warm-blooded mammal, usually via a bite, scratch or lick on an open wound	Two licensed products in the United Kingdom – Rabies vaccine BP and Rabipur. A full course of three doses of rabies vaccine before travel ensures immunity to the rabies virus, although post-exposure treatment would still be required, but treatment is then more achievable. Vaccine schedules are days 0, 7 and 21–28 or days 0, 3, 7 and 365 with a booster dose which may be given from 1 year after the primary course if further risk is considered to be high. Current guidance suggests this is sufficient pre-travel protection for life, remembering that the post-exposure treatment must always be applied after a potential risk exposure.	In times of vaccine shortage, an unlicensed vaccine is sometimes used – Verorab, which is licensed in France. Rabies vaccine can be given intradermally but is not licensed for this route, and it is not usual to give it this way in general practice surgeries; special training for the injection technique would be required. bSee section below for further important information

Table 4.3 Private travel vaccines—cont'd.

Disease	Causative organism	Main transmission	General vaccine information All vaccines must be stored in the cold chain at 2° C–8° C	Comments
Japanese encephalitis (JE)	Virus	Mosquito bite	Only one product available in the United Kingdom – Ixiaro. Licensed schedule of 0 and 28 days in anyone from 2 months of age, with a booster generally at 12–24 months (this varies depending on age and risk – see the Green Book). A rapid schedule of 0 and 7 days is licensed for those aged 18–64 years but is also possible off licence in children from 2 months and in individuals over 65 years, when genuinely no time is available to complete the standard schedule.	Virus is maintained in a life cycle between water fowl and pigs. Human-to-human transmission is not possible. JE is found mainly in rural areas in Southeast Asia, the Pacific islands and the Far East, so rural areas near pig farms and paddy fields are higher risk. Although JE is usually a mild infection, it can be very severe, causing a serious cerebral infection with major life-changing consequences. Primary immunisation should ideally be completed at least 1 week before JE exposure.
Tick-borne enceph-alitis	Virus	Infected tick bite	Only one product is available in the United Kingdom – Tico-Vac, in adult and paediatric formulation (from 1–16 years of age). Schedule of both vaccines – three doses on day 0, 1–3 months after the 1st dose and 5–12 months after the 2nd dose.	This dDisease is rare in travellers and is found in central, eastern and north-ern Europe across Russia to parts of eastern Asia. Risk increases if travellers are undertaking activities particularly in woodland or grassland, e.g., when camping or hiking. A rapid schedule giving the 2nd dose 2 weeks after the 1st dose is possible in adults, but see the Green Book for more information.

Continued

Table 4.3 Private travel vaccines—cont'd.

[a]Further important information regarding the yellow fever vaccine

General practice surgeries can apply to become a yellow fever centre; if located in England, Wales or Northern Ireland they have to apply through NaTHNaC, and in Scotland through Health Protection Scotland. Training needs to be undertaken every 2 years ,and there are a number of regulations that the surgery has to abide by (NaTHNaC, 2016). Serious adverse events identified from yellow fever vaccine are important, particularly in those aged 60 years and over. This is a complex subject, and the practice nurse new to travel health would be better off considering administering the yellow fever vaccine once he/she feels more competent in general travel health first. The Royal College of Nursing competency framework considers yellow fever vaccine administration to be a skill of the nurse experienced in travel health (RCN, 2018). However, all practitioners need to understand the risk assessment for yellow fever vaccine to appropriately refer the traveller to a private travel clinic for further advice.

[b]Further important information regarding the rabies vaccine

Rabies infection is usually fatal. Vaccination is advised for those going to high-risk areas who will be remote from a reliable source of vaccine for post-exposure treatment. A full course of three doses of rabies vaccine before travel ensures immunity to the rabies virus. If the traveller then has an exposure, they still need to get post-exposure treatment of two further doses of rabies vaccine, but this is more achievable. Those who have had no pre-exposure vaccine or an incomplete course, depending on the risk of exposure (i.e., the risk within the country, the type of animal and the severity of the wound) will require a full course of vaccine, which in the United Kingdom is four doses (or five doses in an immunocompromised individual), and they may also need to receive rabies-specific immunoglobulin (RIg). This provides antibodies enabling immediate protection, whereas vaccination will take several days to develop an antibody response. However, there is a global shortage of RIg which may result in the traveller possibly needing to fly to another country to find it or having to return home early. No traveller who has received a full course of rabies vaccine before travel has ever been known to have died from rabies exposure (Warrell, 2012). This information, together with the risk of fake rabies vaccine being found in some countries (NaTHNaC, 2019d), provides compelling reasons for travellers to have a pre-exposure course. However, because of the high cost of vaccine, it is often difficult to persuade travellers to invest in this protection. Whether or not they have vaccine before travel, if they have any animal contact it is absolutely essential that they know to wash the wound thoroughly with soap and running water for a minimum of 15 minutes, add an antiseptic (something like povidone iodine is very effective) and then seek immediate medical help, as described in Box 4.5. If a general practice does not provide rabies vaccine, it is still essential to offer this advice and document that you have done so.

From PHE. (2013). *Immunisation against infectious disease. 'The Green Book'.* https://www.gov.uk/government/collections/immunisation-against-infectious-disease-the-green-book; Electronic medicines compendium. (2019). https://www.medicines.org.uk/emc/.

A private travel vaccine is one that is not funded as an NHS provision, so the traveller will need to fund this. The fee usually covers the basic cost of the vaccine, and an additional sum is included to cover the travel health advisor's time to assess the need for the vaccine, give the vaccine and carry out any accompanying administrative work. The private vaccines are available in private travel clinics but may also be given and charged for in a GP setting.

Administering travel vaccines in a primary care setting

The majority of travel vaccines are given by the IM route into the deltoid muscle or the anterolateral aspect of the thigh. The arm is usually the preferred site for the traveller, but sometimes, if many vaccines are given, additional sites may need to be used. If giving the vaccines in one site, then a distance of 2.5 cm must be left between the injection sites. Sometimes there are also important reasons for not using particular limbs; for example, if someone has had a lymph node clearance, it is recommended this limb is avoided (Chiodini, 2018). Details of the specific route for each vaccine would be found in the Summary of Product Characteristics and the PGD for the individual vaccine, and the GPN should be aware of this detail and work accordingly within the PGD.

Excellent guidance is provided on the administration of vaccines in Chapter 4 of the Green Book found at https://www.gov.uk/government/publications /immunisation-procedures-the-green-book-chapter-4.

One of the commonly asked questions regarding vaccines is the expulsion of an air bubble that may be seen within the vaccine barrel. The clinician should not attempt to get rid of the air bubble. To try to expel it risks accidently expelling some of the vaccine and therefore not giving the patient the full dose. The air bubble is also there for a reason – the air injected into the muscle forms an airlock that prevents the medication seeping out along the needle track into subcutaneous tissue and onto the skin. The small bolus of air injected following administration of the vaccine clears the needle and prevents a localised reaction from the vaccination (PHE, 2014). Vaccine Update is a key resource and tool for the GPN for all immunisation issues. An excellent index of back copies is available electronically at: https://www.healthpublications.gov.uk /ViewArticle.html?sp=Svaccineupdateindex.

Prescribing travel vaccines in a primary care setting

Unless the travel health advisor is a nonmedical prescriber, travel vaccines are usually administered by use of PGD in General Practice. A PGD is a legal document which must be updated every 2 years. It is important that the GPN reads this document fully before signing it, which then allows the practitioner to administer the vaccines which may be advised for a traveller after a careful travel risk assessment. In England, templates for the NHS travel vaccines are written and found at: https:// www.gov.uk/government/collections/immunisation-patient-group-direction-pgd.

However, they cannot be used until signed off (in Section 2, usually found on page 4) by your local organisation that has the legal authority to authorise the PGD. If PGDs are not available (and if private travel vaccines are given within a GP surgery; this will often be the case), then they can be administered under a PSD.

For more details see: https://www.janechiodini.co.uk/help/faqs/faq-1-prescribing-travel/.

Non-vaccine-preventable risks and special-risk travellers

This section describes a few of these risks, but further reading is required to understand the scope of many of the diseases and risks. Further information is available at: https://travelhealthpro.org.uk/.

Other mosquito-borne diseases for which there are currently no vaccines available represent significant risk to the traveller. These include malaria, dengue fever, Zika virus, chikungunya, West Nile Virus and Rift Valley Fever. Mosquito bite prevention is essential in all cases.

Malaria is a parasitic infection spread by the bite of an infected anopheline mosquito. There is currently no vaccine available that is suitable for use in travellers, and prevention is by awareness of the risks, bite prevention, taking the appropriate antimalarial tablets and being aware of the symptoms of malaria to help identify and treat the disease promptly. Common symptoms are those of a flu-like illness with fever, aching, headache and sometimes diarrhoea or cough, and travellers should be advised to seek urgent medical advice if this happens, tell the practitioner they have travelled to a malarious country and ask for a malaria blood test. Malaria is a notifiable disease, which means that a registered medical practitioner has a statutory duty to notify the 'proper officer' at their local council or local health protection team of suspected cases (PHE, 2019a). Each year we see, on average, 1500 travellers returning to the United Kingdom with malaria, of which about six die. Most cases are caused by the most dangerous species to humans, *Plasmodium falciparum,* which can in some circumstances kill a person within 24 hours of developing the symptoms of malaria. Malaria is both preventable and treatable, but those at greatest risk are travellers who are visiting friends and relatives, so it is important they understand the risk and take advice (NaTHNaC, 2019e; PHE, 2019b). The reader is advised to undertake further study on this important topic by reading the UK Malaria Guidelines. An e-learning course covering the topic is available free of charge at: http://bit.ly/2VyaDLN.

Travellers' diarrhoea is the most common infectious disease in travellers for which there is no vaccine; it can be caused by bacteria, parasites or viruses. Prevention relies on the travellers' behaviour, specifically taking care over what they eat and drink and ensuring they wash their hands before eating or preparing food. Travellers' diarrhoea is defined as three or more loose stools in a 24-hour period, often accompanied by abdominal pain, cramps and vomiting. It usually lasts 2 to 4 days and, although it is not a life-threatening illness, it can disrupt your trip for several days. Risk is variable in different countries of the world, with high-risk countries generally including those in North Africa, sub-Saharan Africa, the Indian subcontinent, Southeast Asia, South America, Mexico and the Middle East. The main danger from the illness is dehydration, which, if very severe, can kill if it is not treated. Treatment is therefore by rehydration. In severe cases, and particularly in young children and the elderly, commercially prepared rehydration solution is extremely useful. Antimotility drugs can be used for adults but should never be used in children under 4 years of age, and should only be used on prescription for children aged 4 to 12 years. Commonly used oral agents are loperamide and bismuth subsalicylate. None of these should ever be used if the person has a temperature or blood in his or her stool, and medical help should be sought if the affected person has a fever, blood in the diarrhoea or diarrhoea for more than 48 hours (or 24 hours in children), or becomes confused. In some circumstances, antibiotics are used as a standby treatment for travellers' diarrhoea. Medication advised in antici-pation of a traveller being ill while away is not usually available on the NHS and needs to be prescribed privately. A clinical knowledge summary written by NICE is available on this topic at: https://cks.nice.org.uk/diarrhoea-prevention -and-advice-for-travellers.

Schistosomiasis (sometimes referred to as bilharzia) is a parasitic disease found in freshwater lakes and streams in Africa, South America, some parts of the Caribbean and some parts of Southeast Asia. Larval forms of the parasite live in certain species of snails and are released into infested lakes and rivers. The larvae can penetrate human skin and migrate to internal organs. There may be no symptoms, or symptoms may not become apparent until months or years later. There is currently no vaccine against schistosomiasis. Schistosomiasis is diagnosed by testing urine or stool, as well as by taking blood samples (serol ogy). Screening should be carried out at least 6 weeks after exposure to fresh water and is best done through referral to a specialist infectious diseases unit. Prevention is by avoiding contact with freshwater rivers and lakes in high-risk areas where possible (NaTHNaC, 2018b).

Respiratory illnesses

Middle East respiratory syndrome coronavirus, or MERS-CoV, was first iden-tified in Saudi Arabia in 2012. Symptoms include fever, cough and shortness of breath. Pneumonia is common, but not always present. Gastrointestinal symp-toms, including diarrhoea, have also been reported. Although symptoms can be very mild, approximately 35% of reported patients with MERS-CoV infec-tion have died. Transmission is not fully understood, but there is thought to be a link particularly with camels, so travellers visiting areas where dromedary camels are present are advised to practice general hygiene measures, includ-ing regular handwashing before and after touching animals, and should avoid contact with sick animals. People with diabetes, renal failure or chronic lung disease and immunocompromised persons are considered to be at high risk of severe disease from MERS-CoV infection. These people should avoid being in contact with camels, drinking raw camel milk or camel urine or eating meat that has not been properly cooked (WHO, 2019b). Travellers are at a high risk of contracting influenza, especially those travellers undertaking activities such as cruise ship travel, and it is important to consider influenza and pneumococcal vaccines for travel in addition to those which would be recommended for life in the United Kingdom as part of the national immunisation programme.

Special risk travellers

There are many excellent factsheets to explain additional risks for travellers with underlying medical health conditions and for the more vulnerable travellers such as pregnant women, young children and older travellers. Other travellers, such as lesbian, gay, bisexual, and transgender (LGBTQ+) individuals, could be at greater risk if travelling to a country where such practices are illegal. A risk of travel being undertaken for the purpose of female genital mutilation may be identified within a pre-travel consultation, and it is important to understand the risks to prevent this from happening. Links to helpful information can be found in the resources at the end of the chapter.

The future of travel health provision

In September 2019, NHS England and NHS Improvement published a document, 'Interim findings of the Vaccinations and Immunisations Review', which included travel vaccinations but stated this subject will be considered in the second stage of the review (NHS England, 2019). There has been no further update since that time, but there is debate as to whether travel health would continue to be provided in primary care as an NHS provision. In addition, in Scotland it was decided to remove the provision of travel health in general practice, and a 'Vaccine Transformation Programme' is currently in progress to decide how the service will be delivered, although to date it has been stated that this will remain an NHS service (NHS Health Scotland, 2019).

COVID-19

A completely new coronavirus was identified late in December 2019 in Wuhan City in the Hubei Province of China. At the end of January 2020, the WHO declared the newly named coronavirus-2019 (abbreviated to COVID-19) a Public Health Emergency of International Concern (WHO, 2020b), and in March it was declared a pandemic. The world has been significantly disrupted from both a health and economic perspective. Considerable work was undertaken to develop accurate and time-efficient testing methods, effective treatments and vaccines, and there was still much work to do as of April 2021. The travel industry, aviation and other forms of travel such as cruising were severely affected, and would continue to be so for some time to come because traveller movement was restricted and social isolating measures which helped to stop the spread of the virus limited the scope of travel. However, other pandemics (such as SARS-CoV-2) demonstrate that, individuals would continue to travel once the health crisis was over, and the need for travel health advice would be required again. Hopefully the importance of infectious diseases and the significance of their spread across international borders will enhance the importance of this specialist subject in terms of public health and ensure that travellers are more mindful of the health prevention advice delivered during a consultation.

Conclusion

Travel health is a very broad and challenging subject. However, it is also a very interesting and variable topic that the GPN may find particularly enjoyable once competence is achieved.

The scope of this chapter can only provide an introduction to the subject, and further study will be required. The full impact of COVID-19 on travel and travel health has yet to be determined.

Resources

Essential guidance for travel health practice
- Chiodini, J. H., Taylor, F., Geary, K., Lang S., Moore, J., Ross, D. A., et al. (2020). *Good Practice Guidance for Providing a Travel Health Service.* Faculty of Travel Medicine of the Royal College of Physicians and Surgeons of Glasgow. https:// rcpsg.ac.uk/travel-medicine/good-practice-guidance-for-providing-a-travel-health-service
- Royal College of Nursing. (2018). *Competencies: Travel health nursing – career and competence development.* Royal College of Nursing. https://www.rcn.org.uk/professional-development/publications/pdf-006506. See pages 32–34 for a comprehensive list of resources, including travel risk assessment and management templates which can also be downloaded from items no. 1 and 2 at https://www.janechiodini.co.uk/tools/.
- 'Immunisation against infectious disease' (the 'Green Book') from Public Health England (the online version must be used, and individual chapters are updated regularly): https://www.gov.uk/government/collections/immunisation-against-infectious-disease-the-green-book
- The UK Malaria Prevention Guidelines from Public Health England: https://www.gov.uk/government/publications/malaria-prevention-guidelines-for-travellers-from-the-uk
- To access these and other resources essential for nurses new to travel health: https://www.janechiodini.co.uk/tools/new-to-travel/
- For links to information regarding prescribing for travel health frequently asked questions, a travel health service, vaccine storage resources, general immunisation, female genital mutilation and travel and more: https://www.janechiodini.co.uk/help/

Continued

- Royal College of Nursing (Public Health Forum) travel health resources: https://www.rcn.org.uk/clinical-topics/public-health/travel-health
- Female genital mutilation: RCN guidance for travel health services: https://www.rcn.org.uk/professional-development/publications/pub-005783
- Royal College of Physicians and Surgeons Female Genital Mutilation and pre-travel health consultations: https://rcpsg.ac.uk/elearning/product/female-genital-mutilation

National online travel health websites and helplines for health care professionals
- TRAVAX from Health Protection Scotland (subscription login required if not practising in Scotland): https://www.travax.nhs.uk/
- TravelHealthPro (National Travel Health Network and Centre [NaTHNaC] from Public Health England): https://travelhealthpro.org.uk/
- Malaria Reference Laboratory e-mail service for health care professionals only on complex malaria queries: https://www.gov.uk/government/publications/malaria-risk-assessment-form

Key resources for vaccines and immunisation training
- Public Health England Immunisation Collection (includes links to Vaccine Update and the Green Book): https://www.gov.uk/government/collections/immunisation
- National Minimum Standards and Core Curriculum for Immunisation Training for Registered Healthcare Practitioners: https://www.gov.uk/government/publications/national-minimum-standards-and-core-curriculum-for-immunisation-training-for-registered-healthcare-practitioners
- Yellow Fever Training from NaTHNaC: https://nathnacyfzone.org.uk/managing-your-yfvc#Training; and Health Protection Scotland: https://www.hps.scot.nhs.uk/web-resources-container/yellow-fever-training-programme/
- Electronic Medicines Compendium for details of all the Summary of Product Characteristics of vaccines and malaria chemoprophylaxis: https://www.medicines.org.uk/emc/
- NaTHNaC factsheets for individual diseases and details of the relevant vaccines: https://travelhealthpro.org.uk/factsheets
- Travel vaccine chart tool – item no. 3: https://www.janechiodini.co.uk/tools/; and general immunisation resources: https://www.janechiodini.co.uk/help/immunisation-resources/

Useful travel health sites for the general public
- Fit for Travel: https://www.fitfortravel.nhs.uk/home
- TravelHealthPro: https://travelhealthpro.org.uk/
- Foreign and Commonwealth Office: https://travelaware.campaign.gov.uk/
- NHS Choices: https://www.nhs.uk/live-well/healthy-body/before-you-travel/
- Traveller advice resources: https://www.janechiodini.co.uk/help/tar/

International resources
- Centers for Disease Control and Prevention. (2020). *The Yellow Book 2020 (Health Information for International Travel)*. https://wwwnc.cdc.gov/travel/page/yellowbook-home
- World Health Organisation travel page: https://www.who.int/ith/en/

Cervical cytology by Helen Crowther and Paula Spooner

Introduction

Cervical cancer is one of the leading causes of morbidity and mortality in women worldwide (Chew et al., 2005) and it is the fourth most common cancer to affect women in the western world (Vizcaino et al., 2000). It is of significance then that cervical cancer is generally a preventable disease. This chapter will introduce GPNs who are new to general practice and newly qualified nurses to the national cervical screening programme, provide an overview of challenges that can be posed for patients and practitioners, explore solutions and signpost to appropriate resources for further in-depth reading.

Background

The national cervical cancer screening programme is offered to women aged 25 to 64 years and uses a cytology test based on the examination of cells under a microscope (UK National Screening Committee, 2016). The sample is acquired via cervical screening, which can be undertaken by a registered nurse/midwife or doctor. The test involves taking a small sample of cells from the cervix to check for abnormalities. Since the NHS computerised call and recall cervical screening system was introduced, most cervical samples have been undertaken in primary care, and the majority are carried out by GPNs.

GPNs, as with other health care professionals, must undertake additional training and assessment in competency to perform cervical screening. The consultation and procedure require competency in history taking, clinical assessment, clinical skill and communication skills to perform effectively.

Why is screening so important?

Screening and early detection can save lives. Cervical screening in the United Kingdom has been subject to many media campaigns in recent years, with correlating peaks and troughs in uptake. One key example is that of the death of media celebrity Jade Goody from advanced cervical cancer in 2009, at the age of 27, which heightened a national awareness of the importance of cervical screening. However, despite an increase in awareness, the uptake level of cervical screening remains concerning. Research has indicated that 72% of 25- to 29-year-olds feel uncomfortable getting undressed in front of health care professionals, and 26.2% are too embarrassed to attend for cervical screening (Jo's Cervical Cancer Trust, 2017, updated 2019). Other research also informs us that uptake of cervical screening among women aged 50 to 64 years is declining (Ryan et al., 2019). See Box 4.6 for tips to promote screening and improve uptake.

Box 4.6   Top tips to promote cervical screening and improve uptake

- Use local knowledge of the practice population, look around the surgery whilst putting yourself in the shoes of a woman attending for screening to identify potential barriers.
- Check and document a correct recall date on every female patient registered at your practice, providing the swift opportunity to invite if eligible.
- Provide up-to-date leaflets and displays regarding cervical screening in different languages including information regarding recent changes in screening.
- Ensure the invitation letter which is sent out to patients is up to date and personal and that the wording is appropriate for your service users. This may include using the easy-read leaflet. If language is potentially a barrier it is essential to use a translator to ensure that women understand their invitation.
- Bring cervical screening into conversations with patients opportunistically to reinforce important messages.
- Ask yourself whether the consultation room is accessible, private, convenient, pleasant and well equipped.
- Consider whether appointments can be made online.
- Nominate a practice cancer champion to help convey the message of screening to a wider audience.
- Consider whether women can attend to discuss the screening process before attending for screening.
- Determine whether there appointments out of hours so the woman does not have to miss work.
- See whether the appointment is promoted as child-friendly, or if appointments are available alongside an immunisation clinic.
- Consider sending digital messages, such as a text or email reminder, to patients to prompt them to attend for screening.
- Ensure that your surgery's website is up to date and giving concise, clear information on the screening process and local policy.
- Have a robust policy regarding cervical screening to ensure consistency of information given to patients and high standards of care.
- Have a clear plan for those who may struggle to attend, such as housebound patients and those with learning or physical disabilities who may need additional time and support.
- Involve the whole practice team in promotion, such as midwives, general practitioners, pharmacists and receptionists.
- Ensure that all staff, including receptionists, are aware of the promotional aspects required for screening and have basic knowledge of timings, booking requirements, etc.

Cervical screening in the United Kingdom

Until changes in 2019, screening was designed to detect abnormal squamous cells exfoliated from the cervix. These cells were then examined in a laboratory, and women with abnormal cells were then invited to clinic for further investigation.

Recent developments in our understanding of the link between human papilloma virus (HPV) and cervical cancers (Bosch, 2002) and four large European randomised controlled trials have led to consideration of the use of HPV testing as a primary screening test (Kitchener et al., 2009) and enabled a change in technique to a method of swabbing to detect HPV rather than solely swabbing for abnormal cells. The swab is examined and, if the sample does not contain the HPV virus and no abnormalities are identified by the clinician performing the procedure, the woman is recalled as per the previous invitation structure. This is a much quicker and more cost-effective method of screening at scale (Bains et al., 2019; Kitchener et al., 2014). Randomised trials have shown that screening for HPV is more sensitive than cytology in the detection of cervical intraepithelial neoplasia and provides greater protection against the development of cervical cancer (Ronco et al., 2014). HPV infection can be transient if the woman's immune system is adequate; thus, the clinician's ability to accurately assess the health of the cervix is imperative. Women with chronic immunosuppression are more susceptible to squamous cell carcinoma, as the immune system cannot rectify any transient changes to the cervix, as the virus is active, leading to the persistence of cervical disease and possible progression to malignancy.

HPV is sexually transmitted, and squamous cell carcinoma has a very low prevalence in women who have never had coitus; thus, the more sexual partners a woman has had, the higher the risk of this cancer. HPV types 16 and 18 are recognised by the WHO and the International Agency for Research on Cancer as oncogenic viruses, and HPV DNA has been found in 99.7% of cases of squamous cell carcinoma.

No cervical screening method is 100% effective because an HPV infection or abnormal cells can sometimes be missed (a 'false negative' result), or abnormal cells can develop and turn into cancer in between screening tests. If screening does not find abnormal cells, this does not guarantee they will never develop in the future.

Human papillomavirus vaccines

Currently, both girls and boys are entitled to HPV vaccines in their second year of secondary school, and a catch-up programme is also available in General Practice for eligible cohorts. The HPV vaccine provides protection against the two HPV strains, type 16 and 18, known to convey a high risk of cancers of the cervix and penis, as well as types 6 and 11, which are known to cause genital warts (WHO, 2020c). Evidence is demonstrating that the vaccine also provides protection against other HPV-associated cancers, including those of the mouth, throat and anus. The vaccine is also available for men who have sex with men up until the age of 45 years in genitourinary medicine, sexual health and human immunodeficiency virus clinics.

Reflection

Find out how your workplace promotes human papillomavirus vaccines

The Gardasil HPV vaccine protects against HPV types 6 and 11, which are responsible for 90% of genital warts, with statistics demonstrating that the immunisation has had a dramatic impact since its introduction into the UK immunisation schedule in 2008 and is 99% effective. The WHO reports that the implementation of the vaccination programme will in time eliminate cervical cancer altogether; however, only time will show this (Vaccine Knowledge Project, 2019). The first cohort of eligible women to receive the HPV vaccine were invited for their first cervical screening in 2015. The majority of women requiring screening will therefore not have had the vaccination, so screening must continue. Rozemeijer et al. (2017) documented an increase in cervical cancer in woman over 60 years. Often these cases are in an advanced stage, so considerations relating to menopause and HPV are important.

The role of the general practice nurse

Following appropriate training and assessment of competency, the GPN needs to ensure that there is a robust and up-to-date practice protocol for cervical cytology, including following up non-attenders and the results of screenings which they have undertaken. The GPN will only perform cervical screening after completing a recognised educational training course and being issued with a unique sample-taker personal identification number (PIN). This PIN should only be used by that sample taker, and it will reflect locally agreed arrangements which may use your Nursing and Midwifery Council PIN or other locally agreed identifier.

The www.gov.uk website has all the essential Public Health England (PHE) guidelines for management of the procedure, including video resources, signposting to accredited training organisations and the latest updates in cervical cytology. Information is available here: https://www.gov.uk/government/collections /cervical-screening-professional-guidance.

The call and recall system and process

PHE states that general practices must be able to demonstrate that they offer women cervical screening, which is currently done by the use of a digital system called 'Open Exeter'. After PHE has invited eligible women for their screening, any non-attenders are identified via a document known as a prior notification list. This is electronically sent to practices, prompting a review to invite or defer; actions following this need to be documented in the patient's clinical records. Open Exeter allows sample takers to access the prior notification list to see who is eligible from their practice; this also allows the monitoring of the uptake of cervical screening. This enables a safety mechanism to prevent patients from being missed off the invitation list if, for example, they have moved geographical areas. By having an efficient call/recall process the practice can invite women at the time of the initial national screening, which may help with attendance and reduce the risk of non-attendance.

Preparation for the test

Before the screening is undertaken, the GPN will set up the consulting room with the appropriate equipment and conditions. The room should be prepared to ensure that there is a comfortable environment with sufficient warmth and privacy, and that all the equipment is ready and available to use. The GPN will also check the records for the eligibility of the patient to have the test within the required screening interval.

Examination

Cervical screening can be an uncomfortable and embarrassing experience for some women, so it is very important that the GPN is calm and confident in performing the procedure and is able to offer a full explanation of what to expect and why it needs to be done. Women should always be offered the opportunity to be accompanied by a chaperone for the procedure, and this should be clearly documented in the patient's clinical record.

The examination couch should have good lighting and a privacy curtain, should be positioned away from the wall to allow the knees to drop to the side, and ideally should be easy to raise and lower. The couch should always be covered with a hygienic paper sheet, and the patient should be provided with a modesty sheet to cover herself.

The GPN inserts the speculum into the vagina, and once the cervix is clearly seen and no abnormalities are identified, the sample can be taken (Fig. 4.3).

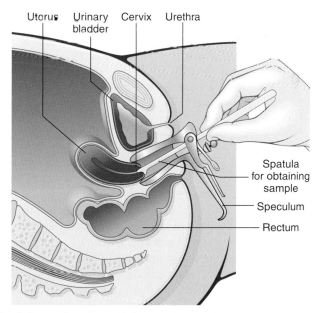

Fig. 4.3   Cervical screening. (From Chabner, D. (2021). *The language of medicine* (12th ed.). Elsevier.)

How to deal with difficult examinations

There are many barriers and challenges that patients may face when attending for their screening. Within their specific training as a sample taker, GPNs will learn about effective communication skills and how to explain the procedure and provide reassurance.

Vaginismus is the body's automatic reaction to the fear of some or all types of vaginal penetration such that, whenever penetration is attempted, the vaginal muscles tighten up on their own. If the patient has vaginismus, the GPN must ensure that the procedure is not rushed. Occasionally it might take a couple of consultations before the actual sample can be taken. It is important to have a range of speculums and a small amount of appropriate lubricant to make the procedure as comfortable as possible.

The process following the examination

After the examination the GPN will discuss the results process with the patient, including what to expect and what to do if she does not receive her results. If the GPN identified any anomalies in the examination and a referral is required to another clinic or clinician, the GPN will explain this process and provide reassurance and a clear explanation of what to expect.

Case study

The Vale practice demonstrated an effective method of increasing screening uptake after its general practice nurse negotiated discounted deals at a local beauty salon for women who were booked for or who had undertaken their cervical screening.

Another practice used pink paper when writing to invite women who were overdue for their test as a visual reminder. This practice led to increased uptake and was nationally recognised.

Audit

Every clinician who undertakes cervical screening is required to keep a log of the patients they have screened. This is to ensure that they are working to a required standard and not having recurrent insufficient sample returns, and to ensure that those patients with positive results do not get lost within the system. It is essential to understand the responsibilities within general practice, including acting on and documenting non-responders and providing urgent results when contacted by the cytology laboratory. On occasions, the sample taker may be required to make a referral to a colposcopy clinic or follow up a patient who fails to attend a colposcopy clinic appointment. A GPN taking cervical smears should have visited a colposcopy department as part of his or her initial training to understand this process.

It is the GPN's responsibility to ensure that he or she personally remains updated by undertaking continued self-evaluation and professional competence training. This may be by face-to-face or online learning, but must include a formal update every 3 years. If a sample taker does not maintain the required standard, he or she must not perform any tests until the appropriate training has been undertaken.

Reflection

Standard process for results

The woman will receive a letter to inform her of one of the four possible outcomes of her cervical screening:

1. A human papillomavirus (HPV)-negative result means that HPV is not currently detected, and it is highly unlikely that there will be any abnormal cervical cells. This will mean the woman is to continue with the current recall process for screening in 3 to 5 years.
2. An HPV-positive result with no abnormal cells will be called in for screening sooner than the routine 3 to 5 years to ensure that the woman's immune system has cleared the transient HPV infection.
3. An HPV-positive result with abnormal cells found can have different levels of concern. There are several 'grades' of abnormal cells, as some are more serious than others. The personalised letter will explain the results for the patient. If a patient has HPV and any grade of abnormal cervical cells, she is referred for colposcopy.
4. Inadequate results may be attributed to a technical problem, for example, if the laboratory cannot get an HPV test result from the sample or cannot see if abnormal cells are present or not. In these cases, the woman is invited for further cervical screening after 3 months. This wait is to ensure that there are enough cells to obtain a sufficient sample.

COVID-19

Once the COVID-19 pandemic began, an increased use of personal protective equipment was essential to offer screening to patients. The pandemic caused a backlog and delay in screening normal recall patients; however, GPNs were innovative, forward thinking and pragmatic in addressing this issue, and patients began to be seen in practices for routine cervical screening again.

Conclusion

All women are susceptible to HPV infection, whether vaccinated or not, and should always undergo cervical screening when invited. Increasing awareness that cervical screening can make a positive difference to health should be opportunistically reinforced. GPNs who perform cervical screening should undergo training with assessment of competence and confidence. There is an imperative for action, regular screening and effective follow-up. Early diagnosis and treatment saves lives and reduces stress and anxiety for the woman and her family.

Wound care by Gill Boast

Introduction

The diversity of the GPN role means that a wide range of assessment skills are needed, and one area where this is particularly important is wound assessment. Whatever commissioning arrangements have been made for wound care in each geographical area, GPNs will find themselves at some point assessing a patient with a wound. This part of the chapter will briefly discuss some of the types of wounds seen in general practice and the current evidence-based management.

The National Wound Care Strategy Programme (NWCSP) was set up to improve wound care across the United Kingdom (Academic Health Science Network, 2020). This was commissioned by NHS England/NHS Improvement in response to the Burden of Wound study undertaken by Guest et al. (2015), which found there were clinical and economic benefits from improving systems of care and raising awareness of the impact of wounds. Remember that wound dressings alone will not heal wounds, and it is vital that GPNs access appropriate education and seek guidance from tissue viability specialists. To help reduce the substantial cost of wound care GPNs need to ensure they can undertake a holistic assessment and make an accurate diagnosis so that evidence-based guidelines can be followed (Wounds UK, 2018).

Types of wounds

The main types of wounds are traumatic injuries, surgical wounds, pressure ulcers and lower limb ulcers, and the NWCSP programme (Adderley, 2020) has focused on three main areas:

1. Surgical wounds
2. Lower limb ulcers
3. Pressure injuries/ulcers

Wound healing

There are two main categories of wound healing:

- Primary intention: minimal tissue loss, wound edges held together by clips, staples and sutures; for example, in post-operative wounds where the progress of healing is more predictable.
- Secondary intention: greater tissue loss, wound edges further apart. Healing takes place through granulation and subsequent epithelialisation (Plester & Montgomery, 2010).

The process of wound healing (Fig. 4.4)

This process can be hindered by biofilms, which are clusters of bacteria in a wound that delay healing. The best indicator of biofilms being present is a non-healing wound despite optimal care. It is thought that the wound healing process gets stuck at the inflammation phase (Wounds International, 2019a; Wounds International, 2019b). Early intervention is required before biofilms become a serious challenge. Further information is available here: http://www.woundinfection-institute.com/resources

Wound assessment

The ability to undertake a comprehensive assessment is a vital skill for GPNs (Table 4.4).

The triangle of wound assessment (Fig. 4.5) divides the assessment into three distinct areas; the wound bed, the wound edges and the periwound (surrounding) area.

Traumatic injuries

GPNs may often encounter patients presenting with traumatic injuries. The following section will focus on:

- Bites (animal and human)
- Insect bites and stings
- Skin tears and lacerations
- Burns and scalds

Bites (animal and human)

Most animal bites in the United Kingdom are from dogs or cats, with injuries often on the hand (GP Notebook, 2019), or from human bites. Unfortunately, there is a high risk of bite wounds becoming infected (NICE, 2018a); therefore,

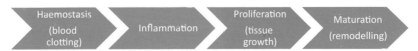

Fig. 4.4 The process of wound healing.

Table 4.4 Conducting a comprehensive wound assessment.

General health information	General health and skin integrity Susceptibility to infection Risk factors for delayed healing Medication Allergies and skin sensitivities Impact of wound on quality of life
Wound baseline information	Number of wounds Wound location Wound type/classification Wound duration Treatment Reassessment date
Wound assessment parameters	Wound size, maximum length, width, depth Undermining/tunnelling Category – pressure ulcers Wound bed tissue type Wound bed tissue amount Description of wound margins/edges Colour and condition of surrounding skin Whether wound has healed
If wound is on the lower limb	Leg skin condition Any oedema Leg shape Ankle circumference General mobility Ankle flexion Palpable foot pulses Ankle brachial pressure index (ABPI)
Wound symptoms	Presence of wound pain Frequency of pain Severity of pain Exudate amount Exudate consistency/colour/type Any odour Signs of systemic infection Signs of local infection Whether wound swab has been taken
Specialists	Investigations, e.g., for lower limb ABPI Referrals to Tissue Viability, hospital consultant, specialist clinics

From Coleman, S., Nelson, E. A., Vowden, P., et al. (2017). Development of a generic wound care assessment minimum data set. *Journal of Tissue Viability, 26*(4), 226–240.

all animal bites should be considered contaminated and receive wound care (BMJ Best Practice, 2018a). It is important to look for any foreign bodies that may be embedded, especially in deep wounds, (e.g., broken teeth). Some useful

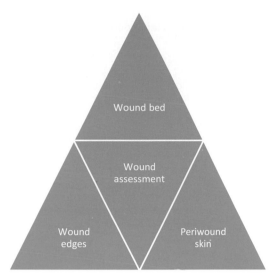

Fig. 4.5   Triangle of wound assessment. (From Dowsett, C., Protz, K., Drouard, M., & Harding, K. G. (2015). Triangle of wound assessment made easy. *Wounds International*. www.woundsinternational .com.)

algorithms are available via BMJ Best Practice (2018a): https://bestpractice .bmj.com/topics/en-gb/280. Log in via an Open Athens account. See Table 4.5 for initial assessment and care.

Insect bites and stings

GPNs may see patients who present with an insect bite, often to the leg. Most insect bites and stings in the United Kingdom are not serious; however, sometimes an allergic reaction develops, which may resemble cellulitis, and a blister may form at the bite (NHS, 2019a). Pain, swelling and itching may be present for several days, so pain relief and antihistamines may be required. Most insect bites will improve after a few days. Carefully remove the stinger or tick if it is still present. Ticks that cause Lyme disease are found all over the United Kingdom, so it is best to remove a tick as soon as possible and be aware of the signs and symptoms of Lyme disease (NHS, 2019a). A cold compress may help to ease the pain from bee and wasp stings. Stings near the eye or in the mouth or throat should be referred for an urgent medical opinion. Occasionally there may be a severe allergic reaction which could cause breathing difficulties and swelling to the mouth or face, with the need for urgent medical attention (NHS, 2019a). The second most common cause of anaphylaxis in the United Kingdom is insect stings (GP Notebook, 2020). Also check whether patients have travelled abroad in case there is a risk of malaria or other insect-borne disease (Chiodini, 2020). A useful guide to the various types of insect bites is available on the NHS website (NHS, 2019b).

Table 4.5 Initial assessment and management of bite wounds.

Bites: initial assessment and wound care	Management
Immediate first aid if required	Control the bleeding if necessary. Refer for specialist assessment if the bite has penetrated a joint or bone or the damage is severe. Patients with multiple bites, severe local infection or evidence of systemic infection or severe underlying illness require hospital admission.
History taking	Document the type of animal and the circumstances, including timing and nature of the bite, with the wound description, and note any erythema. General medical history, including any factors that may impede healing, e.g., immunosuppression, diabetes. Any allergies, especially antibiotics and dressings. Current medications. Consider safeguarding issues if the patient is a child or vulnerable adult.
Clinical examination	Observe and inspect for any sign of damage to blood vessels, nerves, tendons, bones and joints and any lymphadenopathy. Carefully examine wounds overlying a joint and check full range of movement. Check the range of movement in adjacent joints. Look for any embedded foreign bodies, e.g., broken teeth. Baseline measurements of the wound width, length and depth. Photographs or diagrams may be useful. Assess the risk of tetanus or blood-borne virus infections (NHS, 2019a). The following link provides information: https://www.gov.uk/government/publications/tetanus-advice-for-health-professionals. Consider post-exposure tetanus or rabies prophylaxis (PHE, 2018): https://www.gov.uk/government/publications/rabies-the-green-book-chapter-27.
Initial treatment	Irrigate the wound with saline (or running tap water if saline is not available). Irrigate with a solution of povidone iodine if the animal was rabid (BMJ Best Practice, 2018). Wound closure is controversial, but if more than 24 hours has elapsed since the bite or if it is infected, it should be left open. On facial wounds primary closure should be undertaken by plastic surgeons. Cover the wound with a suitable dressing. Elevate the affected limb, especially if the wound was caused by a human bite to the hand or a cat bite with a puncture wound near to a joint.

Table 4.5 Initial assessment and management of bite wounds—cont'd.

Bites: initial assessment and wound care	Management
Ongoing care	Prophylactic antibiotics should be considered in high-risk cases, e.g.: puncture or crush wounds, wounds requiring surgical repair, wounds near to prosthetic joint, when there is impaired circulation or poor lymphatic drainage, etc. Hospital admission should be considered for multiple or severe bites, severe immune compromise or serious underlying illness, signs of severe infection or bone involvement (BMJ Best Practice, 2018). Apply suitable wound dressings and review patient and wound at each dressing change for signs of complications.
Complications	There are many complications to consider when dealing with animal bites. For example: Abscess formation Sepsis Osteomyelitis or septic arthritis Endocarditis Damage to deep structures, including tendons, nerves, vessels.

Skin tears and lacerations

Skin tears differ to lacerations because they occur owing to a variety of mechanical forces, including shearing or friction, and are often misdiagnosed in clinical practice (Wounds International, 2018). These acute wounds frequently occur on the hands, arms or lower limbs. They may result in partial or full skin-flap loss (Wounds International, 2019c). Elderly patients or those with dry/fragile skin are at increased risk of skin tears. Skin-tear risk should be assessed, and there should be a collaborative approach to prevention (Wounds International, 2018). Once a skin tear has occurred, assess the skin, mobility and general health of the patient and categorise the skin tear (Carville et al., 2007; LeBlanc et al., 2013). See Box 4.7 for skin-tear classification systems and Fig. 4.6 for a skin-tear treatment pathway.

Lacerations

A laceration is a break or split in the skin caused by trauma or incision (NICE, 2018b). There is a high risk of infection if the laceration is contaminated with soil, body fluids, pus or faeces, and wound healing may be complicated further by diabetes, frailty, age or other factors (NICE, 2018b). Referral to the accident

Box 4.7 **Skin tear classification systems**

For example:

International Skin Tear Advisory Panel

    Type 1: no skin loss

    Type 2: partial flap loss

    Type 3: total flap loss

    International Skin Tear Advisory Panel: A toolkit to aid in the prevention, assessment and treatment of skin tears using a simplified classification system. https://journals.lww.com/aswcjournal/Fulltext/2013/10000/International_Skin_Tear_Advisory_Panel__A_Tool_Kit.7.aspx.[a]

Skin Tear Audit Research

    1a: no skin loss

    1b: skin flap can be realigned

    2a: skin edges cannot be realigned, but flap is pink

    2b: skin edges cannot be realigned, and flap is dark/dusky

    3: skin flap is completely absent

    A consensus for skin tear classification. *Primary Intention, 15*(1), 18–28.)[b]

[a]From LeBlanc, K., Baranowski, S., Christensen, D., et al. (2013).
[b]From Carville, K., Lewin, G., Newall, N., et al. (2007).

and emergency department is recommended when there is possible nerve or tendon damage, if the wound is extensive, if there is a foreign body present in the laceration, for facial wounds or if there is any associated cellulitis over a joint (NICE, 2018b).

Burns and scalds

Burns and scalds are injuries that are quite commonly seen in general practice but may be challenging for GPNs to deal with. The impact of a burn injury can be enormous, and there may be severe distress for patients and their families (Edwards, 2007). First aid and initial management can significantly affect the outcome (BMJ Best Practice, 2018b). It is therefore particularly important for GPNs to be confident in assessing and managing a burn injury, including measuring the burn area. Suboptimal emergency burn care can lead to multiple adverse consequences, including loss of function, joint restriction and psychological impact (Holdsworth, 2015). Adequate analgesia is also required, as burns are particularly painful injuries. Burn injuries can be classified as noncomplex or complex:

● Noncomplex: burns that will heal spontaneously with conservative treatment
● Complex: burns that require the involvement of specialist burns services

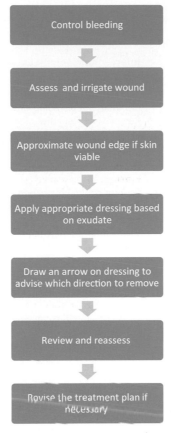

Fig. 4.6 Skin tear treatment pathway.

Referral to burns services

- Any burns where more than 3% of the body is affected (2% in children)
- All full-thickness burns
- All circumferential burns
- All chemical/electrical burns
- Any burn with suspicion of non-accidental injury
- Any burn not healed within 2 to 3 weeks. Burns that take longer to heal are more likely to result in hypertrophic scarring (NHS Specialised Services, 2012)

Consider the size, depth, site and mechanism of injury. Early referral to specialist burns services may be necessary when the face, ears, hands, feet, major joints or genitals have been affected (BMJ Best Practice, 2018b; NICE, 2019a). The Best Practice guidelines for effective skin and wound management in noncomplex burns are a valuable resource for GPNs (Wounds International, 2014). Table 4.6 has been drawn up from the information within these guidelines.

Table 4.6 **Emergency management of burns.**

Emergency management of burns	Intervention
General first aid	Check that it is safe to approach, call for help Stop the burning process (drop and roll, turn off electricity supply if appropriate) Remove any restrictive clothing or jewellery
Cool the burn	Ideally cool with tepid, running water for up to 30 minutes (avoid very cold water or ice) If running water is not available, damp towels or hydrogel sheets can be used on adults Perform cooling of the burn within 20 minutes of the injury to reduce the pain, minimise swelling and clean the wound Chemical burns may require a prolonged period of irrigation, as corrosive agents continue to cause pain until completely removed Cool the burn but not the patient; keep the patient warm
Cover the burn	Cover the burn to prevent bacteria colonising and to relieve the pain from the exposed nerve endings Layers of cling film can be laid in sheets over the wound; do not apply circumferentially Be aware that cellophane film can worsen chemical burns, so apply dressings soaked in saline or water instead Do not apply any creams at this stage because this will hinder assessment
Relieve pain	Cooling may provide some relief, but opioids may be required in the initial stages Superficial burns are especially painful, as the nerve endings remain intact, so a combination of paracetamol and low to moderate doses of opioids initially may be appropriate. Patients with dermal burns should be given intravenous opioids or intra-nasal diamorphine Check tetanus status

From Wounds International. (2014). *International Best Practice Guidelines: Effective skin and wound management of non-complex burns.* www.woundsinternational.com.

Be aware of the possibility of toxic shock syndrome. This may develop around 2 to 4 days post-injury, with rapid deterioration, particularly in those under 2 years of age.

Assessment of burns

The severity and size of the burn is assessed as a percentage of the total body surface area affected and the depth of the burn (first degree to fourth degree) (Table 4.7).

Table 4.7 **Cutaneous burns.**

Classification according to depth	Description of burn	Healing rate
First degree (superficial)	Usually dry and painful Erythema (epidermis only affected) Typical of severe sunburn No blistering	Usually heals within 7 days with conservative treatment No scarring
Second degree (superficial partial-thickness or superficial dermal or deep dermal)	Usually wet and painful Partial thickness involving the epidermis and dermis Typical of scalds Blistering present	Usually heals within 14 days with conservative treatment No scarring if superficial Deep dermal (deep partial thickness) are more difficult to treat and may require surgical intervention. There may be scarring
Third degree (full-thickness)	Usually dry and lack sensation Full thickness involving epidermis, dermis and appendages Typical of flame or contact injuries Underlying tissue may be pale or blackened Remaining skin dry and white, brown or black with no blisters	Seldom heal without surgical intervention
Fourth degree	Involve underlying tendon, bone or muscle Typical of high-voltage electrical injuries	Requires surgical intervention

From BMJ Best Practice. (2018b). *Cutaneous burns.* https://bestpractice.bmj.com/topics/en-gb/412.

Total body surface area

To quickly estimate a small burn: consider the palm of the patient's hand to be 1% of the body surface area. Reddening of the surrounding skin does not need to be included. See Fig. 4.7.

Ensure appropriate assessment and initial management. Decide whether the burn is suitable for management in primary care. Reassess the wound within

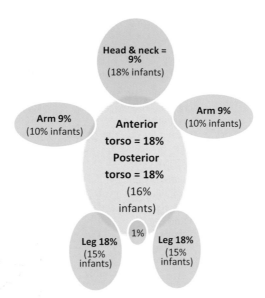

Fig. 4.7 Wallace rule of nines. (From Wallace, A. B. (1951). The exposure treatment of burns. *Lancet, 1,* 501–504. doi:10.1016/s0140-6736(51)91975-7.)

48 hours and arrange ongoing follow up every 3 to 5 days depending on the extent of the wound. Excessive exudate can occur within 72 hours, so may be a normal finding, but observe for other signs of infection, as there is an increased risk in burns (Edwards, 2013). Cleanse, debride and manage exudate if present. Provide analgesia and select appropriate dressings. If there is continued exudate, friable tissue and redness, treat with topical antimicrobials to manage infection and review every 2 to 3 days (Wounds International, 2014).

Most small superficial burns should heal within 2 weeks. If healing is delayed, refer on to specialist burns services. Healed burns often remain sensitive and may develop dry, scaly skin. This delicate new skin is vulnerable to further injury. Protect the area from the sun. Advise patients to use a non-perfumed emollient daily and massage using a circular and downward motion. Emollients should be continued for up to 12 months or more (Wounds International, 2014). A useful algorithm for management of non-complex burns is available in Best Practice Guidelines Wounds International (2014).

A handy patient information leaflet is available via BMJ Best Practice (2018b): https://bestpractice.bmj.com/patient-leaflets/en-gb/pdf/1183564235144/ Burns%20%28minor%29.pdf.

Post-operative/procedure care

Patients may attend to see the GPN after a range of surgical procedures and operations. In general, incision sites should be covered for 48 hours, unless there are signs of infection or excessive exudate warranting inspection of the wound site. Ideally the wound should be photographed and the image recorded in the care record before discharge from secondary care (NWCSP, 2020). Unfortunately, around 5% of people undergoing a surgical procedure develop a surgical site infection; NICE (2019b) guidance provides information, including the importance of pre-operative assessments, to identify those at risk of problems with wound healing and preparation of the patient before surgery.

Patients may present to the GPN for suture or clip removal. The timing of removal varies according to the surgical site. Sutures to the head and neck are usually removed after 3 to 5 days, sutures over joints are normally removed after 10 to 14 days, and sutures to other parts of the body are removed after 7 to 10 days (NHS, 2020).

Red flags include any wound showing signs of infection/sepsis, dehiscence, spreading cellulitis or suspected fistula or tunnelling. Seek review via the surgical team. Wounds that are failing to heal by primary intention after 2 weeks should also be reviewed. Arrange review by tissue viability specialists if there are concerns.

Sepsis

Broken skin is a source of entry for infection. Other comorbidities, for example, diabetes or lymphoedema, may cause infection to spread more rapidly. Cellulitis may develop in the dermis and subcutaneous tissue after any wound (NICE, 2019c). It may be difficult to distinguish cellulitis from lipodermatosclerosis, but usually cellulitis affects just one leg (British Lymphology Society [BLS], 2016). Cellulitis may lead on to sepsis, which is the body's response to overwhelming infection, and may lead to organ failure and death (Sepsis Trust, 2020). However, if caught early enough, sepsis is treatable. It is therefore very important for GPNs to recognise the signs and symptoms, which may vary but can initially present as a chest infection, gastroenteritis or flu (see Box 4.8).

Refer all patients with suspected sepsis to emergency medical care, usually via 999 ambulance. Risk stratification tools (NICE, 2016) and further information are available via: https://www.nice.org.uk/guidance/ng51.

Additional resources specifically for general practice are available on the Sepsis Trust website: https://sepsistrust.org/.

Lower limb wounds

Prevention

There are many risk factors for leg ulceration, including leg injury/trauma, age, female sex, a higher number of pregnancies, physical inactivity and family history or previous history of ulceration (Atkin, 2019; Lim et al., 2018). Venous disease causes skin changes, dryness and thickened areas (Nazarko, 2018), and early intervention and proactive management of these early stages is important to prevent ulceration.

Box 4.8 Signs and symptoms of sepsis

Sepsis in adults
- Slurred speech or confusion
- Extreme shivering or muscle pain
- Passing no urine in a day
- Severe breathlessness
- Feeling like they are going to die
- Skin mottled or discoloured

Sepsis in children
- May be breathing very fast
- Fits or convulsions
- Mottled colour, bluish or pale
- Rash that does not fade on pressure
- Lethargic or difficult to wake
- Abnormally cold to the touch

Sepsis in under-5s
- May not be feeding
- Vomiting repeatedly
- Have not passed urine for 12 hours

From Sepsis Trust. (2020). *What is sepsis.* https://sepsistrust.org/.

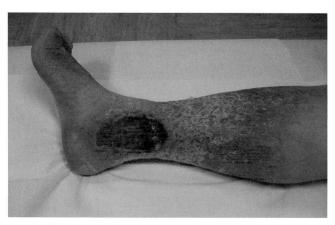

Fig. 4.8 Example of a leg ulcer. (From Harding, M. M. (2020). *Lewis' medical-surgical nursing: Assessment and management of clinical problems* (11th ed.). Elsevier.)

Definition of a leg ulcer

A leg ulcer is a break in the skin below the knee that has not healed within 2 weeks (NICE, 2013). Leg ulcers are a symptom of an underlying disease, and a large proportion are due to venous insufficiency (NWCSP, 2019) (Fig. 4.8).

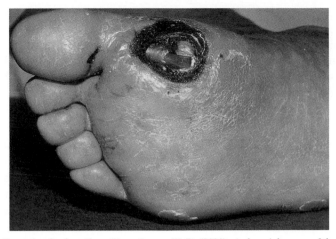

Fig. 4.9   Example of a foot ulcer. (From James, W. D. (2020). *Andrews' diseases of the skin* (13th ed.). Elsevier.)

Definition of a foot ulcer

A foot ulcer is break in the skin below the ankle (malleolus) (Fig. 4.9). In England, seven out of 10 major amputations are in men, and the highest rates are in the Black population (All Party Parliamentary Group [APPG], 2019). People with diabetes are more likely to have an amputation than those without diabetes, and approximately 7000 lower limb amputations are carried out in people with diabetes in England every year (NWCSP, 2019). However, peripheral arterial disease is also related to lower limb amputation and associated with early death (APPG, 2019). GPNs therefore need to be proactive in the prevention, early detection and evidenced-based treatment of those with arterial or venous disease.

Red flags

Immediately escalate:

- Red, hot, swollen leg or foot
- Spreading infection of leg or foot
- Chronic limb-threatening ischaemia
- Suspected deep vein thrombosis
- Suspected skin cancer

Immediate care and early intervention

This should include:

- Wound and skin cleansing
- Wound assessment
- Simple low-adherent dressing with suitable absorbency
- Light/reduced compression (up to 20 mm Hg) if appropriate (NWCSP, 2019)

Any patient with a wound to the foot below the ankle should have a full assessment within 48 hours of presentation (NWCSP, 2019). It is essential to adopt a multidisciplinary approach, as complex interventions may be required, for example, pressure offloading or surgical procedures (NICE, 2015). For lower limb wounds above the ankle a full holistic assessment should be undertaken within 14 days of presentation (NWCSP, 2019).

Assessment

A full holistic assessment includes a thorough assessment of the patient, the limb and the wound. This should include elements of the generic wound assessment shown in Table 4.4 (Coleman et al., 2017), photographs and wound mapping, quality of life assessment (Green, et al., 2018) and a risk assessment of wound healing and the treatment plan. The holistic assessment should follow an established pathway, including vascular assessment and ankle brachial pressure index (ABPI) (Wounds UK, 2019a). Look out for signs of venous disease/oedema/varicosities, skin changes, skin staining (haemosiderin), atrophie blanche, lipodermatosclerosis, lymphoedema, lipodema, malignancy, critical limb ischaemia, cellulitis, infection and untreated deep vein thrombosis (Fig. 4.10).

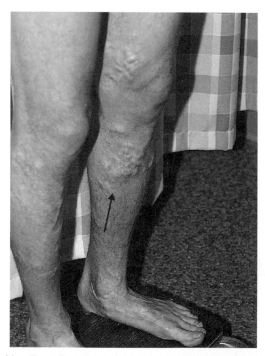

Fig. 4.10   Varicosities. (From Copstead, L. C. (2018). *Pathophysiology* (6th ed.). Elsevier.)

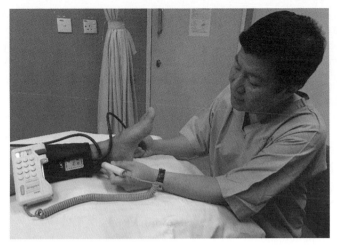

Fig. 4.11   Measuring ankle brachial pressure index. (From Garden, O. J. (2018). *Principles and practice of surgery* (7th ed.). Elsevier.)

Diagnosis

The measurement of ABPI has been recognised as an important element of the holistic assessment to identify the presence or absence of arterial disease (Wounds UK, 2019b) (Fig. 4.11). However, many factors affect ABPI, and there are some limitations to its use, particularly in those with lymphoedema, diabetes, renal disease or rheumatoid arthritis (BLS, 2018). Undertaking a manual ABPI assessment requires a level of expertise, and it may also be difficult to obtain an ABPI in some patients, particularly those with severe swelling or pain, those with a high body mass index or those unable to adopt a recumbent position.

Automated ABPI devices are now available and have been successfully introduced in practice (Boast et al., 2019; Dowsett & Taylor, 2018; Wounds UK, 2019b). If signs of arterial disease are detected, refer for vascular specialist opinion and follow NICE (2018c) guidelines for peripheral arterial disease.

Patients without signs of arterial disease should be cared for in line with national guidelines for venous leg ulcers (NICE, 2019d; Scottish Intercollegiate Guideline Network [SIGN], 2010), including compression therapy (minimum 40 mm Hg). There is evidence that compression hosiery kits, which exert 40 mm Hg of pressure, are an effective alternative to bandaging (Journal of Wound Care, 2016) and are cost effective, but they may not be suitable for some patients (NICE, 2013). Furthermore, early intervention with compression is important, and GPNs may need to access specialist leg ulcer services or undertake additional training to enable the provision of compression therapy. Those patients with leg swelling, abnormal limb shape, very fragile skin or copious exudate should be referred for expert opinion and advice about lymphoedema (NWCSP, 2019). Patients with venous disease should be offered referral for endovenous intervention (Gohel, et al., 2018; NICE, 2013). Duplex scans, computer tomography angiogram, magnetic resonance angiogram or catheter angiogram may also be required.

All patients with leg wounds should be offered:

- Analgesia
- Medicines review
- Advice on skin care and footwear
- Exercise, rest, limb elevation, nutritional advice and self-care guidance
- Written information about the diagnosis and treatment plan (NWCSP, 2019)

Each dressing change should include wound and skin cleansing and review of the treatment plan. Skin care and the use of emollients are particularly important. Assess for reduction in wound size and document using photography ideally. Assess pain/discomfort and reduction in limb swelling. If the aetiology is not certain, refer to tissue viability specialists, and if the ulcer is not showing signs of healing after 2 weeks in full compression, refer on to a vascular specialist.

Case study

Betty's story (NHS Rightcare, 2017) highlighted variation in the management of leg ulcers, offering suboptimal and optimal care pathways. This is the link: https://www.england.nhs.uk/rightcare/wp-content/uploads/sites/40/2017/01/nhs-rightcare-bettys-story-narrative-full.pdf

---

There is a specific commissioning for quality and innovation for the assessment, diagnosis and management of lower leg wounds: https://www.england.nhs.uk/wp-content/uploads/2020/01/FINAL-CQUIN-20-21-Indicator-Specifications-190220.pdf.

The national minimum data set expected that more than 70% of chronic lower leg wounds should be healed by 24 months (Coleman et al., 2017). However, some other underlying conditions can impact on wound healing (Wounds UK, 2019a). Patients may need to be referred on to specialist teams, especially when the following exist:

- Autoimmune disease, particularly rheumatoid arthritis
- Diabetes
- Heart failure
- Haematological disorders
- Immunosuppression
- Previous deep vein thrombosis
- Drug injection into the lower limb
- Renal or liver disease

Ongoing care once healed

Leg ulcers recur unless secondary prevention is maintained. Compression hosiery is therefore recommended to prevent recurrence, and is likely to be required indefinitely (SIGN, 2010). Skin care and emollients remain important aspects of self-care, and patients should be reviewed at least annually (Wounds UK, 2019a).

The Legs Matter campaign is a coalition of health care organisations that provides a wealth of information for patients and health care professionals, available via the following link: https://legsmatter.org/help-information/.

Pressure injuries/ulcers

Pressure injuries/ulcers may arise in several ways when the skin and tissues are damaged as a result of pressure and impaired blood supply (NICE, 2014). All patients are potentially at risk, but pressure injuries/ulcers are more likely to occur in serious illness, when there is lack of mobility, deformity, neurological conditions or poor nutrition (Wounds UK, 2017). Patients may occasionally present to the GPN with a pressure injury/ulcer. These types of wounds are recognised as patient harm (NHS, 2018), and therefore, if there are any omissions to patient care, refer to safeguarding policy. It is important for health care professionals to work collaboratively, and wounds that arise as a result of pressure damage should be reported using the local incident reporting system and referred to Community Nursing Services for full assessment.

The Stop the Pressure programme (NHS Improvement, 2018) recommended a consistent approach to defining, measuring and managing pressure ulcers. The National Wound Care Strategy Programme incorporated the Stop the Pressure programme into their pressure ulcer clinical workstream; further information is available here: https://www.ahsnnetwork.com/about-academic-health-science-networks/national-programmes-priorities/national-wound-care-strategy-programme/clinical-workstreams/pressure-ulcer-clinical-workstream.

Pressure ulcer/injury staging

Stage 1: precursor to ulceration, intact skin but nonblanchable redness
Stage 2: partial-thickness skin loss
Stage 3: full-thickness skin loss, subcutaneous fat/tissue may be visible
Stage 4: full-thickness skin loss with exposed muscle, tendon or bone.

This was developed from the European Pressure Ulcer Advisory Panel, National Pressure Injury Advisory Panel and Pan Pacific Pressure Injury Alliance (2019) guidelines.

The SSKIN mnemonic is a five-step approach to preventing and treating pressure ulcers (NHS Improvement, 2018):

● Surface: does the patient have the right support?
● Skin: inspect the skin

- Keep moving
- Incontinence/moisture
- Nutrition/hydration

Conclusion

This part of the chapter has provided a brief overview of occasions when GPNs may be involved in wound care management, and the complexity that this can present. It is therefore important that GPNs access appropriate education and training so that they can assess, proactively manage and improve outcomes for patients who present with wounds. Suboptimal care increases care costs and extends healing times (NWCSP, 2019). The diversity of the GPN role means that GPNs can make a very valuable contribution in this area so that, where possible, wounds can be prevented or early intervention offered (Atkin, 2019), working collaboratively with a range of other health care professionals.

References

Academic Health Science Network. (2020). *National Wound Care Strategy Programme.* https://www.ahsnnetwork.com/about-academic-health-science-networks/national-programmes-priorities/national-wound-care-strategy-programme.

Adderley, U. (2020). *The National Wound Care Strategy Programme.* https://www.woundcare-today.com/journals/issue/february-2019/article/national-wound-care-strategy-programme.

All Party Parliamentary Group. (2019). *Saving Limbs, Saving Lives: A call to action to reduce inequalities in lower limb amputation rates.* https://www.vvappg.com/new-page-1.

Andre, F., Booy, R., Bock, H. L., et al. (2008). Vaccination greatly reduces disease, disability, death and inequity worldwide. *Bulletin of the World Health Organization, 86*(2), 81–160.

Atkin, L. (2019). Venous leg ulcer prevention 1: Identifying patients who are at risk. *Nursing Times, 115*(6), 24–28.

Bains, I., Choi, Y., Soldan, K., & Jit, M. (2019). Clinical impact and cost-effectiveness of primary cytology versus human papillomavirus testing for cervical cancer screening in England. *International Journal of Gynecologic Cancer, 29*(4), 669–675.

Boast, G., Green, J., Chambers, R., & Calderwood, R. (2019). Improving assessment and management of lower limb wounds. *Journal of General Practice Nursing, 5*(4), 36–39.

Bosch, F., Lorincz, A., Munoz, N., Meijer, C., & Shah, K. (2002). The causal relation between human papillomavirus and cervical cancer. *Journal of Clinical Pathology, 55*(4), 244–265.

Boyne, L., Chiodini, J., Grieve, S. (2018). *Competencies: Travel health nursing: Career and competence development.* Royal College of Nursing. https://www.rcn.org.uk/professional-development/publications/pdf-006506.

British Medical Association. (2018). *Focus on travel immunisation 2018.* https://www.bma.org.uk/advice/employment/gp-practices/service-provision/prescribing/vaccination/travel-immunisation.

BMJ Best Practice. (2018a). *Animal bites.* https://bestpractice.bmj.com/topics/en-gb/280.

BMJ Best Practice. (2018b). *Cutaneous burns.* https://bestpractice.bmj.com/topics/en-gb/412.

British Lymphology Society. (2016). *Consensus document on the management of cellulitis in lymphoedema.* https://www.lymphoedema.org/images/pdf/CellulitisConsensus.pdf.

British Lymphology Society. (2018). *Position paper for ankle brachial pressure index (ABPI).* https://www.thebls.com/public/uploads/documents/document-2062539855354.pdf.

Campbell, H., Van Hoek, A. J., et al. (2015). Attitudes to immunisation in pregnancy among women in the UK targeted by such programmes. *British Journal of Midwifery, 23*(8), 566–573.

Campbell, H., Edwards, A., Letley, L., Bedford, H., Ramsay, M., & Yarwood, J. (2017). Changing attitudes to childhood immunisation in English parents. *Vaccine, 35*(22), 2979–2985.

Carville, K., Lewin, G., Newall, N., et al. (2007). A consensus for skin tear classification. *Primary Intention, 15*(1), 18–28.

Chew, G., Cruickshank, M., Rooney, P., Miller, I., Parkin, D., & Murray, G. (2005). Human papillomavirus 16 infection in adenocarcinoma of the cervix. *British Journal of Cancer, 93*(11), 1301–1304.

Children Act (1989): (Section 2(9) Children Act). http://www.legislation.gov.uk/ukpga/1989/41/section/2.

Chiodini, J. H., Anderson, E., Driver, C., et al. (2012). Recommendations for the practice of travel medicine. *Travel Medicine and Infectious Disease, 10*(3), 109–128.

Chiodini, J. (2018). Travel Health Update. *Practice Nurse.* https://www.janechiodini.co.uk/wp-content/uploads/2018/06/Practice-Nurse-Update-June-2018.pdf.

Chiodini, J. (2020). *Malaria prevention.* https://www.janechiodini.co.uk/help/malaria/.

Chiodini, J. H., Taylor, F., Geary, K., et al. (2020). Good Practice Guidance for Providing a Travel Health Service. *Faculty of Travel Medicine of the Royal College of Physicians and Surgeons of Glasgow.* https://rcpsg.ac.uk/travel-medicine/good-practice-guidance-for-providing-a-travel-health-service.

Coleman, S., Nelson, E. A., Vowden, P., et al. (2017). Development of a generic wound care assessment minimum data set. *Journal of Tissue Viability, 26*(4), 226–240.

Cooper, L. Z., Larson, H. J., & Katz, S. L. (2008). Protecting public trust in immunization. *Pediatrics, 122*(1), 149–153.

Crocker-Buque, T., Edelstein, M., & Mounier-Jack, S. (2016). Interventions to reduce inequalities in vaccine uptake in children and adolescents aged <19 years: A systematic review. *Journal of Epidemiology and Community Health, 71*(1), 87–97.

Department of Health and Social Care Statement of Financial Entitlements (Amendment No. 2). Directions. 2012. https://www.gov.uk/government/publications/the-statement-of-financial-entitlements-amendment-no2-directions-2012.

Donovan, H. & Bedford, H. (2013) Talking with parents about immunisation. *Primary Health Care, 23*(4), 16–20.

Dowsett, C., Protz, K., Drouard, M., & Harding, K. G. (2015). Triangle of wound assessment made easy. *Wounds International.* https://www.woundsinternational.com/resources/details/triangle-of-wound-assessment-made-easy.

Dowsett, C. & Taylor, C. (2018). Reducing variation in leg ulcer assessment and management using quality improvement methods. *Wounds UK, 14*(4), 46–51.

Edwards, A., Bedford, H., Campbell, H., et al. (2017). Promoting influenza vaccine for children. *Practice Nursing, 28*(10), 1–5.

Edwards, J. (2007). The challenge of developing a nurse-led burns clinic. *Wounds UK, 3*(3), 44–50.

Edwards, V. (2013). Key aspects of burn wound management. *Wounds UK, 9*(Suppl 3), 6–9.

Electronic medicines compendium. (2019). https://www.medicines.org.uk/emc/.

European Pressure Ulcer Advisory Panel (EPUAP). National Pressure Injury Advisory Panel (NPIAP) and Pan Pacific Pressure Injury Alliance (2019). *Prevention and Treatment of Pressure Ulcers/Injuries: Quick Reference Guide 2019.* https://www.epuap.org/pu-guidelines/.

Gohel, M. S., Heatley, F., Xinxue, L., et al. (2018). A randomised trial of early endovenous ablation in venous ulceration EVRA trial. *New England Journal of Medicine, 378*(22), 2105–2114.

GP Notebook. (2019). *Animal bites.* http://www.gpnotebook.co.uk/simplepage.cfm?ID=-1831862215.

GP Notebook. (2020). *Bee stings and wasp stings.* https://gpnotebook.com/simplepage.cfm?ID =-1113980861&linkID=19571&cook=no.

Green, J., Corcoran, P., Green, L., & Read, S. (2018). A quality of life wound checklist: The patient voice in wound care. *Wounds UK, 14*(4), 26–30.

Guest, J. F., Ayoub, N., McIlwraith, T., et al. (2015). Health economic burden that wounds impose on the NHS in the UK. *BMJ Open, 5*(12), 1–8.

Holdsworth, S. (2015). Seeking clarity in minor burn management: part 2. *Wound Essentials, 10*(2), 76–82.

Human Medicines Regulations. (2012). http://www.legislation.gov.uk/uksi/2012/1916/contents/made.

JCVI January. (2021). Joint Committee on Vaccination and Immunisation: advice on priority groups for COVID-19 vaccination, 30 December 2020. https://www.gov.uk/government/publications /priority-groups-for-coronavirus-covid-19-vaccination-advice-from-the-jcvi-30-december -2020/joint-committee-on-vaccination-and-immunisation-advice-on-priority-groups-for -covid-19-vaccination-30-december-2020.

JCVI April. (2020). *Statement from JCVI on immunisation prioritisation.* https://www.gov.uk /government/publications/jcvi-statement-on-immunisation-prioritisation/statement-from -jcvi-on-immunisation-prioritisation.

Jo's Cervical Cancer Trust. (2017, updated 2019). *Barriers to cervical screening among 25–29 year olds.* https://www.jostrust.org.uk/about-us/our-research-and-policy-work/our-research/barriers -cervical-screening-among-25-29-year-olds.

Journal of Wound Care. (2016). Management of patients with venous leg ulcers: Challenges and current best practice. A joint document: European Wound Management Association/Wounds Australia. *Journal of Wound Care, 35*(6), S1–S67.

Kennedy, A., Basket, M., & Sheedy, K. (2011). Vaccine attitudes, concerns, and information sources reported by parents of young children: Results from the 2009 healthstyles survey. *Pediatrics, 127*(Suppl 1), s92–s99.

Kitchener, H., Almonte, M., Thomson, C., et al. (2009). HPV testing in combination with liquid-based cytology in primary cervical screening (ARTISTIC): A randomised controlled trial. *The Lancet Oncology, 10*(7), 672–682.

Kitchener, H., Canfell, K., Gilham, C., et al. (2014). The clinical effectiveness and cost-effectiveness of primary human papillomavirus cervical screening in England: Extended follow-up of the ARTISTIC randomised trial cohort through three screening rounds. *Health Technology Assessment, 18*(23), 1–96.

Leask, J., Willaby, H. W., Kaufman, J. (2014). The big picture in addressing vaccine hesitancy. *Hum Vaccin Immunother, 10*(9), 2600–2602. doi:10.4161/hv.29725.

LeBlanc, K., Baranowski, S., Christensen, D., et al. (2013). *International Skin Tear Advisory Panel: A toolkit to aid in the prevention, assessment and treatment of skin tears using a simplified classification system.* https://journals.lww.com/aswcjournal/Fulltext/2013/10000/International _Skin_Tear_Advisory_Panel__A_Tool_Kit.7.aspx.

Lim, C. S., Baruah, M., & Bahia, S. S. (2018). Diagnosis and management of venous leg ulcers. *British Medical Journal, 362*(8167), 326–329.

McDonald, H., Tessier, E., White, J., et al. (2020). Early impact of the coronavirus disease (COVID-19) pandemic and social distancing measures on routine childhood vaccinations in England, January to April 2020. *Eurosurveillance, 25*(19), 2000848.

MHRA Guidance on GOV.UK. (2017). *Patient group directions: Who can use them.* https://www .gov.uk/government/publications/patient-group-directions-pgds/patient-group-directions-who -can-use-them.

MHRA, PHE, NaTHNaC, HPS. (2019). *Yellow fever vaccine: Stronger precautions in people with weakened immunity and those aged 60 years or older.* https://travelhealthpro.org.uk/media_lib /mlib-uploads/full/2019-11-21-yellow-fever-vaccine-precautions-letter.pdf.

National Institute for Health and Care Excellence. (2013). *Varicose veins in the legs. The diagnosis and management of varicose veins. Clinical guideline 168.* https://www.nice.org.uk/guidance /CG168.

National Institute for Health and Care Excellence. (2014). *Pressure ulcers: Prevention and management.* https://www.nice.org.uk/guidance/cg179/resources/pressure-ulcers-prevention-and -management-pdf-35109760631749.

National Institute for Health and Care Excellence. (2015). *Diabetic foot problems: Prevention and management.* https://www.nice.org.uk/guidance/ng19.

National Institute for Health and Care Excellence. (2016). *Sepsis: Recognition, diagnosis and early management.* https://www.nice.org.uk/guidance/ng51.

National Institute for Health and Care Excellence. (2018a). *Bites – human and animal.* https://cks .nice.org.uk/bites-human-and-animal.

National Institute for Health and Care Excellence. (2018b). *Lacerations.* https://cks.nice.org.uk /lacerations#!topicSummary.

National Institute for Health and Care Excellence. (2018c). *Peripheral arterial disease: Diagnosis and management.* https://www.nice.org.uk/guidance/cg147.

National Institute for Health and Care Excellence. (2019a). *Burns and scalds. Scenario: Management of non-complex burns and scalds.* https://cks.nice.org.uk/burns-and-scalds#!scenarioRec ommendation:3.

National Institute for Health and Care Excellence. (2019b). *Surgical Site Infections: Prevention and treatment.* https://www.nice.org.uk/guidance/ng125.

National Institute for Health and Care Excellence. (2019c). *Cellulitis – acute.* https://cks.nice.org .uk/cellulitis-acute.

National Institute for Health and Care Excellence. (2019d). *Leg ulcer: Venous.* https://cks.nice.org .uk/leg-ulcer-venous.

National Travel Health Network and Centre, TravelHealthPro. (2017). *Older travellers factsheet.* https://travelhealthpro.org.uk/factsheet/70/older travellers.

National Travel Health Network and Centre, TravelHealthPro. (2018a). *Venous thromboembolism factsheet.* https://travelhealthpro.org.uk/factsheet/54/venous-thromboembolism.

National Travel Health Network and Centre, TravelHealthPro. (2018b). *Schistosomiasis factsheet.* https://travelhealthpro.org.uk/factsheet/28/schistosomiasis.

National Travel Health Network and Centre, TravelHealthPro. (2019a). *Rabies factsheet.* https:// travelhealthpro.org.uk/factsheet/20/rabies.

National Travel Health Network and Centre, TravelHealthPro. (2019b). *Kenya vaccine and malaria recommendations.* https://travelhealthpro.org.uk/country/117/kenya.

National Travel Health Network and Centre, TravelHealthPro. (2019c). *Yellow fever vaccination recommendations: Persons aged 60 years or older.* https://nathnacyfzone.org.uk/news/85/yellow -fever-vaccination-recommendations-persons-aged-60-years-or-older.

National Travel Health Network and Centre, TravelHealthPro. (2019d). *Philippines: Falsified rabies vaccines and rabies immunoglobulin – update.* https://travelhealthpro.org.uk/news/440 /philippines-falsified-rabies-vaccines-and-rabies-immunoglobulin-update.

National Travel Health Network and Centre, TravelHealthPro. (2019e). *Travelling to Visit Friends and Relatives factsheet.* https://travelhealthpro.org.uk/factsheet/91/travelling-to-visit-friends -and relatives.

National Wound Care Strategy Programme. (2019). *Lower limb ulcers (Draft)*. https://www.ahsn network.com/about-academic-health-science-networks/national-programmes-priorities /national-wound-care-strategy-programme/clinical-workstreams/lower-limb-clinical -workstream.

National Wound Care Strategy Programme. (2020). *Surgical Wounds (Draft)*. https://www.ahsnnetwork .com/about-academic-health-science-networks/national-programmes-priorities/national-wound -care-strategy-programme.

Nazarko, L. (2018). Choosing the correct wound care dressing: An overview. *Journal of Community Nursing, 32*(5), 42–52.

NHS. (2018). *Stop the pressure. Helping to prevent pressure ulcers.* Available at: https://nhs .stopthepressure.co.uk/professionals.html.

NHS. (2019a). *Consent to treatment*. [online] Available at: https://www.nhs.uk/conditions/consent -to-treatment/.

NHS. (2019a). *Insect bites and stings*. https://www.nhs.uk/conditions/insect-bites-and-stings/.

NHS. (2019b). *Symptoms: Insect bites and stings*. https://www.nhs.uk/conditions/insect-bites-and -stings/symptoms/.

NHS. (2020). *How should I care for my stitches?* https://www.nhs.uk/common-health-questions /accidents-first-aid-and-treatments/how-should-i-care-for-my-stitches/.

NHS Health Scotland. (2019). *Vaccine Transformation Programme – travel vaccinations and travel health advice.* http://www.healthscotland.scot/health-topics/immunisation/vaccination -transformation-programme.

NHS Improvement. (2018). *Pressure ulcers: Revised definition and measurement. Summary and recommen- dations*. https://improvement.nhs.uk/documents/2932/NSTPP_summary__recommendations_2.pdf.

NHS England. (2019). *Interim findings of the Vaccinations and Immunisations Review – September 2019*. https://www.england.nhs.uk/publication/interim-findings-of-the-vaccinations-and-immunisations -review-september-2019.

NHS England. (March 2020). *Next Steps on General Practice Response to COVID-19* 19th March 2020. https://www.england.nhs.uk/coronavirus/wp-content/uploads/sites/52/2020/03/preparedness -letter-primary-care-19-march-2020.pdf.

NHS Rightcare. (2017). *Betty's Story: Leg ulcer wound care*. https://www.england.nhs.uk/rightcare /wp-content/uploads/sites/40/2017/01/nhs-rightcare-bettys-story-narrative-full.pdf.

NHS Specialised Services. (2012). *National Network for Burn Care (NNBC) National Burn Care Referral Guidance*. https://www.britishburnassociation.org/wp-content/uploads/2018/02 /National-Burn-Care-Referral-Guidance-2012.pdf.

NMC. (2007). *Nursing and Midwifery council standards for medicines management*. https://www .nmc.org.uk/standards/additional-standards/standards-for-medicines-management/.

NMC. (2015). *The Code: Professional standards of practice and behaviour for nurses and mid- wives*. https://www.nmc.org.uk/standards/code/.

Nursing and Midwifery Council (NMC). (2018). *The Code: standards of conduct, performance and ethics for nurses and midwives*. Nursing and Midwifery Council. https://www.nmc.org .uk/standards/code/.

Office for National Statistics; Travel trends. (2018). https://www.ons.gov.uk/peoplepopulation andcommunity/leisureandtourism/articles/traveltrends/latest.

Okwo-Bele, J. (2015). *Together we can close the immunization gap.* World Health Organization. https://www.who.int/mediacentre/commentaries/vaccine-preventable-diseases/en/.

PHE. (2013). *Immunisation against infectious disease. 'The Green Book'.* https://www.gov.uk /government/collections/immunisation-against-infectious-disease-the-green-book.

PHE. (2014). Air bubbles in syringes. *Vaccine Update.* https://www.gov.uk/government/publications/vaccine-update-issue-222-november-to-december-2014.

PHE. (2015). *National minimum standards and core curriculum for immunisation training of healthcare support workers.* https://www.gov.uk/government/publications/immunisation -training-of-healthcare-support-workers-national-minimum-standards-and-core -curriculum.

PHE. (2016). *The impact of vaccines: infographic.* Public Health England. https://www.gov.uk /government/publications/the-impact-of-vaccines-infographic.

PHE. (2017, December). Vaccine Update. https://assets.publishing.service.gov.uk/government /uploads/system/uploads/attachment_data/file/669418/VU_273_December2017.pdf.

PHE. (2018). National Minimum Standards and Core Curriculum for Immunisation Training for Registered Healthcare Practitioners. *Public Health England.* https://www.gov.uk/government /publications/national-minimum-standards-and-core-curriculum-for-immunisation-training -for-registered-healthcare-practitioners.

PHE. (2018a). *Immunisation training standards for healthcare practitioners.* https://www.gov.uk /government/publications/national-minimum-standards-and-core-curriculum-for-immunisation -training-for-registered-healthcare-practitioners.

PHE. (2018b). *Rabies: The Green Book. Chapter 27.* https://www.gov.uk/government/publications /rabies-the-green-book-chapter-27.

PHE. (2019a). *Notifiable diseases and causative organisms: How to report.* https://www.gov.uk /guidance/notifiable-diseases-and-causative-organisms-how-to-report#registered-medical -practitioners-report-notifiable-diseases.

PHE. (2019b). *Malaria in the UK: Annual report.* https://www.gov.uk/government/publications /malaria-in-the-uk-annual-report.

PHE. (2019c). Attitudinal survey 2018 report. Public Health England. *Vaccine Update.* https://www .gov.uk/government/publications/vaccine-update-issue-294-may-2019.

PHE. (2020). *Immunisation against infectious disease (The Green Book).* https://www.gov.uk /government/publications/immunisation-against-infectious-disease-the-green-book-front -cover-and-contents-page.

PHE. (2021). *Impact of COVID-19 on childhood vaccination counts to week 51, and vaccine coverage to November 2020 in England: interim analyses.* https://assets.publishing.service.gov.uk /government/uploads/system/uploads/attachment_data/file/961538/hpr0121-chldhd-vc _wk51b.pdf.

Plester, G., & Montgomery, C. (2010). *A to Z Handbook for Nurses in General Practice*: Montgomery Plester.

RCN. (2015). *Immunisation Knowledge and skills competence assessment tool.* https://www.rcn .org.uk/professional-development/publications/pub-005336.

RCN. (2018a). *Tools of the trade: Guidance for health care staff on glove use and the prevention of contact dermatitis.* RCN Publishing. https://www.rcn.org.uk/professional-development /publications/pdf-006922.

RCN. (2018b). *Managing childhood immunisation clinics.* https://www.rcn.org.uk/professional -development/publications/pub-007201.

RCN. (2018c). Competencies: Travel health nursing: career and competence development. *Royal College of Nursing.* https://www.rcn.org.uk/professional-development/publications/pdf -006506.

RCN. (2019a). *The role of nursing associates in vaccination and immunisation.* https://www.rcn .org.uk/professional-development/publications/pub-007565.

RCN. (2019b). *Health care support workers administering inactivated influenza, shingles and pneumococcal vaccines for adults and live attenuated influenza vaccine (LAIV) for children.* https://www.rcn.org.uk/professional-development/publications/pub-007441.

RCN. (2020). *RCN guidance on maintaining the National Immunisation schedule during COVID-19.* https://www.rcn.org.uk/-/media/royal-college-of-nursing/documents/clinical-topics/public -health/maintaining-the-national-immunisation-schedule-during-covid-19.pdf?la=en&hash=7F 5D4E8A84C84E9AD1640B1A5A4A99BF.

Ronco, G., Dillner, J., Elfström, K., et al. (2014). Efficacy of HPV-based screening for prevention of invasive cervical cancer: follow-up of four European randomised controlled trials. *The Lancet, 383*(9916), 524–532.

Rozemeijer, K., Naber, S., Penning, C., et al. (2017). Cervical cancer incidence after normal cytological sample in routine screening using SurePath, ThinPrep, and conventional cytology: population based study. *British Medical Journal, 356*, j504.

Ryan, M., Waller, J., & Marlow, L. (2019). Could changing invitation and booking processes help women translate their cervical screening intentions into action? A population-based survey of women's preferences in Great Britain. *BMJ Open, 9*(7), Article e028134.

Sepsis Trust. (2020). *What is sepsis.* https://sepsistrust.org/.

Scottish Intercollegiate Guideline Network. (2010). *Management of chronic venous leg ulcers: A national clinical guideline.* https://www.sign.ac.uk/assets/sign120.pdf.

Taddio, A., Ipp, M., Thivakaran, S., et al. (2012). Survey of the prevalence of immunization noncompliance due to needle fears in children and adults. *Vaccine, 30*(32), 4807–4812.

Taddio, A., Shah, V., McMurtry, C. M., et al. (2015). Procedural and Physical Interventions for Vaccine Injections. Systematic Review of Randomized Controlled Trials and Quasi-Randomized Controlled Trial. *The Clinical Journal of Pain, 31*(Suppl), S20–S37.

The Human Medicines Regulations. (2012). UK Statutory Instruments No. 1916. https://www .legislation.gov.uk/uksi/2012/1916/contents/made.

Vaccine Knowledge Project. (2019). *HPV Vaccine (Human Papillomavirus Vaccine).* http://vk.ovg .ox.ac.uk/vk/hpv-vaccine.

UK National Screening Committee. (2016). *The UK NSC recommendation on Cervical Cancer screening in women.* https://legacyscreening.phe.org.uk/cervicalcancer.

Vizcaino, A., Moreno, V., Bosch, F., et al. (2000). International trends in incidence of cervical cancer: II. Squamous-cell carcinoma. *International Journal of Cancer, 86*(3), 429–435.

Wallace, A. B. (1951). The exposure treatment of burns. *Lancet, 1*, 501–504. doi:10.1016/s0140 -6736(51)91975-7.

Warrell, D. (2012). Animal attacks, rabies, venomous bites and stings in. In R. Dawood (Ed.), *Travellers' Health – how to stay healthy abroad* (pp. 176–201). Oxford University Press.

WHO. (2010). *Best practices for injections and related procedures toolkit.* https://www.who.int /infection-prevention/publications/best-practices_toolkit/en/.

WHO. (2015). *Reducing pain at the time of vaccination: WHO position paper.* https://www.who .int/immunization/policy/position_papers/reducing_pain_vaccination/en/.

WHO. (2019a). *Rabies key facts.* https://www.who.int/news-room/fact-sheets/detail/rabies.

WHO. (2019b). *Middle East respiratory syndrome coronavirus (MERS-CoV) key facts.* https:// www.who.int/news-room/fact-sheets/detail/middle-east-respiratory-syndrome-coronavirus -(mers-cov).

WHO. (2020a). *Guidance on routine immunization services during COVID-19 pandemic in the WHO European Region (2020).* http://www.euro.who.int/en/health-topics/health-emergencies /coronavirus-covid-19/novel-coronavirus-2019-ncov-technical-guidance-OLD/coronavirus -disease-covid-19-outbreak-technical-guidance-europe-OLD/guidance-on-routine-immunization -services-during-covid-19-pandemic-in-the-who-european-region-2020.

WHO. (2020b). *Coronavirus disease (COVID-2019) outbreak.* https://www.who.int/emergencies/diseases/novel-coronavirus-2019.

WHO. (2020c). *Human papillomavirus (HPV) and cervical cancer.* https://www.who.int/news-room/fact-sheets/detail/human-papillomavirus-(hpv)-and-cervical-cancer.

Wounds International. (2014). *International Best Practice Guidelines: Effective skin and wound management of non-complex burns.* www.woundsinternational.com.

Wounds International. (2018). *Best practice recommendations for the prevention and management of skin tears in aged skin.* https://www.woundsinternational.com/uploads/resources/57c1a5cc8a4771a696b4c17b9e2ae6f1.pdf.

Wounds International. (2019a). *Biofilm-based wound care with cadexomer iodine made easy.* https://www.woundsinternational.com/resources/details/biofilm-based-wound-care-cadexomer-iodine-made-easy-us.

Wounds International. (2019b). *More than silver technology made easy.* https://www.woundsinternational.com/resources/details/made-easy-more-than-silver-technology.

Wounds International. (2019c). *Managing skin tears in practice.* https://www.woundsinternational.com/resources/details/managing-skin-tears-in-practice.

Wounds UK. (2017). *How to guide: Pressure ulcer management.* https://www.wounds-uk.com/resources/details/how-to-guide-pressure-ulcer-management.

Wounds UK. (2018). *Best Practice Statement: Improving holistic assessment of chronic wounds.* https://www.wounds-uk.com/resources/all/0/date/desc/cont_type/21.

Wounds UK. (2019a). *Best Practice Statement: Addressing the complexities in the management of venous leg ulcers.* https://www.wounds-uk.com/resources/details/best-practice-statement-addressing-complexities-management-venous-leg-ulcers.

Wounds UK. (2019b). *Best Practice Statement: Ankle brachial pressure index (ABPI) in practice.* https://www.wounds-uk.com/resources/details/best-practice-statement-ankle-brachial-pressure-index-abpi-practice.

Chapter 5

Management of long-term conditions

Beverley Bostock

Learning outcomes

After reading this chapter you should be able to:

1. Evaluate high-quality consultation approaches for managing long-term conditions
2. Consider how to optimise self-care in long-term conditions
3. Describe when to refer on to the wider disciplinary team

Introduction

As the number of people living with long-term conditions (LTCs) increases, the management of these conditions has become a central focus for primary care. General Practice Nurses (GPNs) are increasingly at the forefront of this area of care and require specialist knowledge, skills and competencies to work autonomously in this setting. Many educational organisations now offer courses in specific LTCs, such as asthma, diabetes, cardiovascular disease (CVD) and other conditions at the diploma, degree and master's level, and as a nurse new to practice you may have an ambition to do this in the future. The aim of this chapter, however, is to highlight some of the key LTCs that might be encountered in everyday practise and to signpost the reader to some of the resources that are available to increase knowledge and comprehension of these areas.

The Quality and Outcomes Framework (QOF) was introduced to general practice as a route to improving standards of care in general practice. Points are awarded for meeting targets which are linked to quality outcomes, based on evidence. Practices are incentivised through payments for meeting these standards, and the payments are calculated on how many QOF points the practice earns. In 2019/2020, a QOF point was worth around £187. One of the most important aspects of QOF is the framework it provides for the delivery of care for LTCs. Nurses working in general practice will be responsible for a significant number of the elements of this care, and most general practices will have QOF templates set up on computer systems to allow them to see what needs to be covered in a consultation to achieve the maximum number of QOF points.

However, QOF is based on a basic standard of care, and there are many more elements to a good-quality consultation than simply ticking the QOF boxes. It is important, then, to be aware of the significance of what is measured and recorded for QOF. Knowing why something is done is as important as knowing what needs to be done.

Scotland discontinued the QOF system from 2016, and funding was changed to a global sum. QOF data were no longer used for payment purposes, although they could be accessed for use by practices to measure their performance internally. The future of QOF in other parts of the United Kingdom remains uncertain.

Areas to be addressed in this chapter are:

- Asthma
- Chronic obstructive pulmonary disease (COPD)
- Hypertension
- CVD, including atrial fibrillation (AF) and heart failure
- Diabetes

For each condition, there is a section on:

- Definition
- Diagnosis
- Treatment
- The review appointment
- Supporting self-management

Reflection

Nurses can make a significant contribution to the management of long-term conditions in general practice. Reflect on this statement and jot down your thoughts as to why this is so. Do a brief SWOT analysis (strengths, weaknesses, opportunities and threats) on this aspect of working in general practice in relation to your own role.

Asthma

Asthma is a common respiratory condition encountered in general practice. Many nurses involved in asthma care have completed further accredited training in this subject and as such may be involved at all stages of asthma diagnosis and management. However, all GPNs are expected to only work within their level of competency.

Definition

Asthma is a variable, reversible respiratory condition caused by airway inflammation and hyper-responsiveness. Key symptoms include cough, expiratory wheeze, tight chest and shortness of breath. There is often a personal or family history of atopy (allergic disease such as hay fever or eczema). Family members may also have asthma. People with asthma will usually report that their symptoms are triggered by something specific such as exercise, viral infections, animals (dogs, cats, horses) or chemicals (cleaning fluids, perfume). Asthma attacks can be life threatening (British Thoracic Society/Scottish Intercollegiate Guidelines Network (BTS/SIGN), 2019).

The underlying pathophysiology of asthma is inflammatory in nature. Airways become inflamed as the result of an overreaction to a trigger, as described. The process leads to narrowing of the airways in the lungs, which in turn leads to the symptoms of wheeze, cough, tight chest and breathlessness.

As the inflammation increases and persists, the lungs become more reactive, and symptoms become more severe. Failure to recognise and treat these symptoms can lead to a life-threatening asthma attack. It is also thought that ongoing low-level inflammation can lead to fixed airways disease, which is not reversible (Pascual & Peters, 2009).

Diagnosis

According to the BTS/SIGN guidelines, asthma is predominantly a clinical diagnosis which will be made based on the history, as described earlier, along with lung function tests which can be used to support the diagnosis by demonstrating reversible airflow obstruction (BTS/SIGN, 2019). The gold standard lung function test is spirometry, although peak expiratory flow rate (PEFR) readings and fractional exhaled nitric oxide (FeNO) tests can also be used. Spirometry is discussed in more detail in the section on COPD. FeNO testing is not generally available in most general practice settings, although the National Institute for Health and Care Excellence (NICE) endorses its use (NICE, 2014b; NICE, 2017). PEFR is easy to access and perform and allows individuals with asthma to monitor changes in their lung function at any time.

Treatment

The treatment of asthma, then, targets the underlying inflammation and in most cases will ensure that the effects are reversed so that normal (or near normal) lung function is achieved. As a result, people with asthma should be able to lead full lives with little or no limitation of their day-to-day activities. There are many famous sportsmen and sportswomen who reach the highest levels in their sport despite a diagnosis of asthma.

There are national and international guidelines on the management of asthma which can support evidence-based care. These include the BTS/SIGN – guidelines

(BTS/SIGN, 2019) and the Global Initiative for Asthma guidelines (Global Initiative for Asthma, 2019).

NICE also has a Quality Standard in asthma care, which covers diagnosing, monitoring and managing asthma in children, young people and adults. It describes what high-quality asthma care should look like and comes with a list of quality statements which identify priority areas for improvement. The Quality Standard can be found here: https://www.nice.org.uk/guidance/qs25.

Most people with asthma should be treated with regular inhaled corticosteroid (ICS) to treat and control the inflammation. These inhalers are usually taken twice daily and include Clenil (beclometasone) and Budesonide via the Easyhaler device. Children under 12 should be prescribed 100 mcg twice daily, and adults should have 200 mcg twice daily. If breakthrough symptoms occur, a bronchodilator (blue) inhaler can be used to relieve them. The reliever should not be necessary more than two to three times a week. People using their reliever inhaler more often than this are at risk of asthma attacks, which can be fatal. This should prompt an early review of the current asthma treatment, to improve control and reduce the need for the blue reliever inhaler.

Resources

https://www.asthma.org.uk/advice/resources/
https://www.blf.org.uk/support-for-you/asthma

Assessing Asthma Control

People with asthma should have an annual review which includes assessment of their asthma control and inhaler technique. Asthma control can be assessed with the Royal College of Physicians, three-questions model (Box 5.1) or tools such as this: https://getasthmahelp.org/documents/ACT_AdultEng.pdf.

Inhaler Devices

Inhaler devices come in three main categories: the pressurised metered dose inhaler (pMDI), the dry powder inhaler (DPI) and the breath-triggered (or actuated/activated) inhaler.

Box 5.1 Three questions for asthma control

1. Has your asthma disturbed your sleep?
2. Have you had asthma symptoms in the day?
3. Have your asthma symptoms interfered with your normal activities (going to work, school, doing housework)?

From Pearson M. G., & Bucknall, C. E. (1999). *Measuring clinical outcome in asthma; a patient-focused approach.* Royal College of Physicians.

Stepping up treatment

If asthma control is inadequate, treatment should be stepped up to the next level. In most cases this will be to a combination inhaler which includes an ICS and a long-acting reliever medication (a β2 agonist). Examples of combination inhalers (in alphabetical order) include the following:

Flutiform

Flutiform contains a combination of fluticasone propionate and formoterol. It comes as a pMDI (licensed from age 5 years) or a breath-triggered device (the K-Haler; licensed from age 12 years).

Fostair

Fostair contains a combination of extrafine-particle beclometasone and formoterol. It comes as a pMDI or a DPI (NextHaler). Fostair is licensed from age 18 years.

Relvar

Relvar contains fluticasone furoate and vilanterol. It comes as a DPI (Ellipta) and is licensed from age 12 years.

Symbicort

Symbicort contains budesonide and formoterol. It comes as a DPI (Turbohaler) and is licensed from age 6 years.

Details on different inhaler devices can be found on the RightBreathe website (https://www.rightbreathe.com/) and via the Electronic Medicines Compendium (https://www.medicines.org.uk/emc).

Correct inhaler technique is essential for good asthma control. Failure to prime the inhaler or inhale correctly will mean that the treatment will not reach the lungs and will be unable to work, leaving the individual with poorly controlled symptoms (Bosnic-Anticevich et al., 2018).

There are some excellent videos available on the Asthma UK website to help people achieve the correct technique: https://www.asthma.org.uk/advice/inhalers-medicines-treatments/using-inhalers/.

Other therapies can be used to improve asthma control, including the oral leukotriene receptor antagonist montelukast and the long-acting muscarinic antagonist Spiriva (tiotropium) in the Respimat device.

Self-management

Asthma is a variable condition, and as such symptoms and treatment requirements can change. Asthma attacks can occur when people have not recognised that their symptoms are increasing and have failed to take appropriate action. It is essential, then, that people are supported to self-manage and that they know what to do if their control deteriorates. All people with asthma should be offered a personalised asthma action plan (PAAP) which includes information about their asthma, their current treatments and how to spot poor control. There are several PAAPs available, including through Asthma UK.

The BTS/SIGN guidelines suggest keeping PAAPs simple, with just a few key points such as:

- Recognise poor control (e.g., increased use of reliever, night waking with symptoms)
- Start oral steroids if PEFR is less than 60% best/predicted
- Seek help urgently if PEFR is less than 40% best/predicted

The annual review

This should include an assessment of current symptoms, any exacerbations that may have occurred since the patient was last seen, a review of inhaler use (adherence and technique), a check on short-acting β2 agonist use, lung function tests (PEFR) and a review of the PAAP.

Reflection

Look at the Asthma UK personalised asthma action plans and some of the commercially available plans that are also available. How do they fit with the British Thoracic Society/Scottish Intercollegiate Guidelines Network recommendations? Which do you prefer?

Key learning points

- Asthma is a variable, inflammatory, reversible respiratory condition
- The diagnosis is made based on the history, along with lung function tests which show reversible obstructive airways disease
- ICSs are used to treat asthma, although additional therapies may be needed to achieve complete control of symptoms
- People with asthma (or parents/carers) should be supported to self-manage to recognise how to optimise symptom control, reduce the risk of exacerbations and avoid unnecessary hospital admissions.

Chronic obstructive pulmonary disease

COPD is often thought of as being similar to asthma (not least by patients), but they are completely different conditions. Where asthma is a reversible condition, COPD is a condition where the changes that have occurred in the lungs are irreversible. As a result, in COPD the focus is on improving symptoms and reducing exacerbations, as opposed to asthma, where lung function can return to normal or near-normal with treatment. This will never happen with COPD.

The most important role for general practice is identifying people at risk and ensuring they are diagnosed and treated as early and as effectively as possible.

Definition

The Global Initiative for Chronic Obstructive Lung Disease (GOLD) defines COPD as 'a common, preventable and treatable disease that is characterized by persistent respiratory symptoms and airflow limitation that is due to airway and/ or alveolar abnormalities, usually caused by significant exposure to noxious particles or gases' (GOLD, 2019).

Diagnosis

The diagnosis is made based on:

- Symptoms (some or all of the following: cough, sputum, breathlessness, reduced ability to carry out activities of daily living)
- Risk factors (mainly cigarette smoking in the Western world, although other risk factors may predominate in other areas of the world)
- Evidence of irreversible airflow obstruction.

The diagnosis is made through recognition of the typical symptoms described earlier in people who have risk factors for COPD – especially smoking. A smoking pack-year history of 10 years or more will increase the risk, and a pack-year history of 20 years or more is considered to be significant. For more information on calculating pack-years, have a look at this website: http:// smokingpackyears.com/.

If the symptoms and risk factors suggest the possibility of COPD, the next step would be to carry out spirometry testing to confirm the diagnosis. Spirometry is a complex test which must be carried out in a quality-assured way to ensure that the readings are reliable. There is some useful guidance on how to carry out quality assured diagnostic spirometry in an easy-to-read publication from Primary Care Commissioning (Primary Care Commissioning, 2013).

Reflection

Find out who carries out calibration and verification of the spirometer in your practice. How often are these carried out? Is there a log you can inspect to see how it is done?

The investigation of choice is spirometry. Remember that spirometry is a test which, when performed correctly, should demonstrate a pattern (normal, obstructive, restrictive or combined) and, in the case of an obstructive pattern, a response to treatment (reversible or irreversible). It does not give the diagnosis but will give objective evidence about lung capacity and patterns of airflow

(Primary Care Commissioning, 2013). So, the diagnosis of any respiratory disease, including COPD, is made first and foremost on the history (for example, symptoms, occupation, smoking), which is then supported by postbronchodilator spirometry, which shows evidence of irreversible airflow obstruction:

- A forced expiratory volume in 1 second/forced vital capacity (FEV1/FVC) ratio of less than 70% (0.7)
- An FEV1 which is most often (but not exclusively) less than 80% of predicted
- An FVC which is usually normal (>80% predicted) (Primary Care Commissioning, 2013).

However, some guidelines suggest that a fixed ratio is not appropriate for diagnosing obstructive lung disease. NICE recommends using the lower limit of normal (LLN), whereas GOLD does not endorse the use of the LLN, stating that there is no evidence for using this parameter to confirm airflow obstruction. Interestingly, the BTS/SIGN asthma guidelines also recommend use of the LLN. NICE continues to point out that a normal spirometry result may still be compatible with a COPD diagnosis, whereas an abnormal result in the absence of symptoms does not constitute a diagnosis. GOLD does much the same, pointing out the importance of spirometry while still recognising its limitations. In both guidelines, spirometry is seen as an adjunct to the diagnosis of COPD, not a standalone diagnostic tool. There can be no substitute for good history taking to decide on the likelihood of respiratory symptoms being the result of COPD.

Treatment

Recommendations about treating COPD vary from guideline to guideline. NICE stresses the importance of smoking cessation, flu and pneumonia jabs and pulmonary rehabilitation as the foundation of COPD management. When it comes to inhaled therapies, NICE recommends starting with a short-acting bronchodilator and then moving onto a dual bronchodilator long-acting β2 agonist (LABA) with a long-acting muscarinic antagonist (LAMA), assuming there is no element of reversibility in the history or lung function tests. If there is evidence of reversibility, an ICS will be needed to control the reversible element, in combination with a LABA for symptom relief.

There are four dual bronchodilators on the market at present, and consideration should be given to the relevant devices, as well as the drugs in each product.

GOLD takes a slightly different approach to choosing inhaled therapies. The focus is still on bronchodilation, but GOLD's approach is more nuanced. Rather than recommending a dual bronchodilator across the board, GOLD continues to recommend that people with COPD are categorised using the ABCD algorithm, which measures their symptoms and exacerbation risk and then treats accordingly (Box 5.2).

Box 5.2 Initial treatment choices for chronic obstructive pulmonary disease

A – Bronchodilator
B – Long-acting β2 agonist (LABA) or long-acting muscarinic antagonist (LAMA)
C – LAMA
D – LAMA, dual bronchodilator, inhaled corticosteroid/LABA

From Global Initiative for Chronic Obstructive Lung Disease. (2019). *Global Strategy for the diagnosis, management and prevention of Chronic Obstructive Pulmonary Disease – 2020 report.* https://goldcopd.org/wp-content/uploads/2019/11/GOLD-2020-REPORT-ver1.0wms.pdf.

If an individual does not respond well enough to this initial treatment, GOLD states that there are different factors which will influence which treatment to use next. These include whether the patient:

- Is predominantly breathless
- Is predominantly exacerbating
- Has raised eosinophils
- Has any evidence of an asthma component to his or her condition.

In breathless patients, the following recommendations are made:

- Unless already in use, introduce a LABA or a LAMA
- If already on one of these therapies, move up to a dual bronchodilator (LAMA/LABA).

GOLD suggests that, although an ICS/LABA or triple therapy might be used in this group, eosinophil levels and exacerbation rates should inform their initiation or ongoing use. Eosinophils over 300 cells/µL suggest potential benefit, as do eosinophils over 100 cells/µL in the presence of two or more exacerbations in the past year (or one severe enough to require admission). However, NICE goes on to say that in this breathless group ICS therapies should be used with caution, especially if there is a history of pneumonia, if previous use of an ICS has had no effect or if it was inappropriately prescribed in the past. In these situations, de-escalation of therapy away from ICS-based treatments should be considered.

In people who are exacerbating, the following recommendations are made:

- If on bronchodilator monotherapy, move to a dual bronchodilator
- Consider an ICS/LABA if eosinophils are greater than 300 cells/µL or greater than 100 cells/µL with two or more acute exacerbations of COPD (AECOPD)
- Patients who are still suffering on either of these can be considered for a move up to triple therapy (ICS/LABA/LAMA).

At the time of writing, there are two triple therapies on the market: Trimbow pMDI (extrafine beclometasone with formoterol and glycopyrronium) and

Trelegy in the Ellipta DPI (containing fluticasone furoate with vilanterol and umeclidinium).

NICE (2018a) and GOLD (2019) both recommend caution when using ICS in people with pure COPD, that is, when there is nothing in the history or lung function to suggest that there is any reversible (i.e., asthmatic) element to their condition. NICE therefore recommends that clinicians should be prepared to discuss the risk of side effects (such as pneumonia and diabetes) in people who take ICS for COPD. This will apply to ICS/LABAs, as well as triple therapy.

Reflection

Find three people with chronic obstructive pulmonary disease (COPD) who are taking an inhaled corticosteroid (ICS) as part of their COPD treatment. Have a look and see if they 'qualify' for an ICS based on the information discussed in the text. It is thought that a significant proportion of people on ICS therapy for COPD do not need it.

The clinical review

A COPD review should be carried out at least annually, although it should be performed more often in people with more severe symptoms. Areas that should be covered include symptoms of breathlessness, cough and sputum, oxygen saturations and exacerbation history, along with an assessment of the patient's holistic wellbeing, which might incorporate areas such as nutrition, physical activity, relationships and mental health. The annual assessment should also include a review of vaccination status and a check of inhaler use (adherence and technique).

Supporting self-management

Many people with COPD, as well as their families and carers, will benefit from a self-management plan (SMP) which has been tailored to their individual needs. The British Lung Foundation provides SMPs which can be ordered from their website (https://www.blf.org.uk/), and there are other commercially available plans, but it may also be possible to develop your own.

Reflection

What sort of areas do you think should be covered in a self-management plan? Have a look at some of those available and critique them for use in your area of practice.

Advice on early treatment of an exacerbation can be part of an SMP and will include advice on using a rescue pack. GOLD and NICE both advise that rescue packs, consisting of antibiotics and oral steroids, may be useful for people who have an AECOPD. However, NICE has also published guidance on the use of antibiotics in people with AECOPD, which recommend a cautious approach to the use of antimicrobials (NICE, 2018b). Furthermore, steroid doses differ between the two guidelines. GOLD (2019) recommends a dose of 40 mg prednisolone for 5 days, whereas NICE currently recommends using 30 mg for 5 days (NICE, 2018a).

Asthma/chronic obstructive pulmonary disease overlap

COPD is often thought of as an irreversible condition, where giving a bronchodilator may improve symptoms but will not impact on lung function. However, COPD is also an umbrella term which covers a range of conditions such as emphysema, chronic bronchitis and chronic asthma (NICE, 2018a). It is also recognised that smokers with asthma have an increased risk of developing fixed airways disease on top of the underlying asthma component (Pascual & Peters, 2009). The basis of asthma treatment is the use of ICS, so any asthma element, including evidence of reversibility, must, therefore, be recognised when making treatment decisions in people who have asthma with COPD. It is thought that up to one in three people with COPD has some element of reversibility (Müller et al., 2016). Both the NICE and the GOLD COPD guidelines focus on the importance of establishing any reversible element before deciding on the most appropriate treatment pathway, particularly when it comes to the use of ICS.

Key learning points

- COPD is a chronic, largely irreversible respiratory condition, predominantly caused by smoking.
- It is diagnosed based on the presence of typical symptoms, along with risk factors and evidence of irreversible airflow obstruction.
- Treatment aims are to reduce symptoms and exacerbation risk. This is achieved through smoking cessation and the use of targeted inhaled therapy. Depending on how the individual presents, short- or long-acting bronchodilators will be needed. In some cases ICS will help to reduce exacerbation risk. Pulmonary rehabilitation can have a significant effect on the holistic wellbeing of the person living with COPD.
- SMPs can help people to understand their condition and what they can do to optimise their symptom control and reduce the risk of exacerbation and hospital admissions. The use of rescue packs can be included as part of the SMP.

Hypertension

High blood pressure (BP), also known as hypertension, is a known risk factor for CVD and is also implicated in a range of other conditions including dementia and kidney disease (Abell et al., 2018; Joint British Societies,

2014; Yusuf et al., 2004). Hypertension rarely causes any symptoms, however, which is why it is often known as the silent killer. Many people with high BP will be unaware that they have it, so regular screening (at least once every 5 years) is recommended in those who have not been diagnosed with the condition.

Definition

An adequate BP is essential to life. However, when the force of the pressure in the arteries increases, harm can occur, leading to macrovascular and microvascular damage. Raised BP is not a disease, but it is a risk factor for a range of cardiovascular conditions. Systolic BP is the top number in a BP reading and occurs in the systolic (pumping) phase of the beat. Raised systolic BP is more closely associated with complications than diastolic BP, which is what is measured in the refilling part of the beat. 'Normal' BP readings vary according to age and existing conditions, but in general a BP of 140/90 mm Hg is considered to be acceptable (NICE, 2019).

Diagnosis

NICE recommends that health care workers taking BP should be trained in doing so. Studies suggest that many health care professionals are not familiar with the correct technique, and that misdiagnosis may result, with potential harm resulting from inappropriate drug treatment (Badeli & Assadi, 2014).

Further advice on the correct procedure for recording BP can be found via the British and Irish Hypertension Society webpage at: https://bihsoc.org/resources/bp-measurement/measure-blood-pressure/.

NICE recommends that, if the initial BP in the clinic setting is 140/90 mm Hg or more, a second reading should be taken, with a third taken if the first two readings are significantly different. The lowest reading is then used as the clinic BP. If this clinic BP is 140/90 mm Hg or more, home readings should be used to confirm the presence of hypertension, using either ambulatory BP measurement (ABPM) or, if that is not available or is not suitable, home BP measurements (HBPM) using a standard, validated and calibrated machine.

For ABPM, a minimum of two readings an hour should be taken during normal waking hours. At least 14 good-quality readings should be recorded for the assessment to be valid. The average of these readings should then be used to confirm or refute the diagnosis of hypertension. If HBPM is used, the patient should take two readings at home, 1 minute apart, whilst sitting, in the morning and in the evening for a minimum of 4 days and ideally for 7 days. The first day's reading should then be discarded, and the others averaged out. A clinic reading of 140/90 mm Hg or more plus home readings (ABPM or HBPM) of 135/85 mm Hg or more confirms the diagnosis of hypertension (Box 5.3).

Box 5.3 Hypertension diagnosis

If clinic blood pressure (BP) is between 140/90 and 179/119 mm Hg, check home
    readings
Ambulatory BP measurement (APBM): gold standard, using daytime average
Home BP measurement if ABPM not available/unsuitable
Average readings from 4 to 7 days, omitting day 1 before making the calculation

From NICE. (2019). *Hypertension in adults: Diagnosis and management.* https://www.nice.org.uk
/guidance/ng136.

Reflection

Look at the different types of blood pressure measuring equipment: mercury, aner-
oid, digital and ambulatory monitors. Each has a specific role to play, and each
has advantages and disadvantages. The British and Irish Hypertension Society
(https://bihsoc.org/) has useful information on the correct procedure for measuring
blood pressure, so have a look at this page for more information: https://bihsoc.org
/resources/bp-measurement/.

Stages of hypertension

NICE recommends that, if the home BP readings are between 135/85 and 149/94
mm Hg, the individual should be diagnosed as having stage 1 hypertension. If
the home BP readings are 150/95 mm Hg or more, this is stage 2 hypertension.
The stage diagnosed dictates how the person should be managed.

Unless the person is already known to have cardiovascular or renal disease, or
has a preexisting diagnosis of diabetes, a cardiovascular risk assessment should
be carried out for anyone with stage 1 hypertension using QRisk: www.qrisk.org.

If the 10-year CVD risk score is over 10% according to QRisk, treatment
for hypertension should be initiated. NICE also states that clinicians should
consider treating anyone under 60 years anyway because lifetime risk may be
underestimated using QRisk.

If the home BP readings are 150/95 mm Hg or more, this is stage 2 hypertension and should be treated, irrespective of any other conditions or CVD risk score.

If the clinic BP is 180/120 mm Hg or more, a thorough assessment should be
carried out to determine whether this is an emergency or not. This will include:

● Fundoscopy to look for papilloedema
● Review of the cardiovascular and renal status
● Assessment for any evidence of abnormal gait, confusion or other symptoms
  suggestive of cerebral involvement.

If any of these are positive, the patient should receive urgent treatment,
which is likely to involve hospital admission. If there is no evidence of these

symptoms, the BP should be rechecked within 1 week (maximum), and ideally within 24 hours.

Treatment

All drug treatments should be underpinned by appropriate lifestyle interventions: weight management, dietary changes such as those recommended in the Dietary Approaches to Stop Hypertension approach (see https://dashdiet.org/), keeping alcohol consumption within recommended targets (and avoiding binge drinking) and stopping smoking.

Medication choices are dictated mainly by age, although people with diabetes should always be considered for an angiotensin-converting enzyme (ACE) inhibitor as first-line therapy.

The following treatment strategies should be applied:

Younger than 55 and/or diabetes?	ACE inhibitor or angiotensin receptor blocker
55+ or Afro-Caribbean?	Calcium channel blocker
Not controlled on the above?	Add the other drug class or a thiazide-like diuretic (indapamide)
Before, the next step, check adherence to meds and lifestyle	
Next step	Use all three

If the patient's BP is not controlled by taking all three drugs appropriately, referral should be considered before adding a fourth drug, which can be spironolactone, a β blocker or an α blocker. The general target for BP is less than 140/90 mm Hg in all groups apart from those aged 80 years and older, where the target is 150/90 mm Hg. However, people with other LTCs such as chronic kidney disease may benefit from lower targets. The NICE hypertension guidelines do not recommend tighter BP goals for people with diabetes, however (NICE, 2019).

The annual review

This should include a review of blood tests (particularly renal function) and BP. A lifestyle review should be carried out to ensure that all support is being given to maintain these changes.

Supporting self-management

People with hypertension should be monitored at least once a year, but they can also be encouraged to self-monitor at home, as home readings may offer a more accurate reflection of their BP than clinic readings. They should be offered support and education if they would like to receive this.

Key learning points

● Hypertension is a risk factor for many conditions, but is often asymptomatic.
● Careful BP measurement both in the surgery and at home can confirm the diagnosis to ensure timely treatment.
● Treatment of hypertension should be initiated and titrated to meet the target set based on age or comorbid conditions, and individuals should be monitored to assess the success of the treatment programme, along with any side effects.
● Lifestyle interventions are an essential part of hypertension management.

Cardiovascular disease

CVD is an umbrella term which covers a range of conditions including coronary heart disease, angina, heart attack, congenital heart disease, hypertension, stroke and vascular dementia (NHS UK, 2018). CVD is the leading cause of death and disability in the United Kingdom, and accounts for around 25% of premature deaths (BHF, 2019). As well as obvious risk factors for CVD such as smoking, obesity, hypertension and dyslipidaemia, there are less obvious risks such as having a significant mental health problem or living in an area of high deprivation. People living in the most deprived areas have almost double the risk of dying of CVD compared with those living in the most affluent areas (BHF, 2019).

Definition

CVD is an umbrella term which covers any disease of the heart or blood vessels. Much of this disease is atherosclerotic in nature, driven by atheroma which has resulted from a toxic mix of high BP, dyslipidaemia and other risk factors including age and family history. CVD may occur in small vessels (microvascular disease) affecting the eyes, nerves and kidneys, larger vessels (macrovascular disease) in the heart, cerebral vessels and peripheral vessels (e.g., in the legs). Erectile dysfunction can also indicate the presence of CVD in the medium-sized penile artery.

Diagnosis

The diagnosis of CVD is usually made based on symptoms; for example, the textbook presentation of acute coronary syndrome would be crushing central chest pain radiating to the arms or jaw, with sweating, nausea and pallor. Investigations might include cardiac markers on a blood test and changes on the electrocardiogram (ECG). In stroke (or a transient ischaemic attack, which lasts for less than 24 hours, and typically only a few minutes), classic features could include a drooping face, weakness in the arms or legs or slurred speech. The diagnosis is confirmed with a scan which will identify the area of the brain that has been affected. People with peripheral arterial disease usually describe cramping pain in the lower legs when walking which is relieved by resting. This diagnosis is also confirmed by scan. All these conditions are caused by the same underlying ischaemic process, which is the result of atheromatous plaques, which can sometimes rupture. Microvascular disease is discussed in the section on diabetes.

Treatment

The treatment of CVD is targeted at the risk factors that caused it. This means addressing lifestyle through healthy eating, weight loss, smoking cessation and keeping alcohol within recommended limits. Other risk factors may also need to be treated with medication, including high BP and dyslipidaemia. There is more information on primary prevention of CVD using lipid-lowering therapy in the section on diabetes.

Following a cardiovascular event, many people will be treated with the maximum tolerated dose of ACE inhibitor (or angiotensin receptor blocker and lipid-lowering therapy (ideally atorvastatin 80 mg)). Most people will also benefit from antiplatelet treatment and, based on recent research, they may benefit from dual antiplatelet therapy (DAPT) (Valgimigli et al., 2018). This will depend on what sort of cardiovascular event they have had, and the evidence base for DAPT. Any benefits will need to be weighed against the potential harm from increased bleeding. In some people, surgical treatment may be indicated, such as coronary artery bypass grafts.

Supporting self-management

Many people who have had a cardiovascular event will be offered cardiac rehabilitation. This is a programme of education and support which facilitates recovery and ongoing self-management. Depression is common following a significant cardiac event, and people will need ongoing assistance to get back to work and return to their activities of daily living (Hare et al., 2014). Annual reviews will include monitoring BP, lipid levels and lifestyle changes. The British Heart Foundation (https://www.bhf.org.uk/) has a wealth of resources to support people after a cardiovascular event. The Primary Care Cardiovascular Society aims to offer education and leadership in CVD for health care professionals and can be found at: https://pccsuk.org.

Atrial fibrillation

The NHS Long Term Plan (https://www.longtermplan.nhs.uk/online-version/) has prioritised CVD for the future and has specifically targeted AF, BP and cholesterol as areas that need improvements in terms of diagnosis and management. Stroke risk is increased in the presence of AF, so diagnosing this condition (which can be asymptomatic up until the stroke happens) is important. The best way to check for AF is to carry out a manual pulse check. If an irregular pulse is detected, an ECG should be performed as soon as possible. If nonvalvular AF is diagnosed, stroke risk should be assessed using the CHADsVAsC tool (see https://www.chadsvasc.org/), and anticoagulation initiated. For most people these days, a direct oral anticoagulant will be initiated rather than warfarin. This offers protection from stroke with a low risk of bleeding and does not require regular blood tests, unlike warfarin. Symptoms of breathlessness and palpitations can be controlled by β blockers, which slow the heart rate down. If symptoms persist, rhythm control medication or ablation procedures can be initiated. Useful information can be accessed via the Arrhythmia Alliance (http://www.heartrhythmalliance.org/aa/uk) or the Stroke Association (https://www.stroke.org.uk/).

Reflection

Atrial fibrillation is usually divided into four main types. Using the resources list, identify these types and how they are classified.

Heart failure

Heart failure can be the end product of poorly controlled hypertension, preexisting cardiac or respiratory disease or diabetes (NICE, 2018c). Symptoms are vague and include fluid retention, breathlessness and fatigue. The definitive diagnosis of heart failure is made on echocardiogram, which will confirm the likely underlying cause and mechanism as heart failure with reduced ejection fraction (HFrEF) or heart failure with preserved ejection fraction (HFpEF). Treatment depends on the cause. There is a strong body of evidence for treating HFrEF, where the left ventricle is failing to adequately supply the systemic circulation, but far less for treating HFpEF. In left ventricular systolic dysfunction, treatment focuses on using ACE inhibitors and β blockers, with possible mineralocorticoid receptor antagonist drugs (spironolactone and eplerenone) to supplement this to optimise symptom control and impact on morbidity and mortality (NICE, 2018c). Diuretic drugs are used to relieve symptoms of fluid retention and breathlessness. A new class of drug was included in the NICE 2018 guidelines for initiation by specialists. Entresto is a neprilysin/ACE inhibitor combination which has demonstrated improvements in morbidity and mortality in people with HFrEF (Jhund & McMurray, 2016).

The review appointment

The review will include blood tests and assessment of BP, symptoms and ongoing lifestyle changes. In some people, drug therapy will need to be optimised through 'uptitration', stepping down doses or discontinuing medication (i.e., in those on DAPT), depending on their diagnosis and treatment strategy. Close liaison with secondary care is important in ensuring that patients get the correct treatment for their cardiovascular condition. A useful resource for health care professionals and people with heart failure is Pumping Marvellous: https:// pumpingmarvellous.org/.

Reflection

Reflect on the anatomy of the heart (chambers, valves and electrical activity) and consider how diseases affecting these areas can lead to a diagnosis of heart failure. Think about how heart failure might result from chronic lung disease, as well as from structural problems within the heart. Use online resources to support your learning.

Key learning points

- CVD is an umbrella term which covers diseases of the heart and blood vessels.
- The underlying causes are the same, and include modifiable and nonmodifiable risk factors.
- Modifiable risk factors such as BP and lipids can be treated with a combination of lifestyle interventions and medication.
- Self-management is key in ensuring that these changes are continued. Cardiac rehabilitation can support people to change, and Chapter 3 in this book on motivational interviewing will provide techniques on how to achieve this.
- AF causes symptoms, as well as increasing stroke risk, and so both of these areas require attention.
- Heart failure can occur as a complication of a range of LTCs and has a poor prognosis. Careful diagnosis and management can improve both morbidity and mortality.

Diabetes

Diabetes is a condition where the body is unable to control blood glucose levels. This can lead to significant acute and chronic complications. Diabetes is a CVD in that it causes vascular complications in both large and small vessels (NICE, 2017). This is not just the result of high sugar levels; it is also linked to the raised BP and abnormal lipid profile which often coexist with type 2 diabetes (T2D) and is sometimes referred to as the metabolic syndrome (International Diabetes Federation, 2006). People with T2D are at increased risk of macrovascular complications such as coronary heart disease, stroke and peripheral arterial disease, and they are also at higher risk of microvascular complications including nephropathy, neuropathy and retinopathy (NICE, 2017).

Definition

There are two main types of diabetes: type 1 and type 2. Type 1 diabetes is an autoimmune condition which occurs mainly in children and young adults, where the β cells of the pancreas stop producing insulin, resulting in the rapid onset of symptoms such as weight loss, polyuria, polydipsia and fatigue. T2D, in contrast, is the result of a chronic loss of blood glucose control, often linked to insulin resistance, which takes place over years and which may cause few symptoms. Up to 90% of all cases of diabetes are T2D. Other types of diabetes, such as latent autoimmune diabetes in adults (LADA) or monogenic diabetes in the young (MODY), are far less common.

Diagnosis

In type 1 diabetes, the diagnosis will be made based on the acute symptoms described above, along with high plasma glucose levels. In some cases, diabetic ketoacidosis may be the presenting feature, where the individual has very high sugar and ketone levels, leading to acidosis, which can be potentially life-threatening and requires urgent admission to hospital. Diabetes UK advises clinicians to use the 4Ts approach (toilet, tired, thirsty, thinner) to make a quick assessment of the risk of undiagnosed type 1 diabetes being responsible for any symptoms.

In T2D, symptoms are often far less overt. The recommended diagnostic test is assessment of the haemoglobin A1c (HbA1c) level, which should normally be below 42 mmol/mol. If the HbA1c is over 48 mmol/mol, this is considered to be in the diabetic range (NICE, 2015). If the person being tested has symptoms of diabetes, such as recurrent infections, extreme tiredness, thirst or polyuria, the diagnosis of diabetes can be made on one test. If he or she does not have symptoms, and the test has been carried out as part of a health check or as part of an annual review of another condition, it should be repeated within 2 weeks. If both tests are 48 mmol/mol or more, the diagnosis is confirmed. People who have an HbA1c level between 42 and 47 mmol/mol are considered to be at risk of T2D, a state which is often referred to as prediabetes (NICE, 2015).

Treatment

In type 1 diabetes, where no insulin is being produced, it is essential to inject insulin. Most people will be given long-acting insulin to provide a base level and then take mealtime insulin doses to control potential spikes in glucose that naturally occur after eating a meal.

In T2D, lifestyle is a big factor in metabolic syndrome and insulin resistance, so the focus will be on healthy eating, increasing activity levels, stopping smoking and maintaining alcohol intake within recommended levels. Most people with T2D will be overweight or obese, so supporting people to lose weight is an essential part of diabetes management. There has been an increased level of interest in how health care professionals can support people to lose weight to reduce the risk of diabetes, cancer, CVD and other LTCs. The EatWell plate, which has been used for decades as a model of healthy eating, has been challenged as being out of date and not in line with current research (Unwin, 2016). Dietary approaches which had previously been ignored are now subject to a renewed level of interest. These include very low calorie diets, low carbohydrate diets and the Mediterranean diet.

The DiRECT study was set up to investigate whether weight loss in people with a diagnosis of T2D could lead to diabetes remission (Lean et al., 2017). In a previous 2-year-long randomised controlled trial comparing gastric banding with standard dietary advice, Dixon et al. (2008) found that a 15-kg weight loss was associated with diabetes remission. With that in mind, the DiRECT study offered an intensive weight loss programme aimed at supporting people to lose 15 kg in a 12-week period.

There were two primary outcomes from the study: the number of patients who achieved and maintained a weight loss of 15 kg or more at 12 months and the number of patients who had remission of their diabetes, defined as having an HbA1c level of less than 48 mmol/mol without taking diabetes medication for at least 2 months. Importantly, the study was not carried out in a specialist centre. Instead, the interventions were for the most part carried out by GPNs, all of whom had attended 8 hours of training about the programme and who were also offered mentorship throughout the study. The participants were aged 20 to 65 years, had a body mass index of between 27 and 45 kg/m^2 and had had diabetes for 3 years on average, with an HbA1c of 59 mmol/mol. The Very Low Carbohydrate Diet (VLCD) provided around 830 calories daily. Participants were encouraged to engage in more physical activity by increasing their step rate to 15,000 steps per day.

The results showed that, of the 149 active participants, 36 (i.e., 24% of the study group) achieved a weight loss of 15 kg or more. No one in the control group ($n = 149$) achieved this, making the result highly statistically significant. In terms of the coprimary outcome, remission of diabetes (meaning an HbA1c level of <48 mmol/mol off all blood glucose–lowering medication for at least 2 months), 68 of the 149 participants (46%) achieved this outcome versus 6 out of 149 people (4%) in the control group; another highly statistically significant result.

Diabetes remission occurred throughout the groups, with 6.7% of all study participants achieving diabetes remission with a weight loss of up to 5 kg and 33.9% of participations achieving remission with a weight loss of 5 to 10 kg. Once people had lost 10 to 15 kg, the figure increased to 57.1%, and the group of patients who lost more than 15 kg saw a staggering remission rate of 86.1%. There were no withdrawals attributed to serious adverse events in either group. This suggests that significant metabolic benefits of weight loss can be seen at even relatively low levels of weight loss.

The VLCD is hard work, however, and will not suit everyone. Any support offered to help someone lose weight should take a personalised approach tailored to the individual's lifestyle.

Low carbohydrate diets are proving very popular (and anecdotally effective) at achieving weight loss and improvements in HbA1c (Clifton et al., 2014). The diabetes.co.uk website has offered almost half a million people help with following a low carbohydrate diet, supplemented by a high protein intake and, sometimes, a higher fat intake than the low fat diet normally advocated. Again, significant weight losses and improvements in diabetes control (and lipids) have been reported on this regime. In the long term, a Mediterranean diet is now recommended as the easiest and most effective way to maintain weight and improve health (Franquesa et al., 2019).

Activity levels should be increased so that people are doing some form of physical activity most days of the week. Pedometers or activity trackers work well to motivate some individuals, whereas others will prefer to join in team sports or attend classes. Many areas of the country now have 'ParkRun', where locals can meet up and walk or run around a designated course with others and work on improving their personal best. Any increase on activity levels is a positive, and people should be encouraged to take this view rather than setting high (and sometimes unrealistic) goals.

Medication

All these lifestyle interventions should underpin any medication that may be prescribed to improve glycaemic control, BP and the lipid profile.

The American Diabetes Association and European Association for the Study of Diabetes (ADA/EASD) publishes recommendations on the management of glycaemic levels in people with T2D, including the use of the most appropriate medication for patients with cardiovascular or renal disease (Davies et al., 2018). The ADA/EASD consensus report recommends that, after lifestyle interventions and metformin as the first-line drug treatment, the next step should be based on the 'profile' of the individual concerned:

- For patients with clinical CVD, a sodium-glucose cotransporter-2 (SGLT2) inhibitor or a glucagon-like peptide 1 (GLP-1) receptor agonist with proven cardiovascular benefit is recommended
- For patients with chronic kidney disease or clinical heart failure and atherosclerotic CVD, an SGLT2 inhibitor with proven benefit is recommended
- For people where weight loss is a priority, an SGLT2 inhibitor or a GLP-1 receptor antagonist will be first-line
- If avoidance of hypoglycaemia is key, sulfonylureas and insulin should be avoided unless necessary, but all other treatments come with very little, if any, risk of hypoglycaemia.

Regarding BP management, the previous section on hypertension explained that current UK guidance is to give an ACE inhibitor as first-line therapy for anyone with diabetes. as these are cardioprotective and renoprotective, as well as being good for BP control (NICE, 2019).

Lipid management in primary prevention is usually based on the cardiovascular risk score (see Hypertension section). If the QRisk score is over 10%, a statin should be offered. The usual recommendation is to prescribe atorvastatin 20 mg, although Scottish guidelines advise giving atorvastatin 10 mg. The aim is to reduce non–high-density lipoprotein (HDL) cholesterol by 40% (NICE, 2014 (2014b, updated 2016)) or to 2.5 mmol/L (Joint British Societies, 2014). A non-HDL cholesterol level of 2.5 mmol/L is equivalent to a low-density lipoprotein cholesterol level of 1.8 mmol/L (Joint British Societies, 2014). Here is an example of how this would work:

Case study

Katherine has type 2 diabetes, and her QRisk score is 14%, so she needs a statin.

Her total cholesterol level is 5.2 mmol/L, and her high-density lipoprotein (HDL) cholesterol level is 1.2 mmol/L.

By subtracting her non-HDL cholesterol level from her total cholesterol level, we can calculate that her non-HDL cholesterol level is 4.0 mmol/L.

We need to reduce this either by 40% (1.6 mmol/L) or to 2.5 mmol/L:
4.0 − 1.6 = 2.4 mmol/L.

The target for treatment is either 2.4 or 2.5 mmol/L, depending on the guideline followed.

If targets are not achieved, statin doses can be increased, or additional therapy such as ezetimibe, can be introduced.

The review appointment

People with diabetes should have regular reviews tailored to their needs. HbA1c measurement should be carried out at least twice a year for most people, with a full blood review, including renal function and lipid profile, performed annually. Annual surveillance for any complications of diabetes should be carried out in primary care to include assessment for signs of nephropathy, neuropathy and retinopathy. These microvascular complications are important in themselves but are also predecessors of vascular disease in the bigger vessels, leading to heart disease, stroke and peripheral arterial disease (Table 5.1).

Supporting self-management

Most of the management of diabetes is done by the individual, possibly with the support of family and carers. It is essential that everyone understands the importance of lifestyle changes, as well as adherence to medication. These days, home blood glucose monitoring is less commonly carried out, as fewer drugs are prescribed which are known to cause hypoglycaemia. However, this means that attendance for regular HbA1c testing is even more important. Some

Table 5.1 **Assessing potential complications of diabetes.**

Complication	Tests	Consider
Nephropathy	Estimated glomerular filtration rate and albumin-creatinine ratio	If either test is abnormal, this is a red flag and a risk factor for macrovascular disease
Neuropathy	Test foot pulses and sensation	Feet can be affected by nerve damage and vascular disease
Retinopathy	Annual retinal screen	Advise patients of the importance of attending to identify changes early

people will want to test for reassurance or in case of concurrent illness. In type 1 diabetes, people may be eligible for flash glucose monitoring on the National Health Service.

Reflection

Many General Practice Nurses carry out foot checks to assess for microvascular and neuropathic changes in the feet of people with diabetes. Have a look at these online resources to prepare for further training in this important area:

https://www.diabetes.org.uk/guide-to-diabetes/complications/feet/what-can-i
-expect at-my-annual foot-check

https://www.e-lfh.org.uk/programmes/diabetic foot-screening-interactive
-assessment/

https://www.nice.org.uk/guidance/ng19

Most patients with diabetes seen in primary care will have T2D, although some people with type 1 diabetes will also be seen between hospital appointments. LADA or MODY are far less common.

Type 1 diabetes is diagnosed by the acute onset of osmotic symptoms caused by high sugar levels, sometimes resulting in diabetic ketoacidosis. T2D is diagnosed with an HbA1c test showing a level of 48 mmol/mol or higher. Two tests within 2 weeks are needed in asymptomatic patients.

Type 1 diabetes is treated with insulin. T2D is usually treated with metformin and additional therapies tailored to the individual. SGLT2 inhibitors and GLP1 receptor antagonists are often used as first- and second-line therapies, as they offer significant additional benefits with regard to CVD, renal impairment and weight loss, without the risk of hypoglycaemia.

As with most LTCs, self-management is the key to improved outcomes, so adherence to lifestyle changes and prescribed medication is essential. Home blood glucose testing may help to support this in some cases.

COVID-19

In 2020 and 2021, the coronavirus pandemic caused a sea change in the way we manage LTCs. Those with severe illness were advised to shield to reduce their risk of contracting the virus. Those living with less severe chronic conditions were advised to take extra care in recognition of the fact that people with an LTC were more likely to become significantly unwell if they contracted coronavirus, and outcomes, in general, appeared to be worse. It will be interesting to review the literature postpandemic to see exactly what happened in each LTC.

Conclusion

This chapter has highlighted some of the key LTCs that might be encountered in the everyday practice of a GPN and signposted some of the resources that are available to increase knowledge and comprehension of these areas. Management of patients with LTCs in primary care is complex, as there are many interconnections with individual diseases impacting on each other. Together with the use of individual drugs to manage individual conditions, the complexity of polypharmacy requires GPNs to have expert knowledge of management of patients with these diseases. Consideration must also be given to the emerging evidence surrounding Long Covid and the possibility that this may be viewed as a new and additional LTC.

References

Abell, J. G., Kivimäki, M., Dugravot, A., Tabak, A. G., Fayosse, A., Shipley, M., & Sabia, S. (2018). Association between systolic blood pressure and dementia in the Whitehall II cohort study: Role of age, duration, and threshold used to define hypertension. *European Heart Journal, 39*(33), 3119–3125.

Badeli, H., & Assadi, F. (2014). Strategies to reduce pitfalls in measuring blood pressure. *International Journal of Preventive Medicine, 5*(Suppl 1), S17–S20.

Bosnic-Anticevich, S. Z., Cvetkovski, B., Azzi, E. A., et al. (2018). Identifying critical errors: Addressing inhaler technique in the context of asthma management. *Pulmonary Therapy, 4,* 1–12.

British Heart Foundation. (2019). *Heart statistics.* https://www.bhf.org.uk/what-we-do/our-research/heart-statistics.

British Thoracic Society/Scottish Intercollegiate Guidelines Network. (2019). *Guideline for the management of asthma.* https://www.brit-thoracic.org.uk/quality-improvement/guidelines/asthma/.

Clifton, P. M., Condo, D., & Keogh, J. B. (2014). Long term weight maintenance after advice to consume low carbohydrate, higher protein diets – a systematic review and meta analysis. *Nutrition, Metabolism & Cardiovascular Diseases, 24*(3), 224–235.

Davies, M. J., D'Alessio, D. A., Fradkin, J., et al. (2018). Management of hyperglycaemia in type 2 diabetes, 2018. A consensus report by the American Diabetes Association (ADA) and the European Association for the Study of Diabetes (EASD). *Diabetologia, 61*(12), 2461–2498.

Dixon, J. B., O'Brien, P. E., Playfair, J., et al. (2008). Adjustable gastric banding and conventional therapy for type 2 diabetes: A randomized controlled trial. *Journal of the American Medical Association, 299*, 316–323.

Franquesa, M., Pujol-Busquets, G., García-Fernández, E., et al. (2019). Mediterranean diet and cardiodiabesity: A systematic review through evidence-based answers to key clinical questions. *Nutrients, 11*(3), 655.

Global Initiative for Asthma. (2019). *Pocket guide for asthma management and prevention*. https:// ginasthma.org/pocket-guide-for-asthma-management-and-prevention/.

Global Initiative for Chronic Obstructive Lung Disease. (2019). *Global Strategy for the diagnosis, management and prevention of Chronic Obstructive Pulmonary Disease – 2020 report*. https:// goldcopd.org/wp-content/uploads/2019/11/GOLD-2020-REPORT-ver1.0wms.pdf.

Hare, D. L., Toukhsati, S. R., Johansson, P., & Jaarsma, T. (2014). Depression and cardiovascular disease: A clinical review. *European Heart Journal, 35*(21), 1365–1372.

International Diabetes Federation. (2006). *IDF consensus worldwide definition of the metabolic syndrome*. https://idf.org/our-activities/advocacy-awareness/resources-and-tools/60:idfconsensus -worldwide-definitionof-the-metabolic-syndrome.html.

Jhund, P. S., & McMurray, J. J. V (2016). The neprilysin pathway in heart failure: A review and guide on the use of sacubitril/valsartan. *Heart, 102*, 1342–1347.

Joint British Societies. (2014). Consensus recommendations for the prevention of cardiovascular disease (JBS3). *Heart, 100*, ii1–ii67.

Lean, M. E. J., Leslie, W. S., Barnes, A. C., et al. (2017). Primary care-led weight management. *Lancet, 391*(10120), 541–551.

Müller, V., Galffy, G., Orosz, M., et al. (2016). Characteristics of reversible and nonreversible COPD and asthma and COPD overlap syndrome patients: An analysis of salbutamol Easyhaler data. *International Journal of Chronic Obstructive Pulmonary Disease, 11*, 93–101.

NHS UK. (2018). *Cardiovascular disease*. https://www.nhs.uk/conditions/cardiovascular-disease/

NICE. (2014a, updated 2019). *Measuring fractional exhaled nitric oxide concentration in asthma*. https://www.nice.org.uk/guidance/dg12.

NICE. (2014b, updated 2016). Cardiovascular disease: Risk assessment and reduction, including lipid modification. Available from https://www.nice.org.uk/guidance/cg181.

NICE. (2015, updated 2019). *Type 2 diabetes in adults: Management*. https://www.nice.org.uk /guidance/NG28.

NICE. (2017). *Asthma: diagnosis, monitoring and chronic asthma management*. https://www.nice .org.uk/guidance/ng80/resources/asthma-diagnosis-monitoring-and-chronic-asthma-management -pdf-1837687975621.

NICE. (2018a, updated 2019). *Chronic obstructive pulmonary disease in over 16s: Diagnosis and management*. https://www.nice.org.uk/guidance/ng115.

NICE. (2018b). *Chronic obstructive pulmonary disease (acute exacerbation): Antimicrobial prescribing*. https://www.nice.org.uk/guidance/ng114.

NICE. (2018c). *Chronic heart failure in adults: Diagnosis and management*. https://www.nice.org .uk/guidance/ng106.

NICE. (2019). *Hypertension in adults: Diagnosis and management*. https://www.nice.org.uk/guidance /ng136.

Pascual, R. M., & Peters, S. P. (2009). The irreversible component of persistent asthma. *The Journal of Allergy and Clinical Immunology, 124*(5), 883–892.

Primary Care Commissioning. (2013). *A guide to performing quality assured diagnostic spirometry.* https://pcc-cic.org.uk/sites/default/files/articles/attachments/spirometry_e-guide_1-5-13_0 .pdf.

Unwin, D. (2016). *The big interview.* https://diabetestimes.co.uk/big-interview-dr-david-unwin/.

Valgimigli, M., Bueno, H., Byrne, R. A., et al. (2018). ESC Scientific Document Group 2017 ESC focused update on dual antiplatelet therapy in coronary artery disease developed in collaboration with EACTS. *European Journal of Cardio-Thoracic Surgery, 53*(1), 34–78.

Yusuf, S., Hawken, S., Ounpuu, S., et al. (2004). Effect of potentially modifiable risk factors associated with myocardial infarction in 52 countries (the INTERHEART study): Case-control study. *Lancet, 364*(9438), 937–952.

Chapter 6

Men's health

Mike Kirby

Learning outcomes

After reading this chapter you should be able to:

1. Understand men's health conditions
2. Describe risk factors relating to men's health
3. Identify treatment options related to men's health conditions
4. Learn about approaches to addressing men's health issues

Introduction

One of the ironies about the prevailing lack of attention to men's health is that, at all stages of life, from foetus to old age, the mortality of males is higher than that of females. In the United Kingdom, life expectancy is 5 years longer for women than for men. In early life, much of the excess male mortality is associated with trauma and accidents, related to our attitude to risk-taking behaviour. Later in life, excesses in mortality from cardiovascular disease (CVD) and a number of cancers also start to play a role, and come to dominate the picture.

When one looks at the health of men and women in the context of the various degrees of socioeconomic disadvantage, the starkest contrast is seen in men living in the most deprived circumstances, who lose 9 years of life expectancy compared with men living in the least deprived circumstances. We need to be alert to these differences when dealing with men, and we clearly need new national health policies directed at men's problems.

Loss of working years because of ill health is an important national economic consequence, and many men in retirement find their lives are blighted by preventable ill health. Around 50% of premature deaths in men are considered to be preventable. There is a general lack of awareness of the importance of a healthy lifestyle in maintaining good health, and, in addition, men are often reluctant to seek health care and may have difficulty in addressing their emotions. There is an increasing number of men living alone, either through divorce or the death of their partner, who often have a lack of social networks that they can call on in times of stress and ill health.

The late presentation of men for diagnosis is an urgent area of health research and policy development, and it is also a priority to which health professionals need to pay more attention.

This chapter is written for primary care nurses (General Practice Nurses), who wrestle every day with the consequences of ill health among men. There are many opportunities within routine consultations to pick up the early signs of CVD and cancers, as well as to promote lifestyle advice including smoking cessation, weight control, a sensible amount of exercise and a healthy diet.

The term 'toxic masculinity' is increasingly used in common parlance to describe cultural masculine norms that are harmful to men themselves, and to society in general. In medical care, this term is particularly apt because it encapsulates a variety of factors that have meant that men's health outcomes, despite significant improvements over the last 40 years, remain far poorer than they should be.

There is an attitude of denial. This is partly because the act of admitting a health problem may be perceived as degrading a man's self-image, of being an invulnerable male. Cultural expectations and peer pressure can compound the problem by encouraging men to take unnecessary risks. This includes overindulgence in unhealthy foods, excessive consumption of alcohol and smoking. In addition to this, risk-taking behaviour puts younger men at risk of ill health from trauma, misuse of drugs and sexually transmitted diseases including human immunodeficiency virus (HIV)/acquired immunodeficiency syndrome.

The content of this chapter will alert nurses to the agenda of men's health, and, by doing so, prevent some of the misery that premature deaths among men cause, not only to their families, but to the whole of society.

Issues relating to men's health

Understanding the specific issues that relate to men's health is the first step toward this goal, and is best illustrated by reviewing the case studies in this chapter.

Midlife crisis and depression

Midlife in men is often a peak time for work and family responsibilities. Stresses can be caused by increased responsibilities, financial worries, difficult relationships with children and illness or losses of parents, all of which can have a consequent negative effect on a man's health. In addition to this, reaching the midpoint in the lifespan implies a recognition of declining energy, physical fitness and health, at a time when men have to face up to the current changes in society, such as the changing tradition in men's roles in response to women's changing roles, and the prospect of redundancy and early retirement. Work is an important central role for many men, and its loss can have devastating effects.

Men are three to four time more likely than women to commit suicide, and many of these men will visit the practice before the event. Spotting the symptoms of depression is important. Enquiry should be made about depressed mood, loss of interest or pleasure in life, significant weight loss when not dieting, insomnia or sleeping too much, psychomotor agitation or retardation, fatigue, feelings of worthlessness, excessive or inappropriate guilt, diminished ability to think or concentrate, indecisiveness, recurrent thoughts of death and current suicidal ideation without a specific plan or a suicide attempt or specific plan for committing suicide. The Patient Health Questionnaire–9 (PHQ-9) is a depression assessment tool that has been validated for use in primary care. An online version is available at: https://patient.info/doctor/patient-health-questionnaire-phq-9.

The PHQ-9 scoring system is as follows:

- 0–4: normal range/full remission
- 5–9: minimal depressive symptoms
- 10–14: major depression, mild severity
- 15–19: major depression, moderate severity
- ≥20: major depression, severe severity

Men scoring 10 to 20 or higher would almost certainly benefit from antidepressant therapy or psychotherapy.

Cardiovascular disease

CVD causes more than a quarter of all deaths in the United Kingdom (British Heart Foundation, 2019a). In 2017, 85,395 men died from CVD in the United Kingdom, compared with 83,075 women. Although coronary heart disease (CHD) accounted for the greatest number of deaths in both sexes, mortality attributed to CHD was far greater in men (40,974 CHD deaths in men versus 25,367 in women). However, death rates from other heart diseases, hypertensive diseases, stroke and vascular dementia were lower in men than in women. Death rates from CVD increase with advancing age and are greatest in those aged 85 years and over (British Heart Foundation, 2019b).

In the United Kingdom in 2017, around 45% of CVD cases were attributed to hypertension, 43% to dietary risks, 25% to high levels of low-density lipoprotein cholesterol, 24% to diabetes, 17% to high body mass index (BMI), 11% to cigarette smoking/secondhand smoke, 8% to low physical activity, 7% to impaired kidney function, 5% to air pollution and 2% to other environmental risks such as lead exposure (British Heart Foundation, 2019b).

Hypertension is thought to affect around 27% of United Kingdom adults. However, half of these are not receiving effective treatment, and as many as 4.7 million adults may be undiagnosed. Around 50% of UK adults have elevated cholesterol levels (>5 mmol/L). Adults with diabetes are two to three times more likely to develop CVD than those without diabetes, and are almost twice as likely to die from heart disease or stroke. One-third of UK adults with diabetes die from CVD (British Heart Foundation, 2019a).

Ideally, men should know their numbers for blood pressure, waist circumference, cholesterol and HbA1c.

Case study

Richard, a 34-year-old gay man with a history of unsafe sex with multiple partners, presented with fever, weight loss and muscle pains, together with unexplained and nonpainful enlargement of lymph nodes in his groin and axilla. He had a previous history of an influenza-like illness, which included fever and large, tender lymph nodes, a sore throat, a rash, tiredness and mouth ulcers, together with balanitis. At that time, he also had vomiting and diarrhoea, which lasted 3 weeks.

Richard was referred for human immunodeficiency virus (HIV) testing, which was positive. He was treated with highly active antiretroviral therapy (HAART), with a view to slowing down the progression rather than curing the disease. Current HAART options are combinations consisting of at least three medications belonging to at least two classes of antiretroviral agents.

His initial treatment consisted of a nonnucleoside reverse transcriptase inhibitor plus two nucleoside analogue reverse transcription inhibitors (zidovudine and lamivudine). The clinicians held a protease inhibitor in reserve.

Richard's current male partner tested negative for HIV and was initiated on preexposure prophylaxis.

HIV/acquired immunodeficiency syndrome (AIDS) is not uncommon in men who have unprotected sex with men. It is also a significant risk for drug addicts who inject themselves. HIV causes AIDS by depleting CD4+ T cells. This weakens the immune system and predisposes the patients to opportunistic infections. During the chronic phase of this illness, the consequences of generalised immune activation, coupled with the gradual loss of the ability of the immune system to generate new T cells, accounts for the slow decline in CD4+ T cell numbers.

In this case, unfortunately, the patient did not report any of the symptoms of immune deficiency that are characteristic of AIDS, and presented some years after infection. This underscores the importance of early diagnosis and treatment.

Cancer

Since the early 1990s, the incidence of all cancers has increased by more than 12% in the United Kingdom, with rates for women increasing by 16% and rates for men increasing by 2%. In 2016, there were around 185,000 new cancer cases in men and 178,000 in women, with breast, prostate, bowel and lung cancers accounting for more than half these (Cancer Research UK, 2019).

Thyroid and liver cancers have shown the fastest increases in incidence over the past 10 years in both sexes, whereas the incidence of melanoma skin cancer, kidney cancer and Hodgkin lymphoma has also increased markedly in men (Cancer Research UK, 2019).

According to British Heart Foundation statistics, more men died from cancer than from CVD in the United Kingdom in 2017, with cancer mortality figures of 91,059 for men and 79,705 for women. Lung cancer rates were higher in men, while breast cancer rates were higher in women. Overall, cancer death rates were greatest in the 75- to 84-year-old age group (British Heart Foundation, 2019b). Cancer is more common in White and Black men than in Asian men, and fewer men than women survive cancer (Cancer Research UK, 2019).

Reduced awareness among men of the malignant diseases to which their bodies are prone may also be a factor in the gender gap. Lung cancer, for example, can be largely prevented by not smoking. Colon cancer is more likely when there is a positive family history, and this can be detected early and cured with little morbidity by the use of faecal occult blood testing and flexible colonoscopy. Prostate cancer may have a familial link in up to 9% of cases and can be detected easily be means of prostate-specific antigen (PSA) testing and digital rectal examination, and cured by radiotherapy or surgery. The Prostate Cancer Risk Management Programme (PCRMP) provides much helpful information for men considering having a PSA test.

Case study

John, a 53-year-old farm worker and exsmoker, presented after noticing a significant change in bowel habit and intermittent rectal bleeding. He had not mentioned this to anyone previously because he felt embarrassed and didn't want to cause any bother. His wife had made the appointment for him.

His General Practitioner diagnosed anaemia and the presence of a palpable liver. A computed tomography scan subsequently revealed multiple unresectable hepatic metastases, and at colonoscopy, he had a poorly differentiated adenocarcinoma of the sigmoid colon.

This led to a sigmoid colectomy, with additional chemotherapy. John had a family history of colon cancer, but approximately half of colorectal cancers are the result of lifestyle factors, and about one-quarter of cases are preventable. Being overweight increases the risk of developing and dying from colorectal cancer, as does physical inactivity. A diet high in red meat and processed meat and low in fibre also increases the risk.

Once again, early diagnosis is critical in this disease.

Lifestyle factors

Many premature deaths are linked to unhealthy dietary and lifestyle habits, as well as risk-taking behaviour. In the United Kingdom in 2017, it was estimated that 67% of men and 61% of women were overweight or obese, 19% of men and 16% of women were smokers, 34% of men and 43% of women were not meeting the recommendations for physical activity, 29% of men and 14% of women were exceeding the weekly alcohol consumption guidelines and 74% of men and 69% of women were not meeting the five-a-day fruit and vegetable recommendations (British Heart Foundation, 2019b).

Risk-taking behaviour

Young people are more inclined to engage in risk-taking behaviours than older people. The major causes of mortality among young men in England and Wales are injury and poisoning. This includes homicide, suicide and accidents.

Case study

Trevor, a 54-year-old heavy smoker (more than two packs per day for at least 30 years), presented with a painless swelling on the right side of the neck that he had noticed some months before but completely ignored. A needle biopsy of the lesion was performed, and computed tomography and magnetic resonance imaging scans arranged.

Histology unfortunately confirmed a poorly differentiated squamous cell carcinoma with lymph node metastases. A multidisciplinary team advised surgical resection followed by radiation therapy. This was because of the extensive nature of the disease, with regional lymph node metastases (stage III or IV). Chemotherapy was also recommended, with the objective of creating an inhospitable environment for metastases to establish themselves in other parts of the body.

Smoking combined with high alcohol intake is one of the main risk factors for head and neck cancer. In addition to lung cancer, cigarette smokers have a lifetime increased risk for head and neck cancer, somewhere between 5- and 25-fold in comparison to the general population. Even when men stop smoking, it takes 20 years for the risk level to fall.

The increasing homicide rate seen in recent years has been most pronounced in male victims and the younger age groups, and one-quarter of men who are victims of homicide are killed at the hands of a friend or acquaintance (Office for National Statistics, 2019a).

In 2018, there were 6507 suicides registered in the United Kingdom, three-quarters of which were in men. The 2019 UK male suicide rate of 17.2 deaths per 100,000 reflects a significant increase from 2017. The highest age-specific suicide rates were in men aged 45 to 59 years (Office for National Statistics, 2019b).

Three-quarters of fatal injuries occurring in 15- to 24-year-olds occur in males. Two-thirds of the fatal injuries occurring in young people result from unintentional accidents, such as road traffic accidents, falls, drownings and poisonings, whereas the other third result from intentional, dangerous behaviours, including violence, suicide and self-harm. Alcohol consumption plays a major role in risk-taking behaviour and contributes to around 40% of all injuries, particularly in men (Eurosafe).

Death rates attributed to accidental poisoning by drugs increased in England between 2001 and 2017, with the highest rates in 2017 in 35- to 44-year-olds. Death rates resulting from misuse of drugs also increased over this timeframe, with the highest rates in 2017 in 40- to 44-year-olds (Office for National Statistics, 2018).

Emphasis needs to be placed on discussing and managing specific problems with men, particularly those affected by homelessness and unemployment and those taking drugs or consuming excessive amounts of alcohol.

Social inequalities are a key factor in poor health in men. In England, men living in the most deprived tenth of areas die around 9 years earlier than those in the least deprived tenth, and may spend almost 20 fewer years in good health. Although deprived areas exist across England, most are in the North. There therefore remains a north-south divide in life expectancy and healthy life expectancy (Public Health England, 2017).

The more deprived areas of the United Kingdom also have a higher prevalence of behavioural risk factors. The prevalence of smoking, inactivity and eating less than the recommended five portions of fruit and vegetables per week is greater in the more deprived areas than in the less deprived areas. Men living in the most deprived areas are also more likely to suffer harmful effects from alcohol consumption (Public Health England, 2017).

Male-specific health problems

Around one in three men over the age of 50 years will experience urinary symptoms, with benign prostatic hyperplasia (BPH) being the most common cause (Prostate Cancer UK, 2017). Erectile dysfunction (ED) is another common complaint in men and is a marker of other diseases. ED has now been added to the QRISK III cardiovascular risk calculator, because it increases the risk of a cardiovascular event by approximately 25% on top of the traditional risk factors (Hackett et al., 2018a). Although in the majority of cases ED can be satisfactorily treated, many men do not seek help because of embarrassment, and we need to be proactive in enquiring about sexual function. A complaint of ED should automatically lead to a testosterone blood test, and the British Society of Sexual Medicine has recently updated its guidelines on the management of ED (Hackett et al., 2018a) and testosterone deficiency (TD; Hackett et al., 2018b).

Testicular pain can be because of infection or torsion of the testes, but many men fear it, thinking it is a sign of testicular cancer. The longer a man delays seeing a doctor about a testicular torsion, the worse the prognosis. Testicular cancer is usually detected by the presence of a lump in the testis, rather than pain, and a reluctance among men to self-examine often results in late presentations, a reduced chance of cure and greater morbidity from the treatments.

What can be done?

A campaign of public information seems appropriate, and we should all take the opportunity to make our general practices more male-friendly. Men should be actively encouraged to adopt a health lifestyle in terms of both diet and exercise, and supported to give up smoking. A visit to a dedicated well-man clinic could include a health check for CVD and enquiry about rectal bleeding and symptoms of prostate disease.

A focused examination based on family and clinical history should be conducted. Patients should be asked about erectile function, as well as symptoms and signs of TD. Any man concerned about his risk of prostate cancer should be counselled about the pros and cons of having a PSA test.

It is prudent to perform a dipstick examination of the urine, because bladder cancer is common in men, especially those who have been heavy smokers, and may present as microscopic haematuria.

Regular health checks not only allow the detection of diseases at a stage when they can be treated effectively, but also provide an opportunity for men to be educated about the best ways to stay healthy.

The men's health clinic

There are several reasons why setting up a well-man clinic should be a viable option. It should:

- Be a significant source of information regarding how to prevent ill health, disability and premature death
- Offer patients scope for improvement
- Target identifiable risk factors that can be addressed through health promotion
- Lead to a measurable improvement following health promotion
- Allow the setting of targets for improvement

Introducing a systematic protocol-led approach can be accomplished by incorporating some or all of the following tasks into a clinic plan, addressing those diseases and targeting men exclusively or preferentially (Box 6.1):

- Health information: providing detailed, accurate, current health information
- Early detection: systematically searching for diseases where early detection is important
- Treatment: monitoring and adjusting for chronic conditions
- Surveillance: monitoring borderline abnormalities

A sample protocol may well include the following:

- Personal data, including name, date of birth, address, occupation, marital status, employment situation, smoking status, alcohol consumption, sexual orientation
- Enquiry about:
- skin health (and discuss avoidance of sunburn)
- past history
- therapy history
- family history
- cholesterol
- stress, anxiety and depression
- sexual health
- exercise history
- prostate health

Box 6.1 **Some essential steps to develop an efficient well-man clinic**

1. Develop effective teamwork. This involves shared goals and understanding of each other's role. One way of developing effective procedures and interpersonal relationships is to use a SWOT analysis. With this, the group meets to discuss agreed current strengths (S), weaknesses (W), opportunities (O) and threats (T) in setting up a well-man clinic. Strengths may be a committed team, a clear protocol, a sound knowledge base, convenient appointment times, support from the Clinical Commissioning Group, patient appreciation or having variety in day-to-day work. Weaknesses may relate to premises, including inadequate space, lack of a computer terminal, none of the team having experience in sexual health, staff already having time pressures, the generation of more work and the time not being convenient. Opportunities may be learning about men's health, disease prevention, healthier and happier patients, increased quality of care and an enthusiastic nurse supported by a general practitioner partner. Threats include lack of motivation, a falling practice size, turnover of staff, uncertain funding, political change in the National Health Service, time pressure and the cost of training.

2. Focus on men's health. It is important for members of the team to have a shared understanding of men's health, which may be promoted initially with the use of brainstorming session in which the key areas of men's health are discussed. This would raise awareness of the diseases from which men suffer and lead to a protocol being constructed, together with an action plan.

3. Ensure that practicalities are addressed. A nurse or doctor will need to lead the project.

4. Define the practice priorities. Arrange a literature search and future meetings to learn more about men's health. Establish who will do what, where and when. Agree to the timing of the clinic, and consider working hours, start date and target patient group (e.g., men aged 45–70 years).

5. Estimate the number of patients who need to attend the clinic, define the length of appointments and clarify how staff can get access to a doctor if questions arise during consultation or if prescriptions are needed. Decide how patients will be informed about the clinic. This may be via the practice notice board and/or practice leaflet, practice website, opportunities during consultations, computer searches, disease indexes and local newspaper publicity. Make arrangements for appointments and recall to decide whether nonattenders will be reappointed. Are there any cultural or language implications? Will there be a specific approach to men with disabilities?

6. Develop an audit trail.

- urinary problems (do they have to get up at night to pass urine, or have they noticed a deterioration in their urinary stream? An affirmative answer should lead to the use of the International Prostate Symptom Score (IPSS) (Fig. 6.1) and quality-of-life assessment).
- For testicular health, offer a leaflet on self-examination
- For osteoporosis risk, provide a checklist for risk factors and consider the use of a dual-energy x-ray absorptiometry scan to evaluate a positive examination

International prostate symptom score (IPSS)

Name: Date:

	Not at all	Less than 1 time in 5	Less than half the	About half the time	More than half the	Almost always	Your score
Incomplete emptying Over the past month, how often have you had a sensation of not emptying your bladder completely after you finish urinating?	0	1	2	3	4	5	
Frequency Over the past month, how often have you had to urinate again less than 2 hours after you finished urinating?	0	1	2	3	4	5	
Intermittency Over the past month, how often have you found you stopped and started again several times when you urinated?	0	1	2	3	4	5	
Urgency Over the last month, how difficult have you found it to postpone urination?	0	1	2	3	4	5	
Weak stream Over the past month, how often have you had a weak urinary stream?	0	1	2	3	4	5	
Straining Over the past month, how often have you had to push or strain to begin urination?	0	1	2	3	4	5	

	None	1 time	2 times	3 times	4 times	5 times or more	Your score
Nocturia Over the past month, how many times did you most typically get up to urinate from the time you went to bed until the time you got up in the morning?	0	1	2	3	4	5	

Total IPSS score	

Quality of life due to urinary symptoms	Delighted	Pleased	Mostly satisfied	Mixed – about equally satisfied and dissatisfied	Mostly dissatisfied	Unhappy	Terrible
If you were to spend the rest of your life with your urinary condition the way it is now, how would you feel about that?	0	1	2	3	4	5	6

Total score: 0--7 Mildly symptomatic; 8--19 moderately symptomatic; 20--35 severely symptomatic.

Fig. 6.1   International prostate symptom score. (From Barry, M. J., Fowler, F. J., O'Leary, M. P., et al. (1992). The American Urological Association Symptom Index for benign prostatic hyperplasia. *Journal of Urology,* 148, 1549–1557.)

- Height, weight, BMI and waist circumference (WC)
- Blood pressure
- Cardiovascular risk calculation, using QRISK3
- Digital rectal examination, if appropriate
- Urinalysis
- Peak expiratory flow rate ± spirometry
- Blood tests (may include lipids and HbA1c; HIV and PSA tests should not be requested without suitable pretest counselling)
- Review all the data collected and give appropriate leaflets on diet, exercise, weight control, smoking, lifestyle, avoidance of sunburn, sexual health, family history of CHD, previous cardiovascular events, prostate health, testicular health and bone health
- Ensure the patient is fully immunised according to approved guidelines
- Determine an appropriate follow-up or discharge
- Audit
- The complaints procedure

With regards to a men's health clinic, the things that need to be considered are mainly age-related (see Table 6.1).

Table 6.1 **Age-related considerations for a men's health clinic.**

Age range (years)	Main considerations
0–19	Developmental progress, height, weight, immunisation records, undescended testes or inguinal hernia, blood pressure, skin conditions (especially acne). Accidents and safety regarding risk-taking behaviour, sexuality, avoidance of sexually transmitted infections (STIs) and skin protection. Mental health, including social development, self-esteem, family and school relationships, stress/anxiety.
20–39	Height, weight, body mass index (BMI), waist circumference (WC), blood pressure. Discuss testicular self-examination, and be alert to skin tumours and abnormal naevi. Accidents and risk-taking behaviour, avoidance of STIs, and skin protection. Mental health, depression, family and social relationships, work stress.
40–49	Height, weight, BMI, WC, blood pressure, lipid profile. Consider testing for diabetes with HbA1c, and record family history of cancer (bowel, lung, prostate), cardiovascular disease and diabetes. Discuss skin cancers. Take a baseline prostate-specific antigen (PSA) value in men aged 44–50 years with a family history of prostate cancer. Consider measuring testosterone in men with obesity, type 2 diabetes and symptoms of testosterone deficiency (TD). Accidents and risk-taking behaviour, avoidance of STIs, and skin protection. Mental health, depression, family and social relationships, work stress.

Continued

Table 6.1 Age-related considerations for a men's health clinic—cont'd.

Age range (years)	Main considerations
50–74	Height, weight, BMI, WC, blood pressure, lipids, diabetes testing and cardiovascular risk calculation. Remind men about PSA testing if there is a family history of prostate cancer. Offer occult blood testing if there is a family history of colon cancer. Enquire about urological symptoms. Consider testosterone testing in men with obesity, type 2 diabetes and symptoms of TD. Discuss aortic aneurysm screening, especially in smokers. Mental health, family and social relationships, bereavement issues, flu immunisations, sexual health.
75+	Additional discussions may include memory loss, eye health such as cataracts, hearing loss, arthritis, osteoporosis risk, urological and bowel symptoms. Mental health, depression, dementia, family, caregiver and social relationships, death in the family, retirement issues, flu immunisation, importance of lifestyle and socialisation.

Male sexual health

Sexual health is an important part of overall health, and sexual dysfunctions can have an impact on quality of life and emotional wellbeing. A low libido may present as a component of many conditions and problems. Examples include substance abuse (such as alcohol, opioids and other psychotropic drugs), sleep apnoea, chronic fatigue, acute or chronic pain, heart failure, cancer, chemotherapy, multiple sclerosis, chronic kidney disease, hypothyroidism, partner sexual dysfunction, CVD, neurological disease (such as Parkinson or Alzheimer), lack of time or hectic schedule, depression and gender dysphoria.

A short sexual history may include clarifying the nature of the sexual problem. Questions may include: is it always present, or does it only occur sometimes? What is the quality of the erections? Do night time erections occur? Is masturbation taking place? Is pornography being used? Discuss the quality of the erection, in terms of the ability to achieve and maintain it. Enquire about sexual desire, ability to ejaculate and orgasm, if there are any sexual concerns in the partner, the state of the current relationship, what treatments have been tried, the frequency of sexual activity and how this compares to the desired frequency, if both the patient and their partner are motivated to address the problem.

A typical approach may be: 'Many men with diabetes or heart disease have difficulty getting an erection, is this something you would like to discuss?'

Or: 'Sexual difficulties are often a sign of underlying medical problems, please feel free to discuss them with us.'

Erectile dysfunction

ED is a risk factor for CVD and may precede CVD by 3 to 5 years. The presence of ED should trigger a cardiovascular risk evaluation. The British Society of Sexual Medicine (BSSM) has produced a practical guide on the assessment and management of ED in men. This guide is based on the BSSM's full guideline on the management of ED, published in 2018, and should be read in conjunction with the BSSM's practical guide on the assessment and management of TD in adult men, which is based on the BSSM's full guidelines on TD in adult men, published in 2017. The practical guides and full guidelines can be found at: http://www.bssm.org.uk/resources/.

TD is one of the many causes of erectile difficulties, which are more common in older men, smokers, and those with a sedentary lifestyle, obesity, metabolic syndrome (MetS), diabetes or dyslipidaemia.

Lower urinary tract symptoms (LUTS) and ED often coexist, and the complaint of one should trigger an enquiry about the other. There are two useful questionnaires, the International Index of Erectile Function (IIEF) and the IPSS. Interpretation of the IIEF-5 or the Sexual Health Inventory for Men (Fig. 6.2) is as follows: severe ED: 5 to 7; moderate: 8 to 11; mild-moderate: 12 to 15; mild: 17 to 21 and no ED: 22 to 25.

With regards to the IPSS, 0 to 7 equals mildly symptomatic, 8 to 19 moderately symptomatic and 20 to 35 severely symptomatic. There is also a quality of life because of urinary symptoms or a bother index, which is helpful. This ranges from delighted to terrible (0–6).

Managing comorbidities and identifying treatable causes of ED are clearly important. Any advice should be accompanied by appropriate lifestyle advice.

Treatments for ED include phosphodiesterase type 5 inhibitors (PDE5i) as first-line therapy. If these fail, there are some useful alternatives, including vacuum erection devices, intraurethral alprostadil, intracavernous injections, alprostadil cream and, if all else fails, penile prosthesis, which may be an option for men who have had pelvic surgery for cancer.

Testosterone deficiency

All men with ED should be screened for TD, as should those with consistent and multiple signs of TD, type 2 diabetes, BMI greater than 30 kg/m^2, WC greater than 102 cm and those on long-term opiate, antipsychotic or anticonvulsant medication.

Consider the use of validated questionnaires, such as the Androgen Deficiency in the Aging Male (ADAM) questionnaire. The ADAM questionnaire is included in the Sexual Advice Associations SMART SAA app, which can be downloaded at: https://sexualadviceassociation.co.uk/app/.

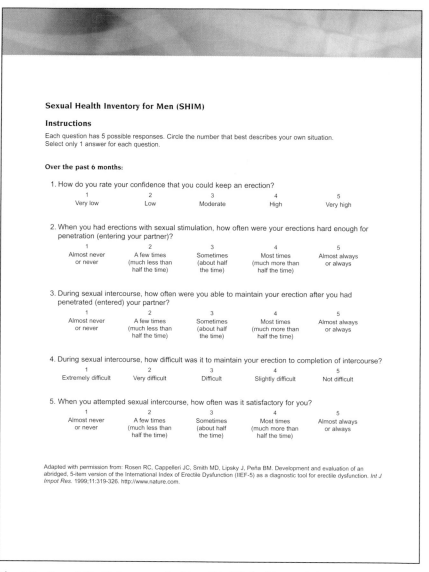

Sexual Health Inventory for Men (SHIM)

Instructions

Each question has 5 possible responses. Circle the number that best describes your own situation. Select only 1 answer for each question.

Over the past 6 months:

1. How do you rate your confidence that you could keep an erection?

1	2	3	4	5
Very low	Low	Moderate	High	Very high

2. When you had erections with sexual stimulation, how often were your erections hard enough for penetration (entering your partner)?

1	2	3	4	5
Almost never or never	A few times (much less than half the time)	Sometimes (about half the time)	Most times (much more than half the time)	Almost always or always

3. During sexual intercourse, how often were you able to maintain your erection after you had penetrated (entered) your partner?

1	2	3	4	5
Almost never or never	A few times (much less than half the time)	Sometimes (about half the time)	Most times (much more than half the time)	Almost always or always

4. During sexual intercourse, how difficult was it to maintain your erection to completion of intercourse?

1	2	3	4	5
Extremely difficult	Very difficult	Difficult	Slightly difficult	Not difficult

5. When you attempted sexual intercourse, how often was it satisfactory for you?

1	2	3	4	5
Almost never or never	A few times (much less than half the time)	Sometimes (about half the time)	Most times (much more than half the time)	Almost always or always

Adapted with permission from: Rosen RC, Cappelleri JC, Smith MD, Lipsky J, Peña BM. Development and evaluation of an abridged, 5-item version of the International Index of Erectile Dysfunction (IIEF-5) as a diagnostic tool for erectile dysfunction. *Int J Impot Res.* 1999;11:319-326. http://www.nature.com.

Fig. 6.2 Sexual Health Inventory for Men. (Modified with permission from Rosen, R. C., Cappelleri, J. C., Smith, M. D., Lipsky, J., & Peña, B. M. (1999). Development and evaluation of an abridged, 5-item version of the International Index of Erectile Dysfunction (IIEF-5) as a diagnostic tool for erectile dysfunction. *International Journal of Impotence Research, 11,* 319–326.)

Information for Clinicians

Scoring instructions

Add the numbers corresponding to the answers for questions 1 through 5. If the patient's score is 21 or less, erectile dysfunction (ED) should be addressed. The SHIM score characterizes the severity of the patient's ED in the following manner:

22–25	No ED
17–21	Mild ED
12–16	Mild-to-moderate ED
8–11	Moderate ED
5–7	Severe ED

Score: _____

Purpose of SHIM

• With the advent of oral therapies for ED, the need for accurate diagnosis is greater than ever.

• The SHIM Questionnaire (also known as the IIEF-5) is an abridged and slightly modified 5-item version of the 15-item International Index of Erectile Function (IIEF), designed for easy use, by clinicians, to diagnose the presence and severity of ED in clinical settings.

• This diagnostic tool may reduce the number of incorrectly diagnosed or underdiagnosed cases. It is intended to complement the physical examination and patient history as a means to detect ED.

Adapted with permission from: Rosen RC, Cappelleri JC, Smith MD, Lipsky J, Peña BM. Development and evaluation of an abridged, 5-item version of the International Index of Erectile Dysfunction (IIEF-5) as a diagnostic tool for erectile dysfunction. *Int J Impot Res.* 1999;11:319-326 http://www.nature.com.

Fig. 6.2 *Continued*

The laboratory diagnosis of TD is made by measuring serum testosterone between 7 am and 11 am, on at least two occasions, preferably 4 weeks apart. Fasting levels should be obtained where possible. If the testosterone level is low or borderline, luteinising hormone and follicle stimulating hormone should also be measured, plus sex hormone binding globulin to calculate free testosterone.

The TD patient should be managed on the basis of action levels rather than laboratory ranges. Total testosterone levels greater than 12 nmol/L are likely to be normal. Levels between 8 and 12 nmol/L are borderline and, if confirmed in the presence of persistent signs and symptoms of testosterone, justify treatment. Levels below 8 nmol/L will almost always benefit from treatment.

Patients taking testosterone replacement therapy should be evaluated at 3, 6 and 12 months, and every 12 months thereafter, to assess serum testosterone (therapeutic levels are in the mid-upper range, 15–30 nmol/L), confirm symptomatic improvement and check for any changes in haematocrit (which should remain <54%) and PSA (an increase of more than 1.4 ng/mL over any one period, or a velocity of 0.4 ng/mL per year warrants urological evaluation).

Testosterone therapy options include testosterone gel and testosterone injections. The gel is delivered transdermally, once daily. Testosterone testing should be done 2 hours after applying the gel, on the opposite arm to which the gel was rubbed, to confirm a satisfactory level.

Testosterone undecanoate is administered via intramuscular injection every 10 to 14 weeks and adjusted to maintain a trough testosterone greater than 12 nmol/L. Administration may be more comfortable if the solution is injected at room temperature, slowly, into the buttock.

Testosterone enanthate is also available as an intramuscular injection but has to be given every 2 to 3 weeks, and the levels fluctuate significantly.

Lower urinary tract symptoms

LUTS is a nonspecific term which refers to any combination of urinary symptoms relating to storage (including urgency, frequency and nocturia) and voiding problems (such as weak or intermittent urinary stream, straining, hesitancy, terminal dribbling or incomplete emptying of the bladder). These symptoms may be related to benign prostatic enlargement, overactive bladder (where the urgency may lead to incontinence), prostatitis, urinary infection, prostate cancer or bladder cancer.

All patients presenting with LUTS need careful examination of the abdomen to check for enlargement of the bladder, a check of the external genitalia to exclude a phimosis, a rectal examination to evaluate the shape and size of the prostate and a basic neurological examination of the lower limbs and perineum.

Investigations include urinary dipstick testing and urea and electrolyte testing if there is a suspicion of renal disease. PSA should be performed after appropriate counselling. A urinary frequency volume chart, filled out over 3 days, can be very helpful. Nocturnal polyuria can be diagnosed if more than one-third of the total 24-hour urinary output occurs at night. It is important to review fluid and food intake and the use of caffeinated drinks, alcohol and spicy foods. Bladder retraining exercises can be very helpful, together with pelvic floor exercises and the avoidance or treatment of constipation.

NICE guidance is available and can be found at: https://www.nice.org.uk/guidance/cg97.

Treatments available for benign prostatic enlargement include α-blocker therapy, which relaxes the bladder neck and prostate smooth muscle, and 5α-reductase inhibitors, such as dutasteride or finasteride, which essentially reduce the size of the gland by about 20%. If symptoms are predominant, an anticholinergic drug, such as tolterodine or solifenacin, can be very helpful, and if ED is present in addition to the LUTS, the PDE5i tadalafil is licensed for this indication. Failure to respond to medications and persistent, bothersome symptoms should trigger a referral to a urologist.

Prostate cancer

This tumour is the most common cancer in men and the second most common cause of cancer death. Risk factors include increasing age, family history and Afro-Caribbean ethnicity. Early prostate cancers are often asymptomatic because they occur in the periphery of the prostate and not close to the urethra. A PSA test can identify prostate cancer, but has significant limitations because the PSA level also increases in the presence of BPH. The advice from the PCRMP (available at: https://www.gov.uk/government/collections/prostate-cancer-risk-management-programme-supporting-documents) is that men over the age of 50 years who request a PSA should be offered balanced information and be able to have the test if they wish to proceed. Multiparametric magnetic resonance imaging (MRI) can be used to identify early prostate cancers and can sometimes avoid the need for biopsy if no tumour is seen. NICE guidance on the identification and management of prostate cancer is available at: https://www.nice.org.uk/guidance/ng131.

In a 2016 publication, Cancer Research UK reported identifying 47,000 diagnosed cases of prostate cancer in 2013 and confirmed that this was the second most common cancer in the United Kingdom, accounting for 13% of all new cases. One in eight men will be diagnosed with prostate cancer during their lifetime. In the United Kingdom, 10,800 men died of prostate cancer in 2012. Survival is improving, partly because of the advent of PSA testing, which has allowed early detection of prostate cancer.

NICE guidance recommends considering a digital rectal examination by a health professional with competency in this procedure and a PSA test for men with any LUTS, such as nocturia, urinary frequency, hesitancy, urgency, retention, ED or visible haematuria. As regards PSA, guidance from the PCRMP in 2016 proposed a single cut-off value of 3 ng/mL to prompt referral for MRI and biopsy if necessary.

Regarding the practicalities of performing the PSA test, the man should not have an active urinary infection, have ejaculated in the previous 48 hours, have exercised vigorously in the previous 48 hours or have had a prostate biopsy in the previous 6 weeks, as these may produce an unreliable result. A baseline PSA value can be helpful in the identification of a rapidly rising PSA in the future, indicating the presence of possible prostate cancer.

The UK National Screening Committee updated its guidance in 2016. Its main message was that it does not currently recommend universal screening for prostate cancer.

Case study

Fred, a 54-year-old unemployed man, had lost motivation of the past few years to find more work. He also reported a lack of energy, feeling tired all the time and dropping off to sleep in the afternoons. He was considerably overweight, with a waist circumference of 110 cm, indicating central obesity. He had lost all interest in sex. His wife was unhappy about this, and concerned about his general health, so she made an appointment for him to have a well-man check.

At this check, his blood pressure and blood lipids were slightly elevated, but his cardiovascular risk calculation was only 8% over the next 10 years. His General Practitioner (GP) did not enquire about erectile function, and the patient did not disclose any issues with this. He was advised to lose weight and take more exercise and to return in 3 months. He went home to tell his wife he was overweight and unfit and needed to go on a diet and take more exercise. He was not motivated to do any of this and failed to attend for further follow up.

If his GP had enquired about erectile function, he would have identified severe erectile difficulties and, as recommended in the guidelines, would have checked his testosterone level, in addition to the other routine tests. In fact, his testosterone level was extremely low, when the diagnosis was eventually made many months later, following a visit to another GP, when he requested a testosterone test himself because he had read up on the signs and symptoms of testosterone deficiency on the Internet.

The prescription for testosterone and a phosphodiesterase type 5 inhibitor significantly improved his erectile capacity and his sex life. The testosterone therapy relieved his symptoms of tiredness and lack of motivation, and over the subsequent year, he managed to lose 2 stone in weight.

At his last check-up, which he attended on his way home from the gym, he told his GP that he was now employed and his wife was happy because she had got the man she had married back.

This case illustrates the importance of early diagnosis and encouraging men to report all their symptoms when they first present, as well as the importance of adopting a healthier, more active lifestyle, reducing alcohol intake and refraining from smoking.

It illustrates the hazards of toxic masculinity and the consequences not only for the man himself, but also for his family.

Testicular cancer

This is the most common solid malignancy diagnosed in men between the ages of 15 and 35 years and accounts for 1% to 2% of all cancers in males. It may present as a nodule or painless swelling of one testicle, although up to one-third of patients do complain of a dull ache or heavy sensation in the lower abdomen, perianal area or scrotum. Periodic palpation of the testes by men themselves ought to lead to the detection of testicular cancers before they cause any symptoms. Early diagnosis, as with all cancers, is important, but testicular germ cell tumours have an overall cure rate of over 90%.

Treatment options include orchidectomy, with or without adjuvant chemotherapy and or/radiotherapy, depending on the stage. Patients who have lost one testicle are at increased risk of developing TD, and this should be borne in mind at follow up, particularly if they have been treated with chemotherapy or radiotherapy, which can damage the remaining testicle.

Metabolic syndrome

According to the International Diabetes Federation consensus worldwide definition, a person is defined as having MetS if he or she has central obesity (WC ≥94 cm in Europid men and ≥80 cm in Europid women, with ethnicity-specific values for other groups) plus two of the following factors:

- Raised triglycerides 1.7 mmol/L (or higher) or specific treatment for this
- Reduced high-density lipoprotein cholesterol less than 1.03 mmol/L in males and less than 1.29 mmol/L in females or specific treatment for this
- Raised blood pressure (systolic ≥130 mm Hg or diastolic ≥85 mm Hg) or treatment for hypertension
- Raised fasting plasma glucose 5.6 mmol/L (or higher) or previously diagnosed type 2 diabetes

Assessment of HbA1c level is also valuable in these patients.

The relationship between low testosterone and obesity is bidirectional. Obesity can give rise to low testosterone, and low testosterone can also promote fat accumulation, insulin resistance and MetS.

MetS is multifactorial, with obesity, a sedentary lifestyle, dietary factors and genetic factors interacting in its occurrence. It is associated with an increased risk of diabetes and stroke in men, as well as the premature development of coronary artery disease. Concomitant low testosterone is also associated with unfavourable levels of several cardiovascular risk factors.

Exercise training can partially reverse MetS, particularly when it is associated with dietary management to reduce weight. A weight loss of more than 5% to 10% is needed for significant improvement in serum testosterone levels.

MetS is often associated with nonalcoholic fatty liver disease (NAFLD), which is an excess of triglycerides in the liver not attributed to excessive alcohol or secondary causes. It is strongly associated with insulin resistance and can progress to advanced liver fibrosis and cirrhosis. NAFLD is usually an incidental finding on liver function tests, or when an ultrasound scan is performed for another reason.

Based on 2016 NICE guidelines, NAFLD should be suspected if a person has risk factors suggestive of MetS, other risk factors for NAFLD, raised liver function tests (LFTs) for 3 months (alanine transaminase level three times higher than normal) or an abnormal ultrasound scan with fatty liver changes.

Management of MetS includes dietary advice, gradual sustained weight loss and regular exercise. Alcohol consumption should be minimal. The management of any comorbidities, such as hypertension, hyperlipidaemia and type 2 diabetes, should be optimised. There should be an annual follow up looking for signs of liver disease that includes measurement of blood pressure, weight, WC, and BMI and blood tests for renal function, HbA1c, lipid profile and LFTs.

Be alert to sleep apnoea in these men. Enquire about excessive daytime sleepiness, choking or gasping during sleep, recurrent awakenings from sleep, unrefreshing sleep, daytime fatigue and impaired concentration. A referral for a sleep study may well be relevant in such men.

There is an inverse and independent association between exercise capacity and the middle-aged population's mortality risk. Men aged 19 to 64 years should accumulate at least 150 minutes of moderate-intensity aerobic physical activity per week. This requirement should be spread across the week, for example, 30 minutes at least 5 days of the week. Alternatively, 75 minutes of vigorous intensity activity provides comparable health benefits, but this should also be spread across the week. Muscle-strengthening activities involving the major muscle groups should be performed at least 2 days per week, in addition to the 150/75 minutes of moderate/vigorous activity.

Greater levels of physical activity are associated with greater health benefits, and patients can be told that, generally, the benefits from performing sufficient physical activity outweigh the risks of injury. These recommendations should, of course, always be tailored to suit the individual's needs and abilities.

Men older than 65 years should also accumulate at least 150 minutes of moderate intensity aerobic physical activity per week and perform muscle-strengthening activities. Older men and those with poor mobility may benefit from physical activity, including balance training on at least 2 days per week to prevent falls. Older men should be advised to gradually increase activity levels over time.

It is important to remind people in all age groups who are overweight that meeting the recommended physical activity criteria will provide numerous health benefits, even if no weight is lost.

Case study

James is a retired information technology consultant who had been drinking more than a bottle of wine a day for the last 20 years, who presented to the practice with tiredness, weakness, skin irritation and marked swelling of the lower legs. There was evidence of jaundice and some signs of bruising. Examination of the abdomen revealed ascites, with diffuse spider naevi present. Blood investigations showed a reduced platelet count, and the aspartate aminotransferase (AST) and alanine aminotransferase (ALT) blood levels were both elevated to 300 IU/L, with an AST:ALT ratio greater than 2.

James was referred to the hospital, where an ultrasound and computed tomography scan suggested a diagnosis of decompensated cirrhosis of the liver, with splenomegaly, associated ascites and early portal hypertension. Following hospital admission, he was treated with diuretics, antibiotics, laxatives, enemas and thiamine. A liver biopsy confirmed the diagnosis. James was advised to avoid alcohol and warned that it may be necessary to have a liver transplant, depending on his progress.

Alcoholic liver cirrhosis is more common in men than in women and may develop in up to 20% of heavy drinkers. Approximately 40% of cirrhosis-related deaths are alcohol-related. Cirrhosis also increases the risk of liver cancer.

A year later, with alcohol withdrawal support, James's liver function had almost returned to normal, and because he had stopped drinking, he had avoided the necessity for a liver transplant.

As far as nutrition goes, combining exercise with dietary advice is the cornerstone of good management. Government-based recommendation on a healthy diet can be found at. https://www.gov.uk/government/publications/the -eatwell-guide.

Weight issues should be addressed in a nonjudgemental and unhurried manner, taking into account the health literacy of the patient. Assess the patient's readiness and ability to change behaviour and incorporate collaborative approaches that involve physicians, nurses, dieticians and other providers in the locality.

Conclusion

To achieve the goal of early diagnosis of diseases relevant to men, there is a need to improve our outreach to men. In part, this can be achieved by making current health centres more accessible, but we must recognise that men will not benefit solely from increasing our opening hours or providing more appointments. In reality, many men would still not access a GP or a General Practice Nurse if they did not feel unwell. There should therefore be investment in finding ways of targeting men more effectively, to identify problems before they become too advanced.

References

British Heart Foundation. (2019a). *UK factsheet (BHF Statistics Factsheet UK).* https://www.bhf
.org.uk/what-we-do/our-research/heart-statistics/heart-statistics-publications.

British Heart Foundation. (2019b). *Heart and Circulatory Disease Statistics 2019 (2019 statistics Compendium (Tables)).* https://www.bhf.org.uk/what-we-do/our-research/heart-statistics
/heart-statistics-publications/cardiovascular-disease-statistics-2019.

Cancer Research UK. (2019). *Cancer statistics for the UK.* https://www.cancerresearchuk.org
/health-professional/cancer-statistics-for-the-uk#heading-Four.

Eurosafe. *Policy briefing 9. Risk taking and injuries among young people.* http://www.euro.who
.int/__data/assets/pdf_file/0006/158181/Policy-Briefieng-9-Risk-taking-and-injuries-among
-young-people.pdf.

Hackett, G., Kirby, M., Wylie, K., et al. (2018a). British Society for Sexual Medicine Guidelines on
the Management of Erectile Dysfunction in Men – 2017. *Journal of Sexual Medicine, 15*(4),
430–457.

Hackett, G., Kirby, M., Edwards, D., et al. (2018b). British Society for Sexual Medicine Guidelines
on Adult Testosterone Deficiency, With Statements for UK Practice. *Journal of Sexual Medicine, 14*(12), 1504–1523.

Office for National Statistics. (2019a). *Homicide in England and Wales: Year ending March 2018.*
https://www.ons.gov.uk/peoplepopulationandcommunity/crimeandjustice/articles/homici-
deinenglandandwales/yearendingmarch2018.

Office for National Statistics. (2019b). *Suicides in the UK: 2018 registrations.* https://www.ons
.gov.uk/peoplepopulationandcommunity/birthsdeathsandmarriages/deaths/bulletins/suicidesin
theunitedkingdom/2018registrations.

Office for National Statistics. (2018). *Deaths registered due to accidental poisoning by drugs, by
age group: England, 2001 to 2017.* https://www.ons.gov.uk/peoplepopulationandcommunity
/healthandsocialcare/drugusealcoholandsmoking/adhocs/009198deathsregisteredduetoacciden
talpoisoningbydrugsbyagegroupengland2001to2017.

Prostate Cancer UK. (2017). *Enlarged prostate.* https://prostatecanceruk.org/prostate-information
/further-help/enlarged-prostate.

Public Health England. (2017). *Research and analysis. Chapter 5: Inequality in health.* https://
www.gov.uk/government/publications/health-profile-for-england/chapter-5-inequality-in
-health#fn:5.

Chapter 7

Women's health

Anne Connolly

Learning outcomes

After reading this chapter you should be able to:

1. Appreciate the importance of the role of the general practice nurse in women's health care
2. Understand the holistic, life-course approach to providing care for women with gender-specific health concerns, which often impact on their physical, social and mental wellbeing, requiring support and empowerment to seek further help
3. Understand the different consultations relating to women's health that frequently present in primary care, appreciating when signposting to information and self-help can be appropriate and when a referral to a more experienced member of the primary care team is required

Introduction

Many essential aspects of women's health care are routinely performed by General Practice Nurses (GPNs), including cervical screening, ring pessary changes and provision of contraception. However, much of the care and support provided is opportunistic.

GPNs are in a privileged position. Women will often find discussing their period problems or other gender-specific concerns with a nurse less embarrassing than when talking to a General Practitioner (GP). Opportunistic encounters can provide women with the support they require, while also providing nurses with an opportunity to signpost them to relevant resources. This empowers women with more of an understanding about their concerns and helps them to make choices about self-care and treatment options.

This chapter begins with an overview of the anatomy of the female genital tract and the menstrual cycle. This is followed with some of the most common concerns that women experience, using a 'life-course' approach. Each section will start with a common scenario, followed by information about how the case can be managed with relevant training or what can be expected following referral on to a clinician with the skills to provide the care required.

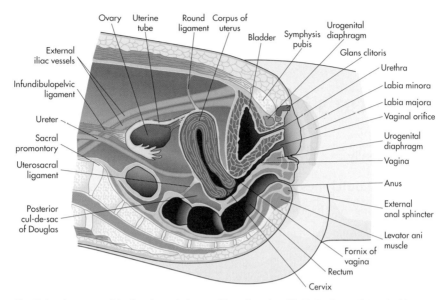

Fig. 7.1 Anatomy of the female genital tract. (From Lowdermilk, D. L., Perry, S. E., Cashion, K., Alden, K. R., & Olshansky, E. F. (2020). *Maternity & women's health care* (12th ed.). Elsevier.)

Anatomy

The anatomy of the female genital tract is shown in Fig. 7.1.

Ovaries

The ovaries are comprised of a central vascular medulla surrounded by an outer cortex. They consist of numerous follicles containing the supply of ova (eggs).

Uterus

The uterus is the shape and size of an inverted, average pear. It is made up of an outer serous layer, a thick muscle layer (myometrium) and a thin glandular layer (endometrium), which surround the central uterine cavity. At the top of each side of the uterus are the fallopian tubes that allow transfer of an egg from the ovary into the uterine cavity.

Cervix

The cervix is a 2.5-cm cylinder that extends from the top of the vagina to become the base of the uterus.

Vagina

The vagina is a fibromuscular 8- to 10-cm-long distensible tube that extends upwards and backward from the introitus at the vulva and is attached to the cervix.

Vulva

The vulva consists of a number of structures, including the mons pubis, labia minora, labia majora and vestibule. The vaginal opening extends from the four-chette posteriorly to the clitoris anteriorly.

Pelvic floor

The pelvic floor is comprised of a number of muscles that support the structures within the lower pelvis.

Menstrual cycle (Fig. 7.2)

The monthly menstrual cycle is reliant on a supply of ova (eggs) being present in the ovary. Women are born with a finite number that gradually reduces until menopause, when the supply is exhausted.

The menarche is the first menstrual cycle, and usually occurs between the ages of 9 and 15 years, about 2 years after the start of puberty (breast bud and pubic hair development).

Menopause is the time when periods end, and typically occurs between the ages of 49 and 52 years.

Between these years, the menstrual cycle is divided into phases.

The proliferative/follicular phase

Follicle-stimulating hormone (FSH) is released by the pituitary gland as a result of stimulation from gonadotrophin-releasing hormone (GnRH) (see Fig. 7.2). This hormone stimulates the ovary, and an ovum develops in a follicle. The developing ovum releases the hormone oestrogen, which blocks further secretion of FSH. Oestrogen causes the endometrial glands to develop so that the endometrium becomes healthy.

Secretory/luteal phase

Luteinising hormone (LH) release from the pituitary gland, also as a result of stimulation from GnRH (see Fig. 7.2), is triggered by the rises in FSH and oestrogen levels. LH completes maturation of the developing follicle, causing release of the hormone progesterone, and stimulates ovulation, when the follicle releases the ovum.

The empty follicle fills with blood and transforms into the corpus luteum, which continues to produce progesterone. Initially, the combination of oestrogen and progesterone stabilises the endometrium, preparing for implantation if a fertilised egg is present. If fertilisation does not occur, the corpus luteum degenerates, and oestrogen and progesterone levels reduce, causing the endometrium to degenerate and shed as menstruation.

The menstrual cycle usually lasts between 24 and 35 days, and the period lasts 4 to 7 days, with an average blood loss of 35 to 70 mL. The first day

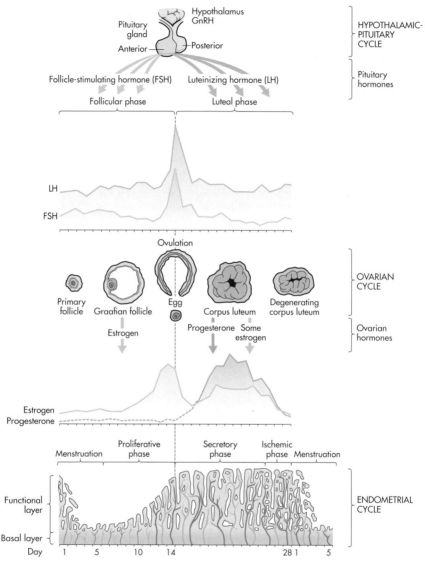

Fig. 7.2   The menstrual cycle. *GnRH*, Gonadotrophin-releasing hormone. (From Lowdermilk, D. L., Perry, S. E., Cashion, K., Alden, K. R., & Olshansky, E. F. (2020). *Maternity & women's health care* (12th ed.). Elsevier.)

of menstruation is counted as day 1 of the cycle, and the cycle length is measured from the first day of one cycle to the first day of the next. Many women track their periods by keeping a diary or using an app, which is useful when needing to find more information about any problem they may describe.

> **Resources**
>
> NHS.UK menstrual cycle animation: https://www.nhs.uk/video/Pages /Menstrualcycleanimation.aspx

> **Case study**
>
> Gemma is a 17-year-old student who attends the local college. She recently started a relationship with Kieran, who is in her art class. She has been taking the 'pill' and wants some more, but she admits that she often forgets to take them and wants to talk about the 'rod' that her friend has.

Contraception

The majority of contraception used in the United Kingdom is provided in primary care clinics by GPNs. This is ideal, as being able to easily access contraception reduces the risks of unplanned or unwanted pregnancy. However, attending training to better understand the risks and benefits of the different contraceptive methods, and therefore be able to offer advice, is necessary.

There are excellent online resources to help advise about contraception for patients and for health care professionals, including those resources found on the sexual health charity Brook's website. Training may be organised locally, but the Faculty of Sexual and Reproductive Health care (FSRH) runs a one-day 'Contraception essentials' course created specifically for primary care nurses that provides a good overview of contraception: https://www.fsrh.org/education -and-training/srh-essentials/.

FSRH also has excellent guidelines, and the UK Medical Eligibility Criteria (UKMEC), the 'safety bible for contraception use', is free to access online: https://www.fsrh.org/ukmec/.

When discussing any method of contraception, it is important to understand:

- Which contraceptive method the patient knows about or has tried before
- How effective of a method she requires
- Which contraceptive methods are safe for her to use
- Whether she can tolerate an unpredictable bleeding pattern
- Whether she wants a method with additional noncontraceptive benefits (i.e., reduced period pains).

Effectiveness

Many women opt to use pills for their contraception, but they do also need to be aware of the long-acting reversible contraceptive (LARC) methods, which are the more effective 'fit and forget' methods that do not require daily administration.

The LARC methods include:

- Copper-containing intrauterine device (Cu-IUD)
- Levonorgestrel-releasing intrauterine system (LNG-IUS)
- Progestogen-only implant
- Progestogen-only injectable

The techniques for inserting intrauterine devices and subdermal implants require additional training, which some GPs and practice nurses undertake to be able to provide these methods to local patients. Further information about this training can be found on the FSRH website under 'Education and training': https://www.fsrh.org/education-and-training/.

The short-acting contraceptive methods are either combined hormonal methods (including pills, patch or vaginal ring) or progestogen-only pills. The barrier methods, including condoms, are less effective at preventing pregnancy but reduce the transmission of sexually transmitted infections (STIs) and should be recommended in conjunction with another, more reliable, contraceptive method. Methods of contraception available in the United Kingdom are noted in Table 7.1.

Table 7.1 Pregnancy rates observed with methods of contraception available in the United Kingdom, excluding emergency contraception

It is clear that some methods are more reliable than others

Method	Typical use (%)	Perfect use (%)
No method	85	85
Fertility awareness–based methods	24	0.4–5
Female diaphragm	12	6
Male condom	18	2
Combined hormonal contraception	9	0.3
Progestogen-only pill	9	0.3
Progestogen-only injectable	6	0.2
Copper-bearing intrauterine device	0.8	0.6
Levonorgestrel-releasing intrauterine system	0.2	0.2
Progestogen-only implant	0.05	0.05
Female sterilisation	0.5	0.5
Vasectomy	0.15	0.1

Modified from Trussell, J. (2011). Contraceptive efficacy. In: Hatcher, R. A., Trussell, J., Nelson, A. L., et al. (Eds.). *Contraceptive technology* (20th ed.). Ardent Media.

Risk assessment

Before providing a method of contraception, it is essential to assess the risks of the different types of contraceptives for each woman on an individual basis. The UKMEC lists all the risks for each method for the majority of conditions (Table 7.2).

Combined hormonal contraception

Combined hormonal contraception (CHC) contains oestrogen and progestogen and can be administered by tablet, patch or vaginal ring. The risks and benefits of CHC are not affected by route of delivery.

One of the benefits of CHC is that the bleeding pattern is predictable and can be prevented altogether if the contraception is taken on a continuous, rather than a cyclical, basis. This noncontraceptive benefit is used in treatment for heavy and/or painful periods.

The disadvantages of CHC include:

- Higher failure rates than LARC methods because of the requirement for regular compliance
- In some women, the experience of hormonal side effects, such as breast tenderness and headaches
- Higher risks than with progestogen-only or nonhormonal methods because of the cardiovascular and thrombotic risks of the oestrogenic component.

Table 7.2 United Kingdom medical eligibility criteria categories

United Kingdom medical eligibility criteria (UKMEC) category	Definition
UKMEC 1	A condition where there is no restriction for the use of the contraceptive method
UKMEC 2	A condition for which the advantages of using the method generally outweigh the theoretical or proven risks
UKMEC 3	A condition where the theoretical or proven risks usually outweigh the advantages of using the method
UKMEC 4	A condition which represents an unacceptable health risk if the contraceptive method is used

From https://www.fsrh.org/standards-and-guidance/uk-medical-eligibility-criteria-for-contraceptive-use-ukmec/.

Table 7.3 Example of United Kingdom medical eligibility criteria guidance

Obesity	Cu-IUD	LNG-IUS	SDI	DMPA	POP	CHC
BMI 30–34 kg/m²	1	1	1	1	1	2
BMI ≥ 35 kg/m²	1	1	1	1	1	3

BMI, Body mass index; *CHC,* combined hormonal contraception; *Cu-IUD,* copper-containing intra-uterine device; *DMPA,* progestogen-only injectable; *LNG-IUS,* levonorgestrel-releasing intrauterine system; *POP,* progestogen-only pill; *SDI,* progestogen-only implant.

From https://www.fsrh.org/standards-and-guidance/uk-medical-eligibility-criteria-for-contraceptive-use-ukmec/.

An individual risk assessment must be made using the UKMEC before recommending use.

See Table 7.3.

Progestogen-only contraception

Progestogen-only contraception has fewer contraindications, meaning these methods are safe for the majority of women to use. Progestogen-only contraception can be provided by pill, injection or subdermal implant, or as an intrauterine system.

When advising a woman on the use of a progestogen-only method, it is impossible to predict how the method will affect her bleeding pattern, and many women may have no bleeding once the method is established (amenorrhoea). This noncontraceptive benefit is an advantage for many but is a concern for other women.

The progestogen-only injection is administered every 3 months, either as an intramuscular or a subcutaneous injection. This method usually produces amenorrhoea after the first few injections. It is important to counsel women that this is the only reversible method that may delay return to fertility on discontinuation, with an average delay of 12 months.

The subdermal implant is the most effective method of contraception currently available and lasts for up to 3 years. This implant is matchstick-sized and is inserted subdermally into the upper arm using local anaesthetic.

The intrauterine devices are either copper-containing (nonhormonal) or progestogen-releasing. These are both extremely effective methods, and both are well tolerated by women who opt to use them.

The Cu-IUD device may last between 5 and 10 years, depending on the device used, and is also the most effective emergency contraceptive method available. As the device is nonhormonal, the bleeding pattern is unchanged, although some women do experience an increase in menstrual flow volume.

The progestogen-releasing intrauterine system may last between 3 and 5 years, depending on device used, and each device has different licensed uses, including contraception, management of heavy menstrual bleeding (HMB) and the progestogen part of hormone replacement therapy.

Other nonhormonal methods

Condoms remain a popular method of contraception; however, efficacy rates are low compared with other methods because of the need for compliance and the failure to apply them correctly. However, they are useful for the prevention of STIs.

Sterilisation offers nonreversible contraception, with the procedure for men (vasectomy) being ten times more reliable than the procedure used for women. Additionally, vasectomy is safer, as this can be performed in the outpatient setting using local anaesthetic, which removes the additional risks of laparoscopic surgery.

Emergency contraception

Emergency contraception requests require advice about the efficacy of the different methods available. Women opting for the more effective Cu-IUD need to know where this can be accessed at short notice.

There are three methods of emergency contraception including, in order of effectiveness (Table 7.4):

- Cu-IUD
- Ulipristal acetate pill
- Levonorgestrel pill

Resources

Brook. Sexual health and wellbeing for under 25s. https://www.brook.org.uk/
NHS UK: Your contraception Guide. https://www.nhs.uk/conditions/contraception/
Sexwise – Contraception advice. https://www.sexwise.fpa.org.uk/contraception
  /which-method-contraception-right-me

Table 7.4 **Three methods of emergency contraception**

	Copper-containing intrauterine device	Ulipristal acetate pill	Levonorgestrel pill
Licensed use after unprotected sexual intercourse (UPSI)	120 hours after UPSI or up to 5 days after anticipated ovulation (day 19 in a 28-day cycle)	120 hours	72 hours

Sexual health

Case study

Natasha is a 22-year-old who has recently finished university. She comes to the surgery to get a new supply of her pills but tells you that she recently went on holiday with her university friends and had sex a couple of times without using a condom. She doesn't have any symptoms but wants to know if she can have a test because she had a chlamydia infection last year and knows it would be good to be tested again.

Sexual history taking is an important skill to gain when working in primary care, with the main challenges being to avoid being embarrassed and to remain nonjudgmental. Women and men are often concerned about discussing their sexual health, but it is important to make sure they appreciate the confidentiality of the consultation, and that they understand that the history is important to be able to make the correct risk assessment and to assess when testing is appropriate.

Many STIs in women are asymptomatic and are transmitted further with a change of partner. Understanding their sexual activity (vaginal, oral, anal) and whether a condom is used on each occasion ensures that, not only is the correct test recommended, but the correct site is tested.

With training, the significant basic questions to ask when discussing possible sexual infections include:

- How long has the problem/concern been going on?
- Does the patient have discharge, and what is it like, including any odour or itch?
- Is there a pattern to any symptoms if she has any?
- Has she taken anything to try to help?
- Does she have any pain?
- And has she had any pain during sex?
- Have her periods changed, including any bleeding between periods or after sex?
- Is she using any contraception, and could she be pregnant (i.e., when was her last normal period)?

To understand the patient's sexual risk, it is important to ask further questions:

- When did she last have sex?
- How long has she been with her partner (be careful not to make assumptions on gender of the partner)?
- When did she have sex with someone other than her current partner?
- And was sex vaginal? Oral? Anal?
- Did they use a condom? And if so, was that for all sex acts?
- Has she been treated for any STIs in the past?

The answers to the questions above help determine when testing is indicated and whether an examination or referral to a more experienced colleague or to the local sexual health clinic is required.

Further training on sexual history taking may be obtained by attending a local training course or FSRH Essentials for primary care: https://www.fsrh.org /education-and-training/srh-essentials/.

Or the STI foundation course: https://www.stif.org.uk/.

Sexually transmitted infections

Chlamydia is a common STI, which is particularly found in younger, sexually active people who have recently changed partner, have had more than one partner in the previous 6 months and do not use condoms. Up to 80% of women who have chlamydia have no symptoms. Those who do have symptoms may notice an increase in vaginal discharge, a change to their bleeding pattern, including bleeding after sex, or pain during and after sexual intercourse. Any woman with symptoms requires examination, but screening is not necessary for asymptomatic women.

Other STIs include:

- Gonorrhoea, which is less frequent and asymptomatic in up to 50% of cases in women. Symptoms are similar to those seen with chlamydia infection, as described earlier
- Genital warts, which are common and may be observed when taking smears, although, since the use of Gardasil for human papilloma virus (HPV) immunisation, the incidence of this infection is decreasing
- Herpes, which causes ulcers similar to those seen with 'cold sores' and can be very painful, especially in the first episode
- Syphilis
- Blood-borne viruses including human immunodeficiency virus (HIV) and hepatitis B and C viruses.

To test for chlamydia and gonorrhoea, it is essential to know which swab is recommended for use in a general practice surgery's respective locality. Testing has become easier with the use of self-taken vulvovaginal swabs. When performing an STI test, a blood test for syphilis and blood-borne viruses should also routinely be offered.

The most common causes of vaginal discharge, however, are caused by non-STIs, including *Candida albicans* infection or bacterial vaginosis (BV). *Trichomonas vaginalis* infection is a STI that can cause a similar discharge to BV, but is rarer in the women seen in primary care. See Table 7.5.

Good guidance for vaginal discharge and other infections can be found on the British Association for Sexual Health and HIV website: http://www.bashh .org.

Table 7.5 Vaginal discharge and other infections

Infection	Bacterial vaginosis	Vulvovaginal candidiasis	Trichomonas vaginalis
	Most common cause of vaginal discharge. Not sexually transmitted	Not sexually transmitted	Sexually transmitted
Symptoms	Watery discharge No irritation Fishy odour	Thick white discharge Itchy vulva No odour	Variable discharge Itchy/soreness/ dysuria Fishy odour
Treatment	Oral/vaginal antibiotics Avoid fragranced products and douching	Topical antifungal treatments If recurrent, consider diabetes and immunosuppression	Oral antibiotics Avoid sexual intercourse Partner testing/ referral

Pelvic inflammatory disease

Pelvic inflammatory disease (PID) is inflammation of the pelvic structures and can be classified as acute or chronic. PID usually results from untreated bacterial STIs, including chlamydia or gonorrhoea.

The presenting symptoms of acute PID include lower abdominal pain, abnormal vaginal discharge or bleeding, deep pain on sexual intercourse (deep dyspareunia) and feeling systemically unwell with fever. In some women, there are no symptoms at all.

Women seen with symptoms suggestive of PID require assessment, including pelvic examination, on the day they present. This is because the symptoms may require urgent treatment if acute but may also mimic other serious concerns (e.g., ectopic pregnancy). Treatment is required with antibiotics, and specialist referral to the local sexual health clinic or admission to gynaecology may be needed if the patient is unwell. If left untreated, the pelvic inflammatory response can lead to scarring and subsequent chronic pelvic pain and infertility.

Resources

Brook. Sexual health and wellbeing for under 25s. https://www.brook.org.uk/
Sexwise – STIs. https://www.sexwise.fpa.org.uk/stis

Cervical screening/human papillomavirus

Case study
Sarah is a 28-year-old mother of twins. She has struggled to find time to attend for her smear test, but her friend has recently had an abnormal result, and she has decided she really needs to have this performed. She has also read online about 'the virus' and wants to know if she has an infection too.

The cervical screening programme started in 1988 and is currently offered to all women every 3 years between the ages of 25 and 50 years, and then every 5 years until the age of 65 years. The prevalence of cervical cancer has significantly reduced since the introduction of screening, which allows early identification of cervical changes and treatment before this progresses.

Over recent years, the importance of the role of HPV as the cause of cervical cancer has been recognised, allowing for the development of an immunisation programme and the inclusion of HPV testing into the National Health Service cervical screening programme (GOV.UK, 2015 updated 2021). These initiatives should reduce further cervical cancer rates and also allow for less frequent screening in women who have been immunised and found to be HPV-negative.

An understanding of the acquisition and role of HPV infection is necessary to help reduce the anxiety and confusion that many women experience when they are informed they may have an infection that is 'sexually acquired'.

- There are more than 100 subtypes of HPV that are divided into those that are high-risk and low-risk for causing cervical cancer. The two most common high-risk HPV (HR-HPV) strains are types 16 and 18, which, along with the other 11 high-risk strains, cause over 99% of cervical cancers.
- HPV infection is common and is transmitted during intimate sexual contact. An estimated 80% of the population contract HPV at some point, which is a useful destigmatising fact that can be used to allay the concern that many women experience when they are informed they are infected with the virus.
- In the majority of women, a normal immune system clears the virus with no requirement for treatment, but some women have persistent infection for many years.
- Some 99% of cases of cervical cancer occur in women with long-term infection with HPV.
- HPV subtypes 6 and 11 are responsible for genital wart infection.
- The HPV vaccine is offered to girls and boys aged 12 to 13 years, offering protection against the HR-HPV strains (16 and 18) and the strains causing genital warts (6 and 11).

The cervical screening programme initially involved sending cervical samples for cytological examination, where abnormal cell structure appearances were identified and, depending on the findings, either the test was repeated

> **Box** 7.1 **Tricks to help with difficult smears**
>
> - Make sure the woman knows what the process involves and how you are going to take the sample
> - Let her know that she can bring a friend with her to help distract or reassure her if she is anxious
> - Have a selection of speculum sizes, as sometimes a smaller one is required
> - Bring the woman to the end of the bed or ask her to put her hands under her bottom to tilt the pelvis if the cervix is very anterior
> - Slide the cut-off finger of a glove (or a condom) over the speculum to allow it to become a tube and to prevent vaginal walls obscuring vision in women with a prolapse.
>
> There are many other tips and tricks that experienced smear takers have, so ask them for advice, because if it makes the experience easier for the woman, it is easier for the smear-taker too.

(low-grade changes), or the patient was referred for colposcopy for further examination and biopsy (high-grade changes).

The programme has continued to change, with the first part of the screening test now involving testing for HPV, and further examination of cell structure abnormalities only being required if the sample is positive for HR-HPV. Approximately 15% to 20% of women with HR-HPV infection will have abnormal cell changes and receive a colposcopy referral for further examination and biopsy/treatment as necessary.

Over the next few years, the combination of immunisation and HPV testing will change the requirements of the programme so that women who have been immunised and who are HPV-negative will require fewer tests. The sample-taking will also change and reduce the need for speculum examination and formal cervical sampling, but this will not stop the need for training in cervical screening for many years, as the immunisation programme only started in 2008.

Performing cervical smear tests can be an important aspect of the work of a GPN and requires extra training, which is comprised of theoretical learning followed by practical training and assessment (Box 7.1).

Details of the training requirements can be found at: https://www.gov.uk /government/publications/cervical-screening-cervical-sample-taker-training.

> **Resources**
>
> NHS.UK What is cervical screening? https://www.nhs.uk/conditions/cervical -screening/
> Jo's Trust (cervical cancer charity). https://www.jostrust.org.uk/

Cervical polyps

> **Case study**
>
> Marie is a 40-year-old receptionist at the local dentist's office. She attends her routine smear appointment. She has no concerns, including no abnormal bleeding or change to her vaginal discharge, has had no problems with previous smears and has always attended on time. On examination you note the cervix appears healthy, other than a small polyp arising from the cervical os.

Cervical polyps vary in size, are usually benign and arise from the cervical canal. They are similar to a skin tag or an extra fold of skin on the inside of the cervix. They may cause no problems or can be symptomatic, with changes to vaginal discharge or postcoital, intermenstrual or postmenopausal bleeding. They can be associated with other polyps inside the uterus, so a decision about referral for further assessment of the endometrium or simple avulsion of the polyp needs to be made.

For newly qualified smear takers who observe any abnormal appearance of the cervix or significant contact bleeding, asking for an opinion from a more experienced colleague is advised.

> **Reflection**
>
> - Discuss with your supervisor how to identify an abnormal cervix and how you may be able to differentiate a normal from an abnormal cervix
> - Identify with your supervisor how you may be able to observe cervical polyps with confidence as part of your smear training
> - How would you describe a polyp to your patient and reassure her in describing this during the consultation?

Preconception

> **Case study**
>
> Ayesha is a 35-year-old diabetic who works in the local supermarket. She is attending the diabetic clinic for her annual follow up and mentions that she and her partner are considering having another baby. She has gained significant weight since her second pregnancy and has a body mass index of 38 kg/m². During her previous pregnancy, she had to use insulin.

To improve the outcome of a pregnancy, it is ideal to optimise the physical and mental health and social wellbeing of the woman before conception.

The GPN is ideally placed to support this work by asking about future pregnancy plans during appointments for other reasons, including long-term condition management, travel immunisations, contraception and cervical screening.

Lifestyle advice, including smoking cessation, dietary changes, weight optimisation (preferably achieving a body mass index between 18 and 30 kg/m^2) and alcohol avoidance, is an important point to cover. If a woman has a long-term condition or mental health concern, it is essential for her to be reviewed by the clinician who normally manages her condition in case medication alteration or further support is required before conception.

Discussing the use of prepregnancy vitamins with a local pharmacist is also a useful suggestion that practice nurses can provide.

Resources

NHS.UK. What is preconception care? https://www.nhs.uk/common-health-questions /pregnancy/what-is-preconception-care/

Planning a pregnancy. https://www.tommys.org/pregnancy-information/planning -pregnancy

---

Fertility

Case study

Amy brings her 4-year-old son for his preschool immunisations. She tells you she is upset because she has been trying for the past 2 years to get pregnant again. She knows that smoking is bad for her, and that she needs to lose some weight, but it is all so hard now that she has the added upset of not conceiving.

Infertility is defined by the World Health Organization as the failure to achieve a clinical pregnancy after 12 months or more of regular, unprotected sexual intercourse.

An estimated one in seven couples has problems with fertility (NICE, 2013, updated 2017), which causes significant upset. The management of fertility problems requires couple-centred care, as the problem may be attributed to issues with sperm production, egg supply or transfer of the sperm to the egg; but often there is no identifiable cause.

It is estimated that:

- One-third of cases of infertility are caused by male problems
- One-third of cases of infertility are caused by female problems
- One-third of cases of infertility are caused by other factors (including same-sex relationships and unknown causes).

The role of the GPN when advising on fertility problems is likely to be opportunistic but provides an opportunity to offer support with smoking cessation and weight optimisation, as well as signposting to support websites for further information and self-care. Lifestyle messages about smoking cessation and weight reduction are important for both partners, as both smoking and excess weight can reduce sperm and egg quality. The charity Tommy's has useful resources for clinicians and people wanting to become pregnant. There is also an online tool that can be downloaded to help with advice and support: https://www.tommys.org/pregnancy-information/planning-pregnancy.

Offering advice about preconception, as above, is important. Encouraging couples to have sexual intercourse 3 to 4 times per week and advising them not to focus on specific times during the cycle is useful in ensuring an adequate supply of sperm for when ovulation (egg release) occurs.

If investigations are indicated, it is important to understand the timing of any blood tests to ensure that the results obtained provide the information required. For the woman, a measurement of FSH is the most useful, as this provides an indication of the woman's remaining egg supply. This test should be performed between day 2 and day 5 of the menstrual cycle for the most accurate results. A man should produce a fresh semen sample to make sure the number and motility of sperm are satisfactory.

Some people with infertility choose not to continue with investigations, but others opt for referral and may require assisted conception, including in vitro fertilisation or similar help. Other options include fostering, adoption or surrogacy.

Resources

NHS.UK. Infertility. https://www.nhs.uk/conditions/infertility/
Infertility and fertility support. https://www.fertilityfriends.co.uk/
Tommy's charity. https://www.tommys.org/pregnancy-information/planning-pregnancy

---

Polycystic ovary syndrome

Case study

Nikki is a 19-year-old student at the local college studying health and social care who attends clinic for her travel immunisations before her summer holiday. She bursts into tears and tells you she is really fed up with the weight gain she has noticed over the past year and the spots and facial hair that she is developing.

On further questioning, she is also worried that she is missing periods – each time she panics that she is pregnant, because she knows she isn't reliable enough with condom use.

Polycystic ovary syndrome (PCOS) is a common endocrine condition, affecting up to 10% of women. It is diagnosed according to the Rotterdam criteria based on the presence of two of three concerns:

- Signs of too much androgen production (acne, hirsutism)
- Infrequent or no periods
- Polycystic ovaries on pelvic ultrasound scan

The condition has:

- Short-term effects including:
  - Acne
  - Hirsutism
  - Male pattern balding
- Mid-term effects including:
  - Subfertility caused by infrequent ovulation (egg release)
- Long-term effects including:
  - Insulin resistance, causing increased risk of diabetes and cardiovascular disease
  - Endometrial cancer because of high oestrogen levels.

The majority of women with PCOS in the United Kingdom are overweight, and the consequences they experience are attributed to insulin resistance. This increases circulating levels of androgens, producing the classical features of acne and hirsutism associated with the condition. In this cohort of women, primary care has an essential role to play in supporting weight reduction and monitoring for other consequences of insulin resistance such as diabetes and cardiovascular disease, similar to the way in which we manage patients with prediabetes.

The weight increase also prevents the hormonal changes required for ovulation to occur, and weight loss is essential to improving ovulation and fertility outcomes. The role of metformin continues to be debated; it is the first recommended treatment for those women who are confirmed as diabetic.

Women who have PCOS and are overweight who do not ovulate in the longer term are at risk of endometrial cancer and require continuous or intermittent courses of progestogens to reduce the risk.

The role of the GPN with regards to women with PCOS is important because they can offer holistic care, including advising on lifestyle improvements to help with weight reduction, signposting to relevant patient information resources and supporting those with poor self-esteem or depression, which is a common concern. In women who can reduce their weight, the fertility outcomes are improved, and long-term health risks are reduced. Occasionally, PCOS is a problem of women who are not overweight, and specialist care is required, especially for fertility advice.

Resources

NHS.UK. Polycystic ovary syndrome. https://www.nhs.uk/conditions/polycystic-ovary-syndrome-pcos/
Verity PCOS (charity). http://www.verity-pcos.org.uk

Premenstrual disorders

> **Case study**
>
> Clare is a 42-year-old English teacher at the school in the neighbouring town and is attending for her smear test. During the procedure she becomes upset, as she is struggling to cope with the challenging behaviour of the students at certain times of each month. She has realised that this is worse before each period. Last month, she went home at lunchtime on one of the days and felt unable to go to school for the next 2 days. She is really worried about what will happen this month.

Premenstrual disorders (PMDs) are a range of common cyclical conditions that occur in the second half (luteal phase) of the menstrual cycle and are relieved by menstruation.

The symptoms experienced by women with PMDs vary in severity, and include:

- Depression
- Anxiety
- Irritability
- Breast pain
- Bloating
- Bowel changes, including constipation and/or diarrhoea
- Sleep problems

The condition is diagnosed from the history and a diary of symptoms. Observing the pattern related to the periods over at least two cycles helps with confirmation.

Women with PMDs require individual support and holistic care. Signposting to relevant online resources so that she can understand the condition and make lifestyle changes will start to help and allow her to be empowered to make choices about any further treatments she may require.

Recommended lifestyle changes include increasing exercise and reducing caffeine and alcohol consumption. Some women finding changing their diet to increase carbohydrate intake in the premenstrual phase helpful. Other women want information about complementary therapies, and a discussion with a pharmacist for further advice may be helpful. As with any long-term condition, holistic individualised support is required.

Some women opt for medical management, which may include first-line treatment via one or both of the following options:

- Cycle suppression to prevent the changes associated with the luteal phase of the cycle:
  - Continuous use of combined hormonal contraceptives (preferably containing drosperinone)
  - Oestrogen patches or cream plus an LNG-IUS or micronised progesterone

- Psychological approach
  - Selective serotonin reuptake inhibitors, either continuously or in the luteal phase
  - Cognitive behavioural therapy

Specialist care may be required if there is no response, or in cases of severe PMDs, for consideration of hormone-blocking treatments to produce a biochemical menopause. Some women with severe symptoms opt for hysterectomy and bilateral salpingo-oophorectomy as a last resort.

Resources

NHS.UK. Pre-menstrual syndrome. https://www.nhs.uk/conditions/pre-menstrual -syndrome/

The National Association of Premenstrual Syndrome. www.pms.org.uk

---

Period problems

Case study

Ciara is a 14-year-old who attends clinic for her asthma review. Her mum asks if it is normal for girls in year 9 to have to miss so much schooling because of their painful periods. She is really worried that if this continues Ciara will struggle with her exams at the end of term. Ciara's periods started when she was 11 and have been painful ever since. The periods are not very heavy, but the pain starts on the day before the bleed starts and becomes unbearable for the first 3 days before starting to improve. Painkillers do not help much.

Endometriosis

Endometriosis is defined as the presence of endometrial-like tissue outside the uterus. The endometrial patches respond to the normal hormonal changes, causing cyclical pain initially, and then, as chronic inflammation and scarring occur, the pain becomes persistent.

An estimated 1 in 10 women of reproductive age suffer from endometriosis, and many do not realise that the pain they experience is not normal, as they have never known anything different (NICE, 2017). Keeping a menstrual diary of symptoms and the pattern associated with menstruation is helpful, as the majority of cases of endometriosis are diagnosed by history alone. Signposting to useful online resources can help by empowering women to understand their condition and the treatment options available to them. The formal diagnosis can only be made by laparoscopy, which may not be required for the majority of women with this condition.

The symptoms women experience vary in type and severity, but may include:

- Painful periods
- Painful sex
- Chronic pelvic pain
- Fatigue
- Depression
- Dysuria
- Dyschezia (rectal pain)

Treatments include:

- Medical:
  - Hormonal: LNG-IUS, combined hormonal contraceptives, oral progestogens, gonadotrophin-releasing hormone analogues
  - Nonhormonal: nonsteroidal antiinflammatories and/or paracetamol and/or codeine, pain modifiers
- Surgical:
  - Laparoscopic ablation/excision of endometriotic lesions
  - Hysterectomy and/or bilateral salpingo-oopherectomy
  - Other surgery if required dependent on involvement of bowel/bladder.

Resources

Endometriosis UK: https://www.endometriosis-uk.org/
NHS.UK. Endometriosis. https://www.nhs.uk/conditions/endometriosis/

Case study

Alice is a 44-year-old teacher at the local secondary school. She attends for her travel vaccines, as she is going to Uganda for the school holiday. She is really concerned about how she will manage when she is away. Her periods have become so heavy that at times she has to take sick leave from work because of the risk of flooding. Her husband has wanted to take her on the trip to see the gorillas for many years, and she doesn't want to let him down.

Heavy menstrual bleeding

HMB is defined clinically as excessive menstrual blood loss which interferes with a woman's physical, social, emotional and/or material quality of life. It can occur alone or in combination with other symptoms (NICE, 2018).

HMB is a common problem that is estimated to affect up to one in three women, particularly women aged over 35 years. This problem causes upset to many women who find that it impacts on their social life, sex life and ability to work, as they worry about the embarrassment of 'flooding'. Many women who suffer with HMB experience tiredness that may be a result of the anaemia they can gradually develop.

In the majority of women, there is no cause found for HMB, but an assessment is important to decide whether examination and investigations are required.

Once again, a menstrual diary is helpful to understand the concern, and a woman can start to keep one while waiting to make an appointment with a GP or nurse practitioner. There are several useful information resources available, including the National Institute for Health and Care Excellence–endorsed shared decision aid for the management of HMB.

The causes of HMB include:

- Dysfunctional uterine bleeding
- Structural causes including:
  Endometrial polyps
  - Fibroids
  - Adenomyosis
  - Malignancy or hyperplasia
- Nonstructural causes including:
  - Coagulation disorders
  - PCOS
  - Iatrogenic (use of anticoagulants).

Investigations depend on the assessment made from the history of the HMB and the examination findings:

- All women require a full blood count to exclude anaemia
- A cervical smear is recommended in women who are due or overdue
- A pelvic ultrasound scan (preferably transvaginal) is usually useful to assess adenomyosis or general uterine enlargement from fibroids but is not useful for assessing endometrial concerns
- Hysteroscopy allows a direct view and assessment of the endometrium and is recommended if there is endometrial pathology (polyps, submucosal fibroids, malignancy)
- Other tests such as thyroid function, coagulation screening, STI screening and pregnancy testing should be performed following individual assessment.

Treatment options depend on whether a specific cause is identified, (e.g., endometrial polyp resection). In women with no identifiable cause, the treatment decisions will be influenced by her imminent and future fertility requirements, as hormonal treatments are usually contraceptive. Surgical treatments are not recommended in women who may want to conceive in the future (Fig. 7.3).

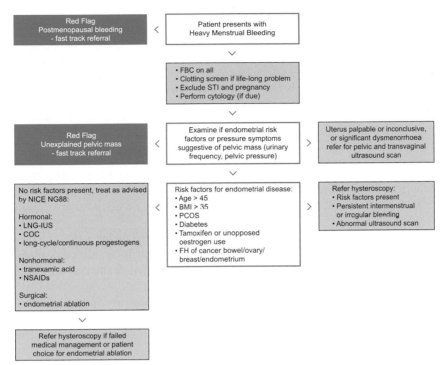

Fig. 7.3 Management of heavy menstrual bleeding flow chart. *COC*, Combined oral contraception; *FBC*, full blood count; *LNG-IUS*, levonorgestrel-releasing intrauterine system; *NSAIDs*, nonsteroidal antiinflammatory drugs; *PCOS*, polycystic ovary syndrome; *STI*, sexually transmitted Infection. (Modified from NICE. (2018). *Heavy Menstrual Bleeding: assessment and management. NG88.* www.nice.org.uk/guidance/ng88.)

Treatment options include:

● Medical
  ● Hormonal: LNG-IUS, combined hormonal contraceptives, oral progestogens
  ● Nonhormonal: tranexamic acid, nonsteroidal antiinflammatory drugs
● Surgical
  ● Endometrial ablation
  ● Myomectomy
  ● Hysterectomy
● Nonsurgical
  ● Uterine artery embolization.

Resources

NHS.UK. Heavy periods. https://www.nhs.uk/conditions/heavy-periods/
National Institute for Health and Care Excellence–endorsed shared decision aid for patients. https://www.nice.org.uk/guidance/ng88/resources/endorsed-resource-shared-decision-making-aid-for-heavy-menstrual-bleeding-6540669613

Incontinence

> **Case study**
>
> Julie, a 65-year-old woman who suffers from chronic obstructive pulmonary disease, attends for her flu jab. She has always avoided having one, but last winter she had a bad chest infection that caused her to cough for months and made her urinary incontinence much worse. She has tried to comply with her inhalers better so that the incontinence is not such a problem.

As with many female-related problems, urinary incontinence is a frequently occurring problem that causes much embarrassment and is underreported. The problem can occur at any age, but it is more common in older postmenopausal women.

There are different types of urinary incontinence, and taking a short history of the problem will help determine which is the main issue, although many women will have a mixed picture, in which case management should be directed to the type causing the most concern (NICE, 2019).

Stress incontinence is caused when abdominal pressure is increased by activities such as coughing, jumping, running or laughing, and the pelvic floor muscles are not strong enough to prevent loss of small amounts of urine. The biggest risk factor for pelvic floor muscle weakness is vaginal childbirth.

Urgency is another problem many women experience as they get older and encounter the need to urinate frequently, with or without episodes of incontinence. This problem often restricts activities, with some women finding they have to map their trips out to be within close reach of a toilet. Urgency is caused by bladder muscle overactivity and can be aggravated by caffeine, fizzy drinks and smoking.

There are other causes of incontinence in women that require different assessment and management. If patients exhibit symptoms such as abdominal bloating or pelvic pressure, then they should be advised to seek further help.

It is good practice to routinely perform a urine dipstix if a woman describes incontinence, as sometimes this is a sign of urine infection, undiagnosed diabetes or bladder cancer, and a simple test can exclude any of these if it is negative.

Once a negative result has been obtained from a dipstix test, women can be signposted to some simple advice and resources that will improve their understanding and start to treat their problem.

Chronic constipation can cause incontinence, and simple dietary advice to increase fibre intake will help. Advising on maintaining an adequate and appropriate fluid intake and restricting caffeine and fizzy drinks, as well as offering weight management and support, can all make a significant difference to the quality of a woman's life by reducing her incontinence and improving her confidence.

The pelvic floor muscles need training to strengthen them and make them work better. There are many websites where these are explained, and

Box 7.2 How to do pelvic floor exercises

- These can be done when lying, sitting or standing, but not when sitting on the toilet passing urine
- Squeeze the muscles as if trying to stop the flow of urine or passing wind
- Make sure the squeeze pulls the muscles up and does not push them down
- Repeat this quickly ten times
- Then repeat slowly, trying to hold each contraction for 10 seconds
- Relax the muscles fully between each contraction, and be careful not to use the stomach muscles
- A woman can check by putting a finger into the vagina and feeling a squeeze.

encouraging women to do these exercises as a daily routine will reduce their problems (Box 7.2).

Bladder diaries, which can be found on the Internet, are useful to help assess drinking habits and measure urine volume and urination frequency. They can also be used to identify if there are any triggers for incontinence, such as running or coughing.

Bladder retraining is another useful management tool, particularly for women suffering with urge incontinence, as it helps the bladder to increase in capacity. The trick is to try to hold on when the urge to urinate starts, including squeezing the pelvic floor muscles to reduce the frequency of bladder empty-ing. Avoiding bladder irritants, including caffeine and carbonated drinks, and increasing intake of water may produce the results your patient is hoping for.

If simple advice is insufficient, then recommended additional treatments include the use of antimuscarinic medication and/or topical vaginal oestrogens.

Resources

Bladder and Bowel UK. https://www.bbuk.org.uk/
Bladder and bowel community. https://www.bladderandbowel.org/
NHS.UK. Urinary incontinence. https://www.nhs.uk/conditions/urinary
  -incontinence/

Pelvic organ prolapse

Case study

Kathy is 65 years old and attends for her last smear test, or so she hopes. She tells you that last time the nurse had a problem taking the smear and had to ask for help from another nurse. She thinks she might have a prolapse because she notices a lump when she goes to the toilet and sometimes she becomes very constipated.

As described, childbirth by vaginal delivery is traumatic to the pelvic floor muscles. As women age and the muscle strength reduces, an estimated 50% of parous women develop a uterine prolapse. There are different degrees and types of prolapse, and they affect women in different ways.

The usual time that a practice nurse will notice a prolapse is when trying to take a cervical smear, as prolapse makes visualisation of the cervix difficult. A useful trick for clinicians who are confident in smear taking is to use the cut-off finger of a glove or a condom, as described earlier (see Box 7.1). If problems are anticipated, then asking an experienced colleague to assist is recommended, in addition to referring on to a clinician who can assess and advise on the pelvic organ prolapse.

Reducing any factors that aggravate the problem will improve some prolapse symptoms, such as encouraging women to increase fibre in their diet to avoid constipation or improving control of chronic obstructive pulmonary disease to reduce coughing. Some women find double urinating helpful (going once, standing up, then passing urine again), and pelvic floor exercises will help relieve symptoms, but sometimes a discussion about use of a ring pessary to support the prolapse or consideration for surgery is required.

Pessaries are varied in type and function, but the ones used most commonly are ring pessaries. These require sizing initially to make sure they sit comfortably in the vagina to support the pelvic floor.

Many GPNs will have learned to change ring pessaries when they need reviewing, which is usually on a 6-monthly basis. Training and assessment of competence is required when reviewing and changing a ring pessary. Having this performed locally at the GP practice is more convenient for women. Traditionally, polyvinyl chloride rings have been used, but the newer milex rings are easier to insert and remove, as they have a notch that allows them to fold. Further information about ring pessary management and the competency required can be found on the Primary Care Women's Health Forum website: https://www.pcwhf.co.uk/resources/conservative-management-of-prolapse-competency-framework-for-primary-care/.

Resources

NHS.UK. Pelvic organ prolapse. https://www.nhs.uk/conditions/pelvic-organ-prolapse/

Vulval problems

The skin of the vulva and perineum can be affected by skin conditions such as psoriasis, problems such as lichen sclerosus or lichen planus or malignancy.

Cancers of the vagina and vulva are rare but will present as abnormal bleeding, persistent irritation of the skin or a lump on the vagina or vulva.

Sometimes when examining women for other reasons, such as a smear test or change of ring pessary, the vulva will look red and excoriated, or the skin may change colour and appear white. Any abnormal appearance or complaint of persistent irritation or a lump should not be ignored and needs to be referred to a clinician in the practice who has more experience of dealing with vulval conditions.

Basic vulval care advice that can be provided for all women who complain of vulval soreness or irritation includes:

- Soap avoidance: including washing with water or soap substitutes and avoiding bathing or washing with soaps or gels
- Use of nonbiological washing powder
- Frequent use of emollients to reduce inflammation and irritation and to act as a barrier cream if there is pain on urination.

Resources

NHS.UK. Lichen sclerosus. https://www.nhs.uk/conditions/lichen-sclerosus/
NHS.UK. Vulval cancer. https://www.nhs.uk/conditions/vulval-cancer/
Primary care dermatology society. http://www.pcds.org.uk

Ovarian cancer

Ovarian cancer survival rates are poor, mainly because women do not recognise early symptoms, resulting in the diagnosis being made at a late stage of the disease. The symptoms are extremely hard to recognise, as they are vague and similar to many less concerning issues, such as irritable bowel syndrome.

The main symptoms of ovarian cancer are abdominal distension, bloating and feeling full quickly after eating (NICE, 2011). Other symptoms include a change in bowel habit, urinary urgency, tiredness and postmenopausal bleeding. If a woman comments on any of these symptoms when being seen for other issues, she should be advised to see someone in the practice who is more experienced with these concerns. Keeping a diary to note any pattern to the symptoms is useful, and examples can be found on the Internet.

Resources

NHS.UK. Ovarian cancer. https://www.nhs.uk/conditions/ovarian-cancer/
Ovarian Cancer Action. https://ovarian.org.uk/ovarian-cancer/
Target Ovarian Cancer. https://www.targetovariancancer.org.uk/

Conclusion

The role of the GPN in women's health care is important but undervalued.

There are opportunities to undertake training to develop skills in provision of care in:

- Contraception
- Sexual health

- Cervical screening
- Ring pessary insertion

There are also enhanced and advanced roles that some GPNs are taking on with additional training, including:

- Intrauterine device and contraceptive implant insertion and removal
- Managing young people's clinics for contraception and sexual health
- Supporting clinics for women with menopause or menstrual problems
- Becoming a cervical screening lead for the practice.

The majority of women will prefer to have their care delivered closer to home in their local primary care setting to avoid having to take time out of their busy lives to attend unnecessary specialist clinics. Training in women's health care is rewarding and an opportunity to provide holistic support and care.

References

Conservative management of prolapse – competency framework for primary care. https://pcwhf.co.uk/resources/conservative-management-of-prolapse-competency-framework-for-primary-care/.

GOV.UK. (2015). *Cervical screening: Programme overview*. https://www.gov.uk/guidance/cervical-screening-programme-overview.

NICE. (2011). *Ovarian cancer: Recognition and initial management. CG122*. www.nice.org.uk/cg122.

NICE. (2013, updated 2017). *NICE Fertility problems; assessment and treatment. CG156*. www.nice.org.uk/guidance/CG156.

NICE. (2017). *NICE Endometriosis: Diagnosis and management*. NG73. https://www.nice.org.uk/guidance/NG73.

NICE. (2018). *NICE Heavy Menstrual Bleeding: Assessment and management. NG88*. www.nice.org.uk/guidance/ng88.

NICE. (2019). *Urinary incontinence and pelvic floor prolapse in women: Management. NG123*. https://www.nice.org.uk/guidance/ng123.

Trussell, J. (2011). Contraceptive efficacy. In: Hatcher, R. A., Trussell, J., Nelson, A. L., et al. (Eds.). *Contraceptive technology* (20th ed.). Ardent Media.

UK Medical Eligibility Criteria (UKMEC). https://www.fsrh.org/standards-and-guidance/.

Chapter 8

Menopause

Louise Newson

Learning outcomes

After reading this chapter you should be able to:

1. Understand the main symptoms of perimenopause and menopause
2. Increase your knowledge of safe hormone replacement therapy (HRT) prescribing, especially with respect to body-identical HRT
3. Learn about alternative ways of managing menopause

Introduction

Menopause is a not an illness but a normal life event for practically every woman who comes through the doors of your practice. However, that is not to say the menopause is usually an easy time for women. Symptoms such as hot flushes, fatigue, low mood, memory problems, muscle pains and vaginal dryness can all impact upon a woman's physical and mental health. The hormonal changes that occur during and after the menopause can also lead to long-term health problems, including an increased risk of osteoporosis, cardiovascular disease, type 2 diabetes, depression, osteoarthritis and dementia.

How much knowledge do you have of the menopause?

Managing women with symptoms of the menopause is a very rewarding aspect of clinical practice, and there are many examples of excellent care.

Yet research and anecdotal evidence show that the effects of the menopause are all too often underestimated or misdiagnosed by health care professionals. For example, diagnostic overshadowing can occur when low mood symptoms associated with menopause are mistaken for depression. Sadly, women do not always receive evidence-based advice and appropriate treatment to manage their symptoms. A recent survey of 203 health care professionals found that, although 86% thought the menopause should be managed in primary care, one-third admitted they were unconfident in managing the menopause among their patients. Tellingly, only half (52%) said they had had specific training in menopause management (Newson & Mair, 2018).

This lack of confidence because of a lack of training has a knock-on effect on patient care. A separate 2019 survey of nearly 5000 women by Newson Health

> **Box 8.1 Menopause: what general practice nurses need to know**
> - An explanation of the stages of menopause
> - Common symptoms and diagnosis
> - Long-term health implications of menopause
> - Benefits and risks of treatments for menopausal symptoms
> - Lifestyle changes and interventions that could help general health and wellbeing
>   This chapter will cover these key points so you can help women make an informed decision about how to manage their menopause.

Research and Education found that one-third of women reported having to wait at least 3 years before their perimenopausal symptoms were correctly diagnosed (Newson Health Research and Education, 2019). Some 59% of women with menopausal symptoms visited their General Practitioner (GP) more than twice, and 18% more than six times, before they received adequate help or advice.

The role of general practice nurses in good menopause care

Women whose lives are being affected by troublesome symptoms should not feel they have to suffer in silence (National Institute for Health and Care Excellence [NICE], 2015). Good menopause care is essential, and that is where you can play a crucial role.

A general practice is often the first port of call for women experiencing menopausal symptoms. This means that, as a General Practice Nurse (GPN), having an understanding of menopause symptoms, long-term health implications and treatments is key to making a prompt diagnosis and helping women in your care.

There are now a number of excellent menopause guidelines and sources of information for health care professionals, including the 2015 NICE guideline on menopause diagnosis and treatment (Box 8.1). Using these guidelines, you can be a powerful advocate for your patients. By offering support and giving clear, evidence-based information, your expertise can help women make informed decisions about treatments and lifestyle changes.

The menopause stages explained

Menopause occurs when a woman stops menstruating. The ovaries stop producing eggs and secreting oestrogen, progesterone and testosterone (NICE, 2015).

There are four stages:

1. Premenopause: the time before any menopausal symptoms occur.
2. Perimenopause: when women experience menopausal symptoms because of hormone changes but still have monthly periods (this is sometimes known as the menopause transition).
3. Menopause: usually defined as when a woman has not had a period for 12 consecutive months (for women reaching menopause naturally).

4. Postmenopause: the time after a woman has not had a period for 12 consecutive months. Women spend on average one-third of their life in the postmenopausal stage (Currie, 2017).

The average age of menopause is 51, and symptoms of the perimenopause often start at around 45 years of age (NHS.uk, 2018).

Oestrogen and progesterone work together to regulate the menstrual cycle and production of eggs. Oestrogen is also an important hormone for a number of functions, including bone health, cognition, mood and skin health. The levels of these hormones fluctuate and decline during perimenopause and menopause, and it is these hormone changes that trigger a range of symptoms throughout the body. Testosterone is also a really important hormone for many women and is actually produced in larger quantities than oestrogen before the menopause.

Early menopause and premature ovarian insufficiency

If menopause occurs when a woman is younger than 45 years, it is known as an early menopause. Menopause in women younger than 40 years is usually referred to as Premature Ovarian Insufficiency (POI).

About one in 100 women in the United Kingdom younger than 40 years have POI, and it affects about one in 1000 women younger than 30 years (Daisy Network, 2019).

For most women, the underlying cause is not known. However, it can be attributed to one of the following:

- Treatment for cancer: radiotherapy (particularly to the pelvic area) and chemotherapy.
- Surgery: including an oophorectomy or a hysterectomy, even when the ovaries remain intact. Menopause because of medical treatment or surgery is known as medical or surgical menopause.
- An autoimmune disease.
- A genetic condition: particularly Turner syndrome.

Diagnosing menopause

If a woman is older than 45 years, is having irregular periods and other typical symptoms and is otherwise healthy, then a health professional should be able to diagnose the menopause on history alone without the need for tests (NICE, 2015). Women should be asked to download the free app balance and create a Health Report from it which will aid the diagnosis. Women then complete the Menopause Symptom Questionnaire included in this app before their consultation and then often make the diagnosis themselves.

In addition, if a woman has had her ovaries removed at any age, she should not need any tests to confirm a surgical menopause.

Diagnosing menopause in women younger than 40 years

The 2015 NICE guideline states that, if POI is suspected, it can be diagnosed based on two factors:

1. Menopausal symptoms, including no or infrequent periods
2. A blood test to measure the levels of follicle stimulating hormone (FSH). If this is raised, then it is very likely a woman is menopausal. However, the test should be repeated 4 to 6 weeks later to confirm diagnosis, because FSH levels vary at different points of the menstrual cycle.

Additional testing for younger women

If POI is suspected, a woman can be referred to a menopause specialist or managed by a GP with an interest in the menopause. After a diagnosis is made, women should also have a dual energy X-ray absorptiometry bone density scan because low levels of oestrogen increase the risk of osteoporosis.

Women younger than 35 years may also be offered a blood test to determine if a chromosomal problem is causing POI.

General signs and symptoms of menopause

About three in four women will experience symptoms during their menopause (NICE, 2015) (Box 8.2). The severity of symptoms varies among women. The average duration of symptoms is about 4 years (Avis et al., 2015), but many women actually experience symptoms for decades. You should also be aware that symptoms can overlap (e.g., cognitive problems and poor sleep). Symptoms can also vary with time, so often women find that their vasomotor symptoms improve, and then they develop symptoms such as low mood and anxiety or

---

Box 8.2 Common Symptoms of Menopause

- Hot flushes and night sweats
- Palpitations
- Low mood
- Anxiety
- Reduced motivation
- Muscle and joint pains
- Fatigue
- Memory problems
- Headaches and worsening migraines
- Reduced libido
- Vaginal dryness
- Urinary frequency and urgency

From: NICE. (2015). Menopause: diagnosis and managment. https://www.nice.org.uk/guidance/ng23.

vaginal dryness. Once a woman has gone through her menopause she is unable to replace the hormones that her body used to produce, so she always has these health risks of the menopause.

Period changes

This is often the first symptom women may present with when perimenopause or menopause is suspected. Women may experience a change in flow, and periods will become less frequent before stopping completely. Some women find that their periods become more frequent and heavier during the perimenopause.

Vasomotor symptoms

Hot flushes are the most common symptom of all, affecting three out of four women (Women's Health Concern, 2015). They can come on suddenly at any time of day, lasting for moments or several minutes. Hot flushes can be accompanied by symptoms such as sweating, dizziness or heart palpitations. Night sweats are another vasomotor symptom, with many women waking up drenched in sweat.

Anxiety, low mood and other mood changes

Mood changes tend to be common if a woman has had premenstrual syndrome in the past.

It is important to distinguish whether these symptoms are a result of menopause-related hormone changes or other forms of depression, as symptoms can overlap.

This will help curb inappropriate prescribing of antidepressants, which are frequently incorrectly prescribed as a first-line treatment for low mood associated with the menopause, despite clear lack of evidence for their efficacy and their unfavourable side effect profile (Leonhardt, 2019).

Fatigue and poor sleep

Poor sleep can be linked to night sweats and low mood.

Brain fog

A collective term for symptoms such as memory slips, poor concentration and difficulty absorbing information. Many women find this presents a challenge not only at work, but also in simple tasks such as reading a book.

Vaginal and urinary symptoms

Low oestrogen can lead to vaginal atrophy or atrophic vaginitis, where the tissues around the vagina become itchy, painful and inflamed.

A lack of oestrogen can lead to thinning and weakening of the tissues around the neck of the bladder and the urethra, which can lead to recurrent urinary tract infections, urge incontinence or cystitis.

Low libido

Testosterone levels also fluctuate and reduce during the perimenopause and menopause, and this can lead to poor sex drive, as well as symptoms of low mood, reduced energy and brain fog. Symptoms of vaginal atrophy can also make intercourse painful and contribute to a lack of libido.

Joint pains and muscle aches

A lack of oestrogen can lead to inflammation in the joints, and muscle pains are also common.

Hair and skin changes

A lack of oestrogen causes reduced blood flow to the epidermis, and this can lead to dry, wrinkled skin. Some women may also develop formication, typified by feelings of numbness, tingling, prickling or a crawling sensation on the skin. Androgens can become more prominent as oestrogen falls, which can lead to increased facial hair and thinning hair on the scalp in some women.

Worsening Migraines

Women many find episodes become more frequent and severe.

Long-term health implications of the menopause

Osteoporosis

Women lose up to 10% of bone density in the 5 years after the menopause.

Other risk factors for osteoporosis to be aware of in your patient include a family history of osteoporosis, high body mass index (BMI), long-term use of high-dose oral steroids, smoking and drinking alcohol.

Cardiovascular disease

Oestrogen helps keep blood vessels healthy because it reduces inflammation in the endothelium and helps control low-density lipoprotein cholesterol levels.

Other risk factors for cardiovascular disease include family history, high BMI, smoking and raised blood pressure.

There is also an increased risk of developing type 2 diabetes, obesity, depression and dementia.

There are also oestrogen receptors on all cells that fight infections, known as immune cells. Oestrogen works to improve the number, genetic programming and lifespan of all these immune cells.

At the time of writing, research into the link between COVID and oestrogen is still emerging. It is likely that oestrogen provides some protection against severity and mortality of COVID infections and is likely to explain some of the gender difference with respect to COVID infections.

An analysis of electronic health records of nearly 70,000 patients who tested positive for COVID-19, from 17 countries, showed that women taking replacement oestrogen (HRT) were more than 50% less likely to die from COVID-19 compared to women not taking HRT. More work is being done in this important area (Seeland, Coluzzi et al., 2020).

Another study from UK has shown that women taking HRT were nearly 80% (OR0.22) less likely to die from Covid compared to women not taking HRT (Dambha-Miller, Hinton et al., 2021 Preprint).

Female hormones are likely to be important for Long Covid also. The largest group of patients with Long Covid are women aged 45-60 and many women are reporting changes or cessation of their periods (Carson et al., 2021). Many of these women will also be perimenopausal or menopausal yet few women are offered or given HRT to replace their missing hormones which will potentially also improve many of their symptoms. The symptoms of Long Covid are very similar to the symptoms of the perimenopause and menopause.

Menopause treatments

The 2015 NICE guideline state that, when a woman speaks to a health professional about her symptoms, she should receive information about the following treatments, all of which will be covered in this section:

- Hormonal treatments, for example, hormone replacement therapy (HRT)
- Nonhormonal treatments
- Nonpharmaceutical treatments, for example, cognitive behavioural therapy.

HRT remains the first-line treatment for the management of menopausal symptoms in most women, improving quality of life and protecting against long-term health risks. Yet a study has shown that in some parts of the United Kingdom only one in 10 women who would benefit from HRT actually take it (Cumming et al., 2015).

There are numerous potential benefits to be gained by women taking HRT. Symptoms of the menopause such as hot flushes, mood swings, night sweats and reduced libido improve. In addition, taking HRT has also been shown to reduce future risk of cardiovascular disease, osteoporosis, type 2 diabetes, osteoarthritis and dementia (Rossouw et al., 2002).

Most benefit is afforded when women start HRT within 10 years of their menopause.

Oestrogen-only and combined hormone replacement therapy

All types of HRT contain oestrogen. Nowadays the National Health Service (NHS) and menopause specialists increasingly prescribe body-identical oestrogen, which is derived from yams and has the same molecular structure as oestrogen produced in the body. The most common body-identical oestrogen is 17β-oestradiol.

Women should only be prescribed estrogen-only HRT if they have had their uterus removed. If the uterus is intact, oestrogen-only HRT can lead to endometrial hyperplasia and can increase the risk of endometrial cancer. Therefore, a combined HRT containing both oestrogen and progesterone is needed, as progesterone reverses this risk. Progestogens, synthetic forms of progesterone, can be used for this element of HRT. However, micronised progesterone, derived from yams, is increasingly being used, as it is body-identical and is associated with fewer side effects and fewer risks to health than progestogens.

Hormone replacement therapy routes of administration

The oestrogen element of HRT is available as a transdermal patch, gel, cream or oral tablet, whereas the body-identical progesterone element is available as an oral tablet (micronised progesterone). Alternatively, the progestogen part can be given as a Mirena coil, which can be used for endometrial protection for 5 years. There are also some patches that contain a combination of oestrogen with a progestogen.

This means that HRT can be altered if necessary to find the optimum dosage and route of administration: for example, some women may find transdermal patches can cause local skin irritation, and for these women the gel is often preferable.

Combined HRT products are available but bear in mind there is less flexibility in altering the oestrogen dose, and they contain older progestogens.

Evidence suggests a combination of transdermal oestrogen and micronised progesterone represents the optimal HRT regimen, particularly in women at risk of cardiovascular events (Newson & Lass, 2018).

Note: Women with POI should take HRT (or the oral combined contraceptive pill) at least up until the age of natural menopause to ease symptoms and to safeguard against an increased risk of long-term health problems such as osteoporosis and cardiovascular disease (NICE, 2015).

Hormone replacement therapy benefits

Symptoms improve

Hot flushes and night sweats usually cease within a few weeks of starting HRT. Vaginal and urinary symptoms usually resolve within 3 months but can take up to a year in some cases.

Other symptoms such as mood changes, difficulty concentrating, joint pain and skin complaints should also improve.

Cardiovascular disease risk reduces

There is some evidence that taking HRT, particularly oestrogen-only HRT, reduces the risk of cardiovascular disease (Boardman et al., 2015). The benefits are greatest in women who start HRT within 10 years of their menopause. HRT also reduces risk of developing osteoporosis, type 2 diabetes, osteoarthritis and depression.

Osteoporosis risk reduces

Taking HRT can help prevent and reverse bone loss, even for women who take lower doses of HRT, so it can reduce risks of bone fracture attributed to osteoporosis. HRT also reduces risk of developing osteoporosis, type 2 diabetes, osteoarthritis, clinical depression and dementia. Women who take HRT for 18 years have a lower risk of all cause mortality, including from cancer (Manson et al., 2017).

Hormone replacement therapy risks

For the majority of women who start taking HRT before the age of 60 years or within 10 years of their menopause, the benefits of HRT outweigh the risks (NICE, 2015).

A thorough consultation is needed to determine the most appropriate HRT preparation and route of administration, taking into account existing conditions, medical history, contraindications, whether a woman still has uterus and if she is still having periods.

Risks of HRT vary depending on the route of administration (oral or transdermal) and on whether the preparation contains a body-identical or synthetic hormone.

It is the possible increased risk of breast cancer with some types of HRT which concerns both women and health professionals the most. However, not all types of HRT are associated with an increased risk of breast cancer, as detailed later, and it is very important that women and health care professionals know this.

Studies have shown that women who take ooestrogen-only HRT have a lower risk of breast cancer and a lower risk of dying from breast cancer (Manson et al., 2017).

In women older than 51 years (the age of natural menopause), taking combined HRT containing synthetic progestogens may be associated with a small risk of developing breast cancer. But to put this risk into perspective, this risk is less than the risk of breast cancer in women who are obese, and is similar to the risk in those women who have never had children and also those women who drink a glass or two of wine each day. Some studies show this risk is lower (or even not at all) in women taking micronised progesterone, and women who take HRT containing micronised progesterone do not have an increased risk of breast cancer for the first 5 years of taking HRT. After this time, the risk of breast cancer is lower than with taking HRT containing synthetic progestogens.

Women with a history of blood clots, liver disease or migraine can still take HRT, but an oestrogen patch or gel or spray is preferable because these methods are associated with no risk of clots. If a woman still has her womb, then she should be given micronised progesterone or a Mirena coil. There is a small risk of clots with the older oral progestogens.

Side effects of hormone replacement therapy

The most common side effects include nausea, some breast discomfort or irregular bleeding. Side effects are most likely to occur when women start taking HRT, but they usually subside.

Different HRT brands contain different oestrogens and progestogens, so changing brands might help with side effects. Switching the route of administration of HRT (e.g., from tablets to the transdermal method), can also help.

The difference between body-identical and compounded bioidentical hormones

Some private clinics offer a type of HRT known as compounded bioidentical HRT. Like body-identical oestrogen, it is derived from plants.

However, bioidentical HRT products are not authorised by the Medicines and Healthcare Products Regulatory Agency (MHRA) (British Menopause Society, 2019a).

They are marketed as natural supplements and do not require approval by the MHRA.

Bioidentical HRT products have not been subject to clinical trials to test safety and efficacy, and there is no evidence that they are more effective than licensed HRT types (British Menopause Society, 2019a). Women should therefore be dissuaded from going to these clinics and using these products. They are potentially dangerous and very expensive (Newson & Rymer, 2019).

Other treatments

Testosterone levels fluctuate and reduce during the perimenopause and menopause, playing a role in regulating sex drive as well as other symptoms including mood, energy and motivation.

The 2015 NICE guidance states that testosterone supplementation for menopausal women with low sexual desire can be considered if HRT alone is not effective.

Although not all women will need testosterone, it is worth considering testosterone if HRT alone is not helping with symptoms, particularly for women with POI, where testosterone production decreases by more than 50% (British Menopause Society, 2019b), and also women who have had an oophorectomy.

Testosterone is usually given as a cream or gel, or sometimes as an implant. Testosterone is not currently licensed for women in the United Kingdom. There are preparations licensed for men which can be used in lower doses, or many clinics now prescribe a female testosterone cream called AndroFeme which is regulated and is available on a private prescription (British Menopause Society, 2019b).

Treatments for vaginal dryness and urinary symptoms

Local oestrogen in the form of a cream, vaginal tablet, vaginal pessary or inserted vaginal ring can help ease symptoms. There is also a pessary called prasterone which contains dehydroepiandrosterone, which converts to oestrogen and testosterone in the vagina.

Using oestrogen in this way is not the same as taking HRT, so it does not have the same associated risks. It can be safely used by most women on a regular basis for a long period of time (so can safely be put on a repeat prescription), which is important as symptoms can persist when women are postmenopausal and often return when treatment is stopped.

Nonhormonal vaginal moisturisers and lubricants to be used during intercourse can be bought over the counter and used alongside hormones or on their own.

Symptoms should improve within a few weeks or months of treatment. Any women who use vaginal oestrogen also need to take HRT to fully optimise their symptoms. It is quite safe for women to use HRT as well as local preparations of vaginal oestrogen. In addition, women who have had an oestrogen receptor positive cancer can still usually safely be given vaginal oestrogen preparations (Newson, Kirby et al., 2021).

Nonhormonal treatments

If there are contraindications (such as a history of a hormone-dependant cancer), or a woman chooses not to take HRT, there are other treatment options for menopausal treatments.

These include citalopram, venlafaxine or gabapentin for vasomotor symptoms, but they are limited by side effects such as nausea. It is important to know that antidepressants are not effective for improving low mood associated with the perimenopause and menopause. They should therefore not be offered for this reason. There are very few women who cannot have HRT. Women with a history of oestrogen positive cancers in the past may still choose to take HRT because of the health benefits and improvements to quality of life that taking HRT gives women.

Cognitive behavioural therapy

Cognitive behavioural therapy is a talking therapy and recommended by NICE as a treatment for low mood associated with menopause (NICE, 2015). It focuses on changing the way a person thinks and behaves, with sessions delivered either in groups or one to one with a therapist.

Alternative and complementary therapies

Some women consider taking herbal medicines alongside or instead of conventional medicines, but natural does not necessarily mean safer.

The 2015 NICE guideline notes that St John's wort, black cohosh and isoflavones can ease vasomotor symptoms. However, potency can vary between preparations, and interactions with other medicines have been reported.

It is always worth asking patients if they use, or are planning to use, herbal medicines for their menopausal symptoms so this can be recorded.

It is also worth pointing out that, although some herbal medicines may help with some symptoms, they will not address changing hormone levels, protect against osteoporosis or reduce the risk of cardiovascular disease in the way that HRT can.

The MHRA oversees a scheme called the traditional herbal registration certification mark. Patients should be advised to look out for this logo if they choose to buy herbal medicines, as it means they have been deemed to be safe when used as intended, manufactured to set quality standards and have reliable and accurate product information (NHS.uk, 2018).

Nonpharmacological treatment options: promoting a healthy lifestyle

Maintaining a healthy lifestyle is important for women of all ages, but particularly during the menopause. Patients should be advised to:

- Eat a healthy, balanced diet: a diet rich in calcium helps protect bone health and reduce the risk of osteoporosis.
- Get regular exercise: NHS guidelines state that adults should aim for 30 minutes of moderate exercise five times a week. Weight-bearing exercises, such as walking or running, also help maintain bone strength.
- Limit alcohol and/or smoking: alcohol can interrupt sleep and exacerbate vasomotor symptoms. If a patient smokes, discuss smoking cessation services and online resources.
- Take vitamin D: vitamin D helps maintain bone health. Most people should get all the vitamin D they need from sunlight and the small amounts found in food, but supplementation is often needed during the autumn and winter months.
- Promote relaxation: the physical and psychological symptoms of the menopause can take their toll on a woman's home and work life. Taking time out can help, be it spending time with friends, exercising or taking quiet moments alone. Although little is known about the effect of aromatherapy on symptoms of menopause (Royal College of Obstetricians and Gynaecologists, 2018), anecdotally some women say an aromatherapy massage or using oils can be relaxing and uplifting.

Box 8.3 Top tips on making every contact count

1. Always ask yourself 'could it be menopause?'
   Consider the possibility of perimenopause and menopause if women present with typical symptoms, and remember that there is more to the perimenopause and menopause than vasomotor symptoms. Do not rule out women on account of age: premature ovarian insufficiency (POI) affects one in 100 women aged 40 years and younger.
2. Make time to talk
   Brief reception staff in your workplace to try to offer a double appointment if a woman discloses menopausal symptoms when calling to book an appointment.
3. Get a full picture of menopausal symptoms
   The Menopause Symptom Questionnaire (available on menopausedoctor.co.uk) is a checklist which lists a range of symptoms, allowing women to score their severity before and during treatment.
4. When discussing lifestyle changes to help manage menopause symptoms, structure your conversation to get the best out of the appointment and defuse difficult conversations
   Motivational interviewing (MI) is a popular approach to 'health coaching', which involves helping people to change their lives to improve their health (Procter-King, 2019).
   There are four areas of MI:
   - Open questions
   - Affirmations demonstrating belief your patient has the skills and attributes needed to bring about behaviour change
   - Reflections, statements on what you have heard to build rapport
   - Summaries to keep patients on track and reflect what they have said about change (Procter-King, 2019)
5. Know when it is appropriate to suggest referring a woman for specialist care
   According to the National Institute for Health and Care Excellence (NICE) 2015 guideline, these circumstances could include suspected or confirmed POI; if treatments do not improve a woman's menopausal symptoms or she has ongoing troublesome side effects; if a woman has menopausal symptoms and contraindications to hormone replacement therapy (HRT); or if there is uncertainty about the most suitable treatment options for a woman's menopausal symptoms.
6. Don't forget about contraception
   HRT is not a form of contraception. Contraception is required until 1 year after the last period in women aged 50 years and over, and for 2 years in those younger than 50 years (Faculty of Sexual and Reproductive Healthcare, 2017). All women can stop contraception at age 55 because pregnancy at this age is extremely rare.
7. Be aware of the impact vaginal dryness can have on cervical smears
   Smear tests can be very uncomfortable for women suffering from vaginal dryness, and this may be a barrier to attending screening appointments. It is important that a good quality lubricant such as YES is used if your patient has discomfort. The screening appointment is also an ideal time for women to be asked if they have had any change to their periods and to be given a Menopause

Continued

Symptom Questionnaire to complete. It is very important that nurses are picking up perimenopausal and menopausal women and then signposting women to the correct information.

8. Signpost sources of information

This can include the NICE menopause guideline, NHS.uk, mymenopausedoctor.co.uk, womens-health-concern.org (the patient-facing arm of the British Menopause Society) and balance-app.com, a free app for perimenopausal and menopausal women.

Common hormone replacement therapy myths busted for your patients

Women do not have to wait for symptoms to be unbearable before seeing a health professional about HRT.

Women can start taking HRT from when symptoms start, even during the perimenopause.

Taking HRT does not delay the menopause.

If women experience menopausal symptoms after stopping HRT, they would have experienced them even if they had never taken HRT.

Women do not need to stop taking HRT after 5 years. There is no maximum amount of time a woman should take HRT for. It depends on your individual circumstances, risks and benefits and personal choice. Most women continue to take it throughout their lives.

HRT can be suitable for women who present with migraines.

If your patient has a history of migraines, transdermal HRT should be given instead of oral. Women who have migraines with aura have a small increased risk of stroke when taking oestrogen in tablet form, but not transdermal. Women with a history of migraines should be given oestrogen as a patch, gel or spray.

Conclusion

Management of the menopause has previously been considered a complex area that has been viewed as having many risks, particularly when it comes to prescribing HRT. The increase in research and myth-busting by leading professionals in the field of menopause management, in addition to NICE guidance, will help GPNs to confidently support women who seek help with menopause symptoms.

References

Avis, N. E., Crawford, S. L., Greendale, G., et al. (2015). Duration of menopausal vasomotor symptoms over the menopause transition. *JAMA Internal Medicine, 175*(4), 531–539.

Boardman, H. M., Hartley, L., Eisinga, A., et al. (2015). Hormone therapy for preventing cardiovascular disease in post-menopausal women. *Cochrane Database Syst Rev*, 2015:CD002229.

British Menopause Society. (2019a). *Bioidentical HRT.* BMS Consensus Statement. http://www.thebms.org.uk/publications/consensus-statements/bioidentical-hrt.

British Menopause Society. (2019b). *Testosterone replacement in menopause.* http://www.thebms.org.uk/publications/tools-for-clinicians/testosterone-replacement-in-menopause.

Carson, G., Long Covid Forum Group., Carson, G. et al. (2021). Research priorities for Long Covid: Refined through an international multi-stakeholder forum. *BMC Medicine, 19,* 84. https://doi.org/10.1186/s12916-021-01947-0.

Cumming, G. P., Currie, H., Morris, E., et al. (2015). The need to do better: Are we still letting our patients down and at what cost? *Post Reproductive Health, 21*(2), 56–62.

Daisy Network. (2019). *What is POI?* www.daisynetwork.org/about-poi/what-is-poi.

Dambha-Miller, H., Hinton W., Joy, M., Feher, M., & De Lusignan, S. (2021). medRxiv (Preprint). doi: https://doi.org/10.1101/2021.02.16.21251853.

Faculty of Sexual and Reproductive Healthcare. (2017). *FSRH guideline: Contraception for women aged over 40 years.* http://www.fsrh.org/news/updated-clinical-guideline-published-contraception-for-women.

Leonhardt, M. (2019). Low mood and depressive symptoms during perimenopause – Should General Practitioners prescribe hormone replacement therapy or antidepressants as the first-line treatment? *Post Reproductive Health, 25*(3), 124–130.

Manson, J. E., Aragaki, A. K., Rossouw, J. E., et al. (2017). Menopausal hormone therapy and long-term all-cause and cause-specific mortality: The Women's Health Initiative Randomized Trials. *Journal of the American Medical Association, 318*(10), 927–938.

Newson Health Research and Education. (2019). *Millions of NHS money wasted with delays in diagnosing the menopause.* www.menopausedoctor.co.uk/news/millions-of-nhs-money-wasted-with-delays-in-diagnosing-the-menopause.

Newson, L., Kirby, M., Stillwell, S., Hackett, G., Ball, S., Lewis, R. (2021). Position Statement of Genitourinary Syndrome of the Menopause (GSM) British Society for Sexual Medicine. http://www.bssm.org.uk/wp-content/uploads/2021/03/GSM-BSSM.pdf.

Newson, L. & Lass, A. (2018). Effectiveness of transdermal oestradiol and natural micronised progesterone for menopausal symptoms. *British Journal of General Practice, 68,* 499–500.

Newson, L. & Mair, R. (2018). Results from the BJFM menopause survey. *British Journal of Family Medicine, 6*(1). https://www.bjfm.co.uk/results-from-the-bjfm-menopause-survey.

Newson, L., Rymer, J. (2019). The dangers of compounded bioidentical hormone replacement therapy. *British Journal of General Practice, 69*(688), 540–541. doi: 10.3399/bjgp19X706169. PMID: 31672802; PMCID: PMC6808563.

NHS.uk. (2018). *Herbal medicines.* http://www.nhs.uk/conditions/herbal-medicines.

NHS.uk. (2018). *Menopause: Overview.* http://www.nhs.uk/conditions/menopause.

NICE. (2015). *Menopause: Diagnosis and management.* https://www.nice.org.uk/guidance/ng23.

NICE. (2015). *Women with symptoms of menopause should not suffer in silence.* https://www.nice.org.uk/news/article/women-with-symptoms-of-menopause-should-not-suffer-in-silence.

Procter-King, J. & McLean, C. (2019). Activities to encourage nurses to learn more about motivational interviewing. *Primary Health Care, 29*(1), 44–49.

Rossouw, J. E., Anderson, G. L., Prentice, R. L., et al. (2002). Risks and benefits of estrogen plus progestin in healthy postmenopausal women: Principal results from the Women's Health Initiative randomized controlled trial. *Journal of the American Medical Association, 288,* 321–333.

Royal College of Obstetricians and Gynaecologists. (2018). *Treatment for symptoms of the meno-pause. Information for you.* http://www.rcog.org.uk/en/patients/patient-leaflets/treatment-symp-toms-menopause.

Seeland, U., Coluzzi, F., Simmaco, M. et al. (2020). Evidence for treatment with estradiol for wom-en with SARS-CoV-2 infection. *BMC Medicine, 18,* 369. https://doi.org/10.1186/s12916-020-01851-z medRxiv 2020.

Women's Health Concern. (2015). *The menopause.* http://www.womens-health-concern.org/help-and-advice/factsheets/menopause.

Chapter 9

Mental health

Alison Oldam

Without mental health there can be no true physical health

Dr Brock Chisholm (1954)

Learning outcomes

After reading this chapter you should be able to:

1. Understand the diagnosis and treatment of the most common mental health problems
2. Describe common presentations and mental health difficulties in primary care, as well as ongoing care and monitoring of patients with mild and moderate mental health problems

Introduction

The relationship between the mind and the body has been a source of debate for many years. This is important, as the way we view the relationship impacts upon how we treat people who have an illness. Originally, religious teaching preached that the body and soul were one, and so illness was believed to be related to a person's sins or evil spirits. Then, in the 17th century Rene Descartes proposed that the mind and body were separate and functioned entirely independently of one another, a theory known as mind-body dualism (Descartes, 1952). One of the consequences of this theory was that research became focussed on the body, independent of the mind (Mehta, 2011). It is this that fundamentally underpins the medical model and subsequent medical research. This view predominantly focuses on what has biologically gone wrong that therefore requires fixing. It is a disease-based model that continues to underpin much of the medical model today. A person's physical health impacts upon their mental health, and a person's mental health impacts on their physical health, and therefore any treatment needs to be holistic. In 2016, NHS England published the Five-Year Forward View for mental health, and this supported the view that both physical health and mental health must be considered in a holistic fashion. The report committed to parity of esteem for mental and physical health. We cannot look after one without looking after the other, and knowledge of mental health and the confidence to ask and talk about mental health must be an essential part of any General Practice Nurse's (GPN) core competencies.

Creating services that represent equal parity for mental health and physical health

The National Health Service (NHS) is increasingly recognising the importance of considering the mind and the body together, but there is still a long way to go. The medical model has been dominant for so many years, but there is increasing recognition of the importance of, for example, multidisciplinary services that treat the 'whole' person, for example, diabetes clinics with a Consultant Physician, Specialist Nurse, Dietician and Clinical Psychologist or specialist mental health professionals based in primary care. In addition, one of the many aims of the 'New ways of working' (NHSE, 2019a) is to promote more holistic care and allow general practices to do more to 'tackle obesity, diabetes and mental ill health'. There is a long way to go, but GPNs are in a unique position to provide holistic care that considers a person's physical and mental health. However, the Clinical Commissioning Group (CCG) guidance on 'Improving physical healthcare for people living with severe mental illness (SMI) in primary care' (2018a) found that although 'primary care staff are likely to have the required skills and expertise in relation to physical health assessments, many feel that they lack the knowledge and confidence in relation to working with people who are living with a serious mental illness'. This was based on a 2014 survey of GPNs, which found that '82% have responsibilities for aspects of mental health and wellbeing for which they had no training, and 42% have had no training in mental health and wellbeing at all' (Fig. 9.1).

General statistics

Data from Mind (2017) and the Mental Health Foundation (2016) report 'Fundamental Facts About Mental Health' show that:

- Approximately one in four people in the United Kingdom will experience a mental health problem each year
- Every week, one in six adults experiences symptoms of a common mental health problem such as anxiety or depression
- Approximately one in ten children experiences mental health problems
- Depression affects approximately one in 12 people in the whole population
- For those receiving Employment and Support Allowance, the figures are higher, with two-thirds reporting common mental health problems and the same percentage reporting suicidal thoughts
- 450 million people worldwide have a mental health problem

Most people represented in those statistics will be supported in primary care. Only those with more severe ongoing difficulties will be treated by specialist mental health services, and this is likely to last for only a limited period of time. Once these patients' mental health is stable, their ongoing support will most commonly happen in primary care.

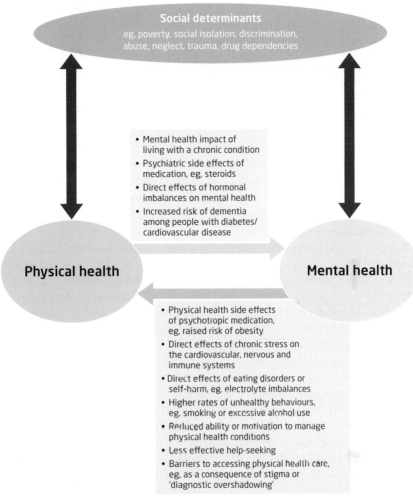

Fig. 9.1   Mechanisms through which physical and mental health interact. (From The King's Fund. (2016). *Bringing together physical and mental health.* https://www.kingsfund.org.uk/publications /physical-and-mental-health.)

The impact of stigma

It is well documented that there is a great deal of stigma around mental health. The Mental Health Foundation (2016) states that nearly nine out of ten people with mental health problems report that stigma and discrimination have a negative effect on their lives. We know that, because of this stigma, it is hard for people with mental health difficulties to talk about this topic with friends, colleagues and, importantly, medical professionals.

Many experienced GPNs find it difficult to ask and talk to their patients about their mental health. From experience, these are some of the reasons that nurses have given as to why this is the case:

● Some felt anxious, concerned and worried
● Some said they did not want to 'open a can of worms'
● Some were worried that they would make it worse
● Some were worried by what the person might say and whether they would know how to respond or what to say
● Some were worried that patients would become angry about being asked because they would find it intrusive or offensive

The evidence from experienced nurses was that they found it hard to ask and talk about mental health. This is not surprising, given the 2014 survey of GPNs (cited in CCG guidance on 'Improving physical health care for people living with SMI in primary care', 2018a) which noted that 42% of nurses have had no training in mental health. This, coupled with the fact that mental health is hard to talk about for patients, means that patients may not disclose their difficulties and may fail to get the support that they need. The Mental Health Foundation (2016), for example, notes that, despite some increase in people accessing treatment, around one-third of all people with a mental health problem have sought no professional help at all. This could have a significant negative impact on both their mental and physical health. It may affect their mental health because they are not receiving any treatment, and we know that mental health difficulties can have a negative impact on a person's physical health (see Fig. 9.1). GPNs need to be as competent and confident in asking about and recognising mental health problems as they are about physical health difficulties. This is supported by Mind, which states: 'Mental health is core business for primary care services. GPs and GPNs play a vital role in supporting the one in four people who experience a mental health problem in any given year. However, these professionals are likely not to have been given enough training and support to enable them to provide the best possible care for people with mental health problems'.

The number of people living with a long-term condition has increased, and this can also result in experiencing mental health difficulties. It is estimated that 17.5 million people have a long-term condition (Department of Health, 2005). The King's Fund (2012) stated that people with long-term conditions now account for about 50% of all General Practitioner (GP) appointments, 64% of all outpatient appointments and over 70% of all inpatient bed days. The Department of Health (2012) estimated that treatment and care for people with long-term conditions accounts for around £7 of every £10 of total health and social care expenditure.

Caring for people with long-term conditions is also a central part of Primary Care, and GPNs have become experts in the management of chronic and complex health conditions. The next step is ensuring this expertise also covers the mental health of people with long-term conditions, a new frontier for integrated care (Bringing together physical and mental health, 2020).

Patients with mental health difficulties

A survey of more than 1000 GPs carried out by Mind (2018) revealed a rising demand for mental health support in primary care, with GPs estimating that 40% of their appointments involve patients' mental health. This study also found that 66% of the GPs questioned felt that the proportion of patients needing help with their mental health had increased in the previous 12 months. A report by Layard et al. (2006) estimated that 33% of all patients visiting their GP had mental health problems, representing an increase over the previous 14 years. These figures suggest that primary care professionals should be routinely asking patients about their mental health. If we compare this with physical health, we know that smoking increases the risk of cancer, and we know that being overweight has significant health risks, such as increasing the risk of type 2 diabetes. We know that drinking above the daily recommended levels of alcohol can have a negative impact on a person's health in several ways. We routinely ask a patient about risk factors that impact on their physical health, such as whether they smoke and how much they drink, but we also need to ask about mental health in the same manner. It could be added as a question to a routine questionnaire, or we can just ask, as long as we do it routinely.

If we explain that we have started asking routinely, then it becomes expected and accepted, and we ensure inclusivity. Routine asking results in normalising conversations around mental health, which is an accepted way of reducing stigma (Time to Change). We did not routinely ask about smoking 20 years ago, but this is now an expected, and in most cases accepted, part of any health check. We are also normalising the fact that we know that physical and mental health are linked. We know mental health can have an impact on how a person feels physically, and we know that having a physical health problem can impact on a person's mental health, as discussed earlier. By asking about mental health in a routine way we are normalising and even promoting or educating patients about these links.

Asking patients about their mental health

For nurses new to general practice, asking patients about their mental health might be unfamiliar or uncomfortable. There are resources within your practice to help you with this. There are also three questionnaires recommended within the National Institute for Health and Care Excellence (NICE) guidelines on depression which are validated for use in primary care. These can be used where there is an indication that the patient is struggling with his or her mental health. These are the Patient Health Questionnaire–9 (Agency Medical Directors, 2015), which is free to use, the Hospital Anxiety and Depression Scale (available from Svri.org, 2019) and the Beck Depression Inventory–II (Beck, 1996), both of which have a charge attached.

The King's Fund Bringing together physical and mental health report (2020) notes the importance of communication and communication skills. It states that the 'way information and reassurance is given, the kind of questions that are asked,

> **Box 9.1 How to ask patients about their mental health**
>
> Here are some example questions:
> - How would you describe your mental health right now?
> - Is there anything about your mental health that is impacting upon your physical health problems at the moment?
> - I can see that you are struggling with long-term health problems. One of the things we know from research is that long-term health conditions can affect how a person feels, so we like to routinely ask about mental health. How do you feel in yourself day to day? How would you say your mental health is?

and the quality of listening a professional is able to offer all have the effect of either narrowing or broadening the scope of a clinical encounter'. It recognised that an open question is more likely to 'open up a discussion about psychosocial wellbeing'. Box 9.1 includes some examples of open questions relating to mental health.

Common mental health problems

When a relevant professional carries out a mental health assessment and a patient is found to have a diagnosable mental health disorder, then a diagnosis is made using either the Diagnostic Statistical Manual of Mental Disorders, 5th Edition (DSM-5; American Psychiatric Association, 2013) or the International Classification of Diseases, 10th Revision (World Health Organization, 1992). The DSM-5 is an American publication, but both are used in the United Kingdom. The diagnostic criteria cited below for anxiety and depression use the DSM-5 criteria.

Depression

Depression is the most common mental health problem worldwide. It is therefore important to be aware of the symptoms and treatment of depression.

The NICE Guidelines for Depression (NICE, 2009) recommend that clinicians assess for the two 'core' symptoms of depression by asking:

- During the last month have you often been bothered by feeling down, depressed or hopeless?
- Do you have little interest or pleasure in doing things?

If either of the two 'core' symptoms have been present most days, most of the time, for at least 2 weeks, then it is important to ask about other typical symptoms of depression (Box 9.2).

Symptoms of atypical depression include reactive mood, increased appetite, weight gain, excessive sleepiness and sensitivity to rejection.

A symptom is counted as significant if it is sufficiently severe and/or persistent to be causing significant distress or functional impairment.

Depression is diagnosed from a positive response to either one (or both) of the core questions, together with at least four of the symptoms listed in Box 9.2.

Box 9.2 Symptoms of depression

- Fatigue/loss of energy
- Worthlessness/excessive or inappropriate guilt
- Recurrent thoughts of death, suicidal thoughts or actual suicide attempts
- Diminished ability to think/concentrate or indecisiveness
- Psychomotor agitation or retardation
- Insomnia/hypersomnia
- Significant appetite and/or weight loss

From American Psychiatric Association. (2013). *Diagnostic and statistical manual of mental disorders* (5th ed.). Washington, DC: Author.

Box 9.3 Severity of depression

- Mild depression: few, if any, symptoms in excess of the five required to make the diagnosis, and symptoms result in only minor functional impairment.
- Moderate depression: symptoms or functional impairment are between 'mild' and 'severe'.
- Severe depression: most symptoms, and the symptoms markedly interfere with functioning. Can occur with or without psychotic symptoms.

(National Institute for Health and Care Excellence. (2009). *Depression in adults; Recognition and Management. (NICE guideline CG90.)* https://www.nice.org.uk/Guidance/CG90.)

As the NICE guidance (2009) notes, it is not only about counting the number of symptoms present: it is essential to consider the 'degree of functional impairment and/or disability associated with the possible depression and the duration of the episode'.

A diagnosis is then made regarding the severity of depression, and this then impacts on treatment choice (Box 9.3).

Treatment

If, following an assessment, the patient is diagnosed as being depressed, then they can be offered talking therapy or, if indicated, medication with follow-up both of which have been found to be effective treatments. For example, for people with moderate to severe depression, Anderson et al. (2008) found that, if no treatment was given, 20% recovered; whereas when a placebo was given, 30% recovered, and where an antidepressant was given, 50% recovered.

NICE guidance (2009) recommends low-intensity psychological treatments known as talking therapies for 'treating subthreshold depressive symptoms and mild-to-moderate depression, based on consideration of effectiveness and cost'. In terms of moderate to severe depression, the NICE guidance cites evidence that 'high-intensity psychological treatments were effective both alone and in combination with antidepressants'.

Self-help materials are also very helpful for people struggling with mental health difficulties; materials recommend by NICE (2009) can be found here: https://cks.nice.org.uk/depression-!scenarioRecommendation:20.

There are also a range of self-help leaflets available from Northumberland, Tyne and Wear NHS Trust (2019) which are very useful and can be found here: https://web.ntw.nhs.uk/selfhelp/.

Generalised anxiety disorder and panic disorder in adults

This is the second most common presentation in primary care. The following is taken from the NICE guidelines (NICE, 2011). The key symptoms of Generalised Anxiety Disorder (GAD) are:

1. Excessive anxiety and worry about several events or activities
2. Difficulty controlling the worry.

For a diagnosis the worry should occur on most days for at least 6 months. The focus of the worry should not be confined to features of another anxiety disorder (e.g., worrying about having a panic attack, social embarrassment, a traumatic event, fear of being contaminated by dirt, germs, viruses, blood, etc. or worrying about having a serious illness).

If the two key symptoms are present, ask about the following associated symptoms:

- Restlessness
- Being easily fatigued
- Difficulty concentrating
- Irritability
- Muscle tension
- Disturbed sleep

Additional information about how long the symptoms have been present, how much distress they cause and how much they impact on functioning are also important in determining whether a diagnosis will be made. If the symptoms have been present on most days for 6 months or more and are causing considerable distress, and are having a significant impact on functioning, then consider a diagnosis of GAD.

Treatment

Psychoeducation is the provision of education and information to those seeking or receiving mental health services. One of the treatments for people suffering from anxiety that NICE (2011) recommends is psychoeducation about anxiety, that is, teaching patients what symptoms are associated with anxiety and the physical reactions people can have, as well as explaining what people can do to help themselves. Self-help and active monitoring are also indicated when the anxiety is less serious (fewer symptoms, shorter duration, lower level of impact, no comorbidity, etc.) NICE (2009) also recommends self help, and provides guidance with a lot of information about GAD and Panic Disorder: https://www.nice.org.uk/guidance/cg113/ifp/chapter/About -this-information.

Northumberland, Tyne and Wear NHS Trust has leaflets specifically on anxiety, social anxiety and panic, which can be found here: https://web.ntw.nhs .uk/selfhelp/.

Long-term conditions and mental health

Background information

There is significant evidence (Department of Health, 2012) that having a long-term condition impacts upon a person's quality of life, and, not surprisingly, there is a strong relationship between having a long-term condition and comorbid mental health difficulties.

There is also a very significant financial impact for the NHS. As Naylor et al. (2012) explained, comorbid mental health problems raise total health care costs by at least 45% for each person with a long-term condition and a comorbid mental health problem. This equates to between £8 billion and £13 billion each year that is spent on long-term conditions linked to poor mental health and wellbeing.

Randall and Ford (2011) outlined the following areas of a person's life which are often impacted by having a long-term condition:

- Work
- Relationships
- Home
- Family
- Social
- Hobbies

Statistics about chronic conditions and mental health

Some 49% of patients with chronic pain have a diagnosis of depression (Chronic Pain Policy Coalition, 2006).

Davies et al. (2004) found that people who had suffered a myocardial infarction had a 30% chance of developing depression.

Goldney et al. (2004) estimated that 24% of people with diabetes also suffered from depression, whereas Boehm et al. (2004) found that people with diabetes were three times more likely to have depression than the general public.

'Compared with the general population, people with diabetes, hypertension and coronary artery disease have double the rate of mental health problems, and those with chronic obstructive pulmonary disease, cerebro-vascular disease and other chronic conditions have triple the rate' (Department of Health, 2012).

People with three or more long-term conditions are approximately four times as likely to suffer from anxiety or depression than the general population (Department of Health, 2012).

Impact of mental health and depression on the physical health of those with long-term conditions

The relationship between physical health and mental health is not linear. Just as our physical health impacts on our mental health, so does our mental health impact upon our physical health (Bringing together physical and mental health, 2020). Having a mental health problem as a primary diagnosis or as a result of a long-term physical health condition can increase the prevalence of comorbidities, increase negative illness outcomes and ultimately increase the morbidity rate. For example, Frasure-Smith et al. (2000) found that people who have suffered a myocardial infarction are three times more likely to die if they have depression than if they do not.

Implications for general practice nurses

It is vital for people with a long-term condition that a holistic view of health and wellbeing is taken. Assessing and addressing a patient's psychological needs can improve his or her quality of life, as well as health outcomes, and can therefore result in a reduction in health care consumption (Bringing together physical and mental health, 2020). Despite this, evidence suggests that mental health difficulties in those with a long-term condition are more likely to be missed than in those presenting with a mental health problem alone. For example, Bridges and Goldberg (1985) found that, although more than 90% of people with depression alone were diagnosed in primary care, depression was detected in less than one-quarter of cases of people who also had a long-term condition. Coventry et al. (2011) suggest that, when someone has a diagnosed long-term condition, physical symptoms, rather than more holistic wellbeing, tend to be the focus of consultations for both the patients and practitioners. If patients with a long-term condition are routinely asking about mental health, and a holistic approach to health is taken, then mental health problems are more likely to be diagnosed. Anxiety and depression can be successfully treated, and this can support people with long-term conditions to have a better quality of life and better health outcomes, and reduce costs for the NHS (Naylor et al., 2012). As part of the personalised care planning process, patients with one or more long-term conditions should be assessed for anxiety, depression and any other mental health problems.

'Social prescribing' can also be very effective in supporting a patient who, as determined by a holistic assessment, seems to be struggling with isolation or loneliness. Social prescribing is a system where health care professionals can

---

Box 9.4 Holistic Open Questions

- One of the things we know from other people is that having a long-term condition such as diabetes/heart disease/arthritis, and so on can have a real impact on a person's mood and mental health. I'm wondering if your diabetes/heart disease/arthritis is having any impact on your mental health at the moment?
- You are struggling with long-term problems with your diabetes/heart disease/ulcers, and so on. Is this having any impact on how you feel in yourself day to day, on your mental health?

From The King's Fund. (2016). *Bringing together physical and mental health.* https://www.kingsfund .org.uk/publications/physical-and-mental-health.

---

refer patients to local, nonclinical services to meet their wellbeing needs. This can cover a number of different activities depending on the patient's preference and what is available locally.

How to ask patients with long-term conditions about their mental health

As noted previously, asking routinely normalises the relationship between long-term conditions and mental health difficulties. The King's Fund Bringing together physical and mental health report (2020) emphasises the important of holistic, open questions. Example questions are outlined in Box 9.4.

The King's Fund Bringing together physical and mental health report (2020) states: 'Integrated care initiatives in England and elsewhere have paid insufficient attention to the relationship between physical and mental health. This aspect of integration should be a major part of efforts to develop new models of care in NHS England's vanguard sites and elsewhere'. This is one of the key drivers of Primary Care networks which are looking to provide fully integrated community-based services (Baird, 2019).

Integration of services

The management teams for chronic diseases need to be better integrated with mental health specialists, as service users often report 'a lack of communication or co-ordination between different components of care. There was particular fragmentation between support for physical and mental health' (King's Fund, 2020). Care for large numbers of people with long-term conditions could be improved by better integrating mental health support with primary care and chronic disease management programmes, with closer working between mental health specialists and other professionals.

The NICE guidance (2015) recognises integration as high-quality care. For example, in relation to children and young people's diabetes services, it states:

'Children and young people with type 1 or type 2 diabetes are able to see mental health professionals who understand the types of problems people with diabetes can have. The mental health professional should be one of the main members of the diabetes team'.

This is an example of an organisational structure that encourages a holistic and generalist approach to health and wellbeing. The King's Fund (2012) has argued that developing more integrated forms of care for people with comorbid mental and physical health problems should be 'one of the top 10 priorities for clinical commissioning groups'.

Case study

Rachel is 25 and lives alone. She works full time as a secretary. She comes in for a prediabetes clinic and blood test. She says she thinks her blood sugars will be a bit high. She explains that she worries that she will become hypoglycaemic at night, and so she tries to ensure her blood sugars are high before bedtime. She worries that she will go into a diabetic coma and no one will know and that she won't be found. When Rachel was in her teens her mum used to take her blood sugars in the night, and she would frequently wake her to give her some food if her blood sugars were low.

You look back in Rachel's notes and see that Rachel's blood sugars have been consistently high for the last few years and, despite several conversations about this and repeated advice regarding her diet, there has been no positive change.

Rachel went away to university aged 18 but struggled with moving away from home and was feeling very anxious and homesick. She came home after one term. She moved into her own house 6 months ago.

You pick up on Rachel's anxiety and ask her a bit more about this. She tells you she is having a lot of stomach aches and feeling very stressed. She has recently been off sick from work quite frequently. She says she just feels overwhelmed and worried by how much work she must do, and that she struggles to concentrate when she is at work. She has been put on an automatic absence monitoring programme after more than three periods of absence in three months. This is making her feel more stressed and is impacting on her ability to sleep.

Notes

The health care practitioner could continue to see Rachel in the diabetes clinic and keep explaining to her why it is so important to reduce her blood sugars to recommended levels, as well as the physical risks of her not doing so. However well this is explained, and however well Rachel is educated on her diet and the risk of complications, it is unlikely anything will change without any support for Rachel's anxiety. The case study information would suggest that underpinning Rachel's behaviour is a very strongly held belief that she is keeping herself safe at night by ensuring her blood sugars are high before bed. The information also indicates that this belief means that Rachel would be anxious that a change in her eating behaviour could result in a diabetic coma and ultimately death. It is likely that help regarding this belief, and support in introducing safe gradual alterations to her diet and behaviour, would be essential for any change to occur.

Rachel is also suffering from more general anxiety. It is highly likely she would benefit from a referral for psychological support. The sooner this was picked up, the more likely she would be to recover. Psychological therapy could potentially reduce Rachel's anxiety, help her manage her work stress better and sleep better, and work toward allowing her to change her diet in a way that would feel psychologically safe for her.

On the other hand, no intervention at this stage is likely to result in Rachel continuing to experience the same level of stress and anxiety, continued absence at work, potential job loss in due course and in the long-term, diabetes complications caused by high blood sugars. This case study illustrates the difference that a holistic assessment, diagnosis and referral can make.

Psychological therapy

In relation to the impact of psychological therapy for people with a long-term condition, research by De Lusigman et al. (2011) found that psychological therapy was associated with reduced emergency department attendance. A metaanalysis carried out by Chiles et al. (1999) found that psychological interventions in hospitals and other settings reduced length of stay by 2.5 days, and overall health care costs per patient were also reduced by about 20%.

The Five-Year Forward View for mental health (2016) and the NHS Long Term Plan (2019b) have both clearly recognised the need for psychological therapy to be available for those with long-term conditions, and the positive impact that this can have on a person's quality of life, as well as physical health. Services such as the Improving Access to Psychological Therapies (IAPT) programme provide talking therapies specifically for people with long-term conditions. Most general practices will have a referral route for these services, and it is important that GPNs become familiar with referral pathways. In some areas people can self-refer or be referred to services by a health professional.

All IAPT services have a national waiting time target which states that 75% of people referred to IAPT services should start treatment within 6 weeks of referral, and 95% should start treatment within 18 weeks of referral.

NICE (2011) guidelines for depression in adults with chronic physical health problems recognise both the prevalence and impact of mental health. They recommend that patients with long-term conditions should receive a complete assessment of depression by a competent health care professional.

NICE also recommends treatment for depression, including stepped care and cognitive behavioural therapy (a type of talking therapy usually provided by IAPT). Stepped care is a system comprising a hierarchy of interventions, from the least to the most intensive, matched to an individual's needs. It also recommends a collaborative approach to care which includes all sectors of care, an identified coordinator who leads on a joint care plan and an agreed plan for short- and long-term follow-up. Collaborative care is recommended for patients who have moderate to severe depression and a chronic physical health problem whose depression has not responded to initial high-intensity psychological interventions, pharmacological treatment or a combination of both.

Serious mental illness and its impact on physical health

What is a serious mental illness?

The NHS England (2018) 'Improving physical healthcare for people living with severe mental illness (SMI) in primary care' guidance for CCGs defines individuals with an SMI as those who have received a diagnosis of schizophrenia or bipolar affective disorder, or who have experienced an episode of nonorganic psychosis. GPNs are strongly encouraged to consider the physical health needs of people with other diagnoses, including, for example, personality disorder.

Research (e.g., NHS England 2018 report) suggests that people with an SMI are more likely to suffer from:

- Respiratory disease
- Endocrine disease
- Cardiovascular disease
- Certain types of cancer

GPNs should be vigilant when consulting patients whose primary long-term condition is a SMI and consider these and other physical health-related conditions.

The NHS document 'Improving physical healthcare for people living with severe mental illness in primary care' (NHSE, 2018) also states that the life expectancy for people living with an SMI is 15 to 20 years shorter than that of the general population, and that two-thirds of these deaths are from avoidable physical illnesses. It is understood that this relates partly to lifestyle factors; for example, people with a SMI are more likely to smoke, and are also more likely to be obese (NHS England, 2018). Additionally, the report highlights that they can struggle to reliably access health care, leading to physical health care needs being overlooked. In addition, the medications taken by patients with an SMI such as antipsychotics can result in higher levels of physical health risks, for

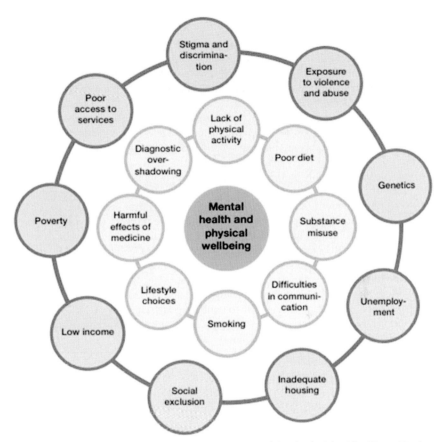

Fig. 9.2 Interrelated dynamic elements affecting people's physical health. (From Nursing, Midwifery and Allied Health Professions Policy Unit. (2016). *Improving the physical health of people with mental health problems: Actions for mental health nurses*).

example, an increased risk of sexual dysfunction, postural hypotension, cardiac arrhythmia and sudden cardiac death (Muench & Hamer, 2010).

Fig. 9.2 outlines the interrelated dynamic elements affecting people's physical health and is taken from the Nursing, Midwifery and Allied Health Professions Policy Unit (2016).

The Five-Year Forward View for mental health report committed to ensuring that, by 2020/2021, 280,000 people living with severe mental illness would have their physical health needs met by increasing early detection and expanding access to evidence-based physical care assessment and intervention each year. Consequently, annual health checks for people with an SMI have commenced, and GPNs may be expected to provide these annual health checks (Box 9.5).

Box 9.5   Carrying out a health assessment with a person with a severe mental illness: areas to cover

- Ask patients about what health issues (if any) they have any concerns about.
- Listen carefully to patients and identify any concerns or worries that they have.
- Identify what is important to them and help them prioritise areas of behavioural change.
- Help them set their own realistic and achievable targets. This is very important because people tend to set unachievable targets and soon get demoralised.
- Help them access services that can support them in the area that they have identified.
- Help patients identify barriers to accessing support and work with them to think about how best to overcome these barriers (supporting patients in identifying their own solutions rather than advising them of what they should do).
- Talk to them about friends, family and health care workers who can support them in looking after their physical health. Offer to liaise with other health care professionals to communicate any plans if the patients feel this would be helpful. Ensure that patients know that family or friends can attend appointments with them if they would find this supportive.
- Ensure that follow-ups take place as required and that reviews record progress and work in a patient-centred way to consider goals, etc.
- Use motivational interviewing when looking at any lifestyle-change approach for people with a serious mental illness.

From NHS England. (2018a). *Improving physical healthcare for people living with severe mental illness (SMI) in primary care. Guidance for CCGs.*

Supporting primary care staff in their role with patients with a severe mental illness

The NHS England (2018a) report 'Improving physical healthcare for people living with severe mental illness in primary care' recognises that primary care staff may need access to training and knowledge regarding mental health to be confident to undertake health assessment of a patient with an SMI. Specifically, it outlines the following competencies that staff should have:

- Understand what an SMI is and how it might be experienced.
- Understand the excess risks of poor physical health and how best to support people with an SMI to engage and access appropriate physical health care.
- Feel confident and empowered to talk about health holistically, including mental health, healthy lifestyles, risk reduction and physical health.
- Have the technical skills and expertise to carry out physical health assessments and obtain and communicate the results.

It outlines several ways that staff can be supported in their development, including ensuring that they have the space and time to access mental health training. They also recommended that staff have access to appropriate

---

Box 9.6 Risk factors for suicide

Risk factors for suicide can include (but are not limited to):

- Gender: in the United Kingdom, men are three times more likely to die by suicide than women
- Young age (<30 years) or advanced age
- Previous attempts at suicide or self-harm
- Expressed feeling of hopelessness or being a burden
- Expressed feelings of isolation or being alone
- Poor social support
- Family history of suicide
- Self-harm such as cutting
- History of substance or alcohol abuse or increased recent use
- Severe depression or recently started on antidepressants

---

supervision, the opportunity for reflective practice and access to multidisciplinary team structures.

Suicide

It would not be appropriate to discuss the area of SMI and mental health without touching on the subject of suicide. Suicide is the biggest killer of both males and females between the ages of 5 and 34 years. Suicide remains the biggest killer of men aged 34 to 49 years, whereas breast cancer is the biggest killer amongst women in this age range. According to a report by the Mental Health Foundation (2016) one person kills him or herself approximately every 2 hours. In 2018, deaths by suicide rose by 11.8%. These shocking statistics indicate that there is much more that needs to be done in the prevention and detection of suicide. Health professionals routinely ask about lifestyle factors that have a critical causal relationship to death and ill health (smoking, weight, alcohol, diet, etc.), yet the same is not consistently true of mental health factors, and rarely is suicide mentioned, despite the figures (Box 9.6).

What can general practice nurses do?

If, during a consultation with someone, there is any indication that a patient might be at risk of suicide (see Box 9.6), then the GPN should ask him or her about this directly (see Zero Alliance and NHS e-learning module cited in resources). The training modules cited explain that suicide survivors and those that experience suicidal thoughts have explained that it is harder for them to talk about suicidal feelings when people are not direct. Passive statements such as 'You are not thinking about doing anything stupid, are you?' avoid directly addressing the issue, whereas using words such as 'suicide' can reduce patients' fear or anxiety about talking about their feelings (Box 9.7).

Box 9.7 Examples of questions to ask to ascertain suicide risk

- Do you ever feel that life is hopeless and not worth living?
- Do you ever think about suicide?
- Have you made any plans for ending your life?
- If the answer is yes, ask what those plans are.
- If patients have a plan, for example, of taking an overdose, explore if they have tablets available to them. If they say they think about harming themselves with a knife, find out if they have access to knives, that is, find out if they have the means available to kill themselves.

Reflection

A suicide prevention training video is provided by Zero Alliance Suicide (2020) and is easily accessible and free to view. It takes about 20 minutes to watch and is available here: https://www.zerosuicidealliance.com/.

As the video explains, it is important to ask directly about suicidal thoughts and intent. It explains that health care professionals should not avoid the word 'suicide'.

There is also a National Health Service e-learning for health care module on suicide prevention which can be found here: https://www.e-lfh.org.uk/programmes /suicide-prevention/.

Treatment

If, at the end of the consultation, the GPN assesses that there is a risk of suicide, then the following services can provide support:

- The Crisis Resolution and Home Treatment team. A voluntary admission or compulsory admission (via a mental health section) to hospital may be required.
- Accident and Emergency (A&E). A crisis mental health service can also be accessed via A&E.

Some practices will have policy guidance on managing patients at risk of suicide, and all GPNs should be aware of any local guidance.

Public Health England and the National Suicide Prevention Alliance have produced a guide for patients who have been bereaved by suicide. This guide is entitled 'Help is at Hand – Support after someone may have died by suicide'. It is available to download in PDF format at the following link: https://www.nhs .uk/Livewell/Suicide/Documents/Help%20is%20at%20Hand.pdf.

Remember, people bereaved by suicide are at increased risk of considering suicide themselves (Samaritans: https://samaritanshope.org/get-help/warning -signs-risk-factors/).

Conclusion

GPNs, in their consultations and encounters with patients, need to consider patients' mental health as a routine part of primary care practice. Having a mental health problem still carries significant stigma in society (Mental Health Foundation, 2016), so health care professionals need to be proactive in enabling patients to talk to professionals about their mental health. Having routine conversations about mental health with all patients is vital to recognising and assessing mental health problems, and thus enabling treatment. Helping patients get the appropriate treatment for their mental health has the potential to have a positive impact on their quality of life, their management of any long-term condition and their general physical health. GPNs must recognise their scope of practice in managing patients with mental health conditions, and if they do not feel confident or competent to identify or manage mental health issues, they should seek to undergo appropriate training.

References

Agency Medical Directors. (2015). *The Patient Health Questionnaire (PHQ-9) – Overview*. http://www.agencymeddirectors.wa.gov/Files/depressoverview.pdf.

American Psychiatric Association. (2013). *Diagnostic and statistical manual of mental disorders* (5th ed.). Washington, DC: Author.

Anderson, I. M., Ferrier, I. N., Baldwin, R. C., et al. (2008). Evidence-based guidelines for treating depressive disorders with antidepressants: A revision of the 2000 British Association for Psychopharmacology guidelines. *Journal of Psychopharmacology, 22*, 343–396.

Baird, B. (2019), Primary care networks are about much more than general practice. *Health Service Journal*.

Beck, A. T., Steer, R. A., & Brown, G. K. (1996). *Manual for the Beck Depression Inventory-II*. Psychological Corporation.

Boehm, G., Racoosin, J., Laughren, T., & Katz, R. (2004). Consensus development conference on antipsychotic drugs and obesity and diabetes: Response to consensus statement. *Diabetes Care, 27*(8), 2088.

Bridges, K. W. & Goldberg, D. P. (1985). Somatic presentation of DSM III psychiatric disorders in primary care. *Journal of Psychiatric Research, 29*, 563–569.

The Chronic Pain Coalition. (2006). The chronic pain coalition. *Annals of the Royal College of Surgeons of England, 88*, 279.

Coventry, P. A., Hays, R., et al. (2011). Talking about depression: A qualitative study of barriers to managing depression in people with long term conditions in primary care. *BMC Family Practice, 12*, 10.

Davies, J. C., Jackson, P. R., Potokar, J., & Nutt, D. J. (2004). Treatment of anxiety and depressive disorders in patients with cardiovascular disease. *British Medical Journal, 328*, 939–943.

De Lusignan, S., Chan, T., Tejerina-Allen, M., Parry, G., & Dent-Brown, K. (2011). Referral for psychological therapy of people with long term conditions improves adherence to antidepressants and reduces emergency department attendance: Controlled before and after study. *Behaviour Research and Therapy, 51*(7), 377–385.

Department of Health. (2005). *Supporting people with long-term conditions*. Department of Health.

Department of Health. (2012). *Long-term conditions compendium of Information* (3rd ed.).

Descartes, R. (1952). Meditations on the first philosophy. In R. M. Hitchins (Ed.), *Great Books of the Western World.* Encyclopaedia Britannica.

Frasure-Smith, N., Lesperance, F., Gravel, G., et al. (2000). Social support, depression, and mortality during the first year after myocardial infarction. *Circulation, 101*, 1919–1924.

Goldney, R. D., Phillips, P. J., Fisher, L. J., & Wildon, D. H. (2004). Diabetes, depression, and quality of life: A population study. *Diabetes Care, 27*(5), 1066–1070.

The King's Fund. (2012). *Long term conditions and multi-morbidity.* https://www.kingsfund.org .uk/projects/time-think-differently/trends-disease-and-disability-long-term-conditions-multi -morbidity.

The King's Fund. (2016). *Bringing together physical and mental health.* https://www.kingsfund.org .uk/publications/physical-and-mental-health.

Layard, R., Bell, S., Clark, D. M., Knapp, M., Meacher, M., & Priebe, S. (2006). The depression report: A new deal for depression and anxiety disorders. *London School of Economics.*

Mehta, N. (2011). Mind-body dualism: A critique from a health perspective. *Mens Sana Monographs, 9*(1), 202–209.

Mental Health Foundation. (2016). Fundamental Facts About Mental Health 2016. *Mental Health Foundation.*

Mind. (2017). *How common are mental health problems?* https://www.mind.org.uk/information -support/types-of-mental-health-problems/statistics-and-facts-about-mental-health/how -common-are-mental-health-problems/#.XYtq-VVKjIU.

Mind. (2018). *40 percent of all GP appointments about mental health.* https://www.mind.org.uk /news-campaigns/news/40-per-cent-of-all-gp-appointments-about-mental-health/.

Mind. (2017). *Better equipped, better care.* Improving mental health training for GPs and practice nurses. https://www.mind.org.uk/media-a/4501/find-the-words-report-better-equipped-better-care.pdf.

Muench, J. & Hamer, A. (2010). Adverse effects of antipsychotic medications. *American Family Physician, 81*(5), 617–622.

National Institute for Health and Care Excellence. (2009). *Depression in adults; Recognition and Management. (NICE guideline CG90.)* https://www.nice.org.uk/Guidance/CG90.

National Institute for Health and Care Excellence. (2009). *Depression in adults with a chronic physical health problem: Recognition and management. (NICE guideline CG91.)* https://www .nice.org.uk/guidance/cg91.

National Institute for Health and Care Excellence. (2011). *Generalised anxiety disorder and Panic Disorder in Adults. (NICE guideline CG113.)* https://www.nice.org.uk/guidance/cg113.

National Institute for Health and Care Excellence. (2015). *Diabetes (Type 1 and Type 2) in children and young people: Diagnosis and management. (NICE guideline NG18.)* https://www.nice.org .uk/guidance/ng18.

Naylor, C., Parsonage, M., McDaid, D., Knapp, M., Fossey., M., & Galea, A. (2012). *Long-term conditions and mental health: The cost of co-morbidities.* The Kings Fund, ISBN: 978-1-85717-633-9.

NHS England. (2018). *Improving physical healthcare for people living with severe mental illness (SMI) in primary care. Guidance for CCGs.*

NHS England. (2019a). *New ways of working to free up doctors as part of the NHS Long Term Plan.* https://www.england.nhs.uk/2019/07/new-ways-of-working-to-free-up-doctors-as-part-of-the -nhs-long-term-plan/.

NHS England. (2019b). *The NHS long term plan.* https://www.longtermplan.nhs.uk/wp-content /uploads/2019/08/nhs-long-term-plan-version-1.2.pdf.

Nursing, Midwifery and Allied Health Professions Policy Unit. (2016). *Improving the physical health of people with mental health problems: Actions for mental health nurses*. https://assets. publishing.service.gov.uk/government/uploads/system/uploads/attachment_data/file/532253 /JRA_Physical_Health_revised.pdf.

Randall, S. & Ford, H. (2011). *Long-term conditions: A Guide for nurses and healthcare professionals*. Wiley-Blackwell.

Svri.org. (2019). *Hospital and anxiety depression rating scale*. https://www.svri.org/sites/default /files/attachments/2016-01-13/HADS.pdf.

West, M., Eckert, R., Stewart, K., & Pasmore, B. (2014). *Developing collective leadership for health care*. https://www.kingsfund.org.uk/sites/default/files/field/field_publication_file /developing-collective-leadership-kingsfund-may14.pdf.

World Health Organization. (1992). *The ICD-10 classification of mental and behavioural disorders: clinical descriptions and diagnostic guidelines*. Geneva: Author.

Chapter 10

Leadership in general practice nursing

Karen Storey

You don't need a title to be a leader or to accomplish amazing things.
See yourself as a leader, now, without changing who you are.

Jo Miller (Women of Influence)

Learning outcomes

After reading this chapter you should be able to:

1. Describe how general practice nurses can contribute as leaders in general practice
2. Understand the principles of leadership
3. Consider the factors that are barriers to effective leadership

Leadership is not about titles, positions or flowcharts.
It is about one life influencing another.

John C. Maxwell

Introduction

As the quote from Maxwell suggests, leadership has little to do with an individual's position or title in an organisation. Although being senior in an organisation might be an indicator that someone has leadership skills, it is not a guarantee of this. Many people who never rise to a position of power or authority in an organisation consistently act as leaders in their day-to-day work. The quote suggests that leadership is about one person being able to influence another. If leadership is thought of in this way, then it becomes something that everyone can achieve, and General Practice Nurses (GPNs) can start to believe that they can be leaders.

The author has experienced that GPNs do not readily consider themselves leaders or consider that they could be leaders in the future. GPNs are in fact leading in their roles every day as they influence people in their care. GPNs use their expert nursing and clinical knowledge to provide patients with information about their health conditions, and influence and empower patients to make the right choices about their health and wellbeing. Leadership thought of in this context becomes something that everyone can achieve, because daily life involves individuals influencing each other.

Reflection

- Take a few moments to think about who you have provided care for in the last few days. What did you do?
- How did you ensure that the care you decided on was appropriate for the patient in your care, and was accepted and adopted by the patient?
- How did you influence the patient's decision to agree to participate in the treatment?

A previous lack of nursing leadership

It has been recognised that there has been a lack of nursing leadership within general practice (Hall, 2007; Howie, 2006). The lack of nursing leadership influences the quality of patient care and impacts on the organisational culture (Sfantou, 2017). General practices in which nurses can develop leadership skills are ones that have a culture where staff members offer each other mutual support and have a positive interest in performance, access to good communication networks and opportunities for professional growth. The challenges are further compounded by the views of GPNs themselves, who do not consider clinical leadership a priority in their role, and suggest that the importance of developing such leadership skills is not always recognised by General Practitioners (GPs) or the nurses themselves (Hughes, 2006). The lack of leadership development has affected GPNs' ability to influence situations within their practice, especially if they have no authoritative or positional leadership role within the practice. Therefore, although GPNs might be assured that the workplace will provide opportunities for them to develop their clinical skills, there appears to be a need to raise awareness of the importance of clinical leadership development amongst GPNs themselves and the GPs who employ them. It has been identified that nurses empower their patients regularly, yet they do not empower themselves, and cite significant barriers that contribute to this (Thyer, 2003).

Development of general practice nursing leadership

Nurses in general practice are highly educated and skilled professionals who are extremely clinically competent in care delivery. However, a survey conducted by the author revealed that, across the country, GPNs have a poor understanding of policy related to health care, wider nursing, primary care and general practice nursing.

Health care policy can be described as a set of rules and regulations that are put into effect to assist in the operation and the shape of health delivery. Health care policy covers a range of issues, including public health, chronic illness and disability, long-term care, the financing of health care, preventive health care and mental health care. This lack of awareness of policy hinders GPNs' ability to contribute to the current changes and development in primary care, and downplays the professional image and contribution of GPNs in the system (While, Webley-Brown, 2017).

The lack of GPNs' ability to influence the system often results in them feeling frustrated with decisions that are made about them, not with them. Scott (2016) suggests that there are many reasons why the nursing voice is either not heard or ignored by those in power, and that by the time staff are consulted on a proposed change it is far too late. Historically, GPNs often report that their voices are not heard, but this does not have to be the case, and new GPNs such as yourself can make this change by asking the following questions: 'What can I do to change this?' and 'How can I help others to understand and pay attention to the valuable role and contributions of GPNs in primary health care?'

With the advent of wider usage of social media, where information can be accessed instantly, it is possible to access firsthand information regarding changes in primary care. Paying attention to these changes and showing an interest in how the profession is developing puts GPNs in the driving seat so that they can influence change for patients, their practices in which they work and much wider decisions about general practice nursing within their Primary Care Networks (PCNs). Having an awareness of and paying attention to the policy changes as they are introduced, and being able to contribute to discussions in a way that gets their voices heard, requires GPNs to invest in development of their leadership skills and to consider this of equal importance to developing their clinical skills. If GPNs have a wider awareness of primary care policy and can share their opinions as general practice nursing experts in this profession, policymakers will start to listen, especially if that voice becomes a collective voice, as a collective voice is difficult not to hear.

Reflection

- As a new general practice nurse, consider how the nursing voice is heard within your practice.
- How can you ensure that the professional opinions of the nurses or the nursing team can contribute to the decisions that are made in the practice?
- Is there a collective professional voice that is able to contribute to clinical team meetings to speak on behalf of nursing care delivery in the practice?

Suzanne Gordon's book 'From Silence to Voice' (Gordon & Buresh, 2013) and the Queens Nursing Institute (QNI, 2016) have helped to strengthen individual GPNs' voices to enable them to speak positively about the expert, often complex, work that they do with patients, communities and the populations that they serve. GPNs must continue to strengthen their voices and connect to the key policy drivers that have shaped general practice nursing, such as the NHS

England General Practice Nursing Ten-Point Plan. Being able to speak about the positive changes that have led to the increased professionalisation of general practice nursing enables other health professionals, policy makers and patients to understand the valuable role that GPNs can play in the primary care system.

Background

Looking back, there have been significant policy achievements affecting general practice nursing since the 1990s. In the United Kingdom the GPN workforce has evolved from playing a lesser and almost invisible role in health care to taking on a leading position in achieving the reforms required for the modernisation of the UK National Health Service (NHS). The evolution of the general practice nursing profession has happened 'organically' over the past decades, and the role of GPN has moved away from being a task-orientated position to being a key player within an integrated, multidisciplinary primary care team. GPNs have considerable autonomy in decision-making, can take a history, make a diagnosis and decide on treatment options in conjunction with the patient, and can prescribe medications. Many nurses are leading the development of new services and working with other members of the primary care team to develop different models of care and service delivery.

The expansion and progression of general practice nursing into advanced practice has raised the profile of general practice nursing, and has given nurses autonomy and increased decision-making scope, putting their knowledge in some instances on a par with that of GPs. This is supported by a recent Cochrane review (Laurant, 2018) of advanced nursing roles in primary care and suggests that care delivered by nurses, compared to care delivered by doctors, probably generates similar or better health care outcomes for a broad range of patient conditions. Nurses in advanced roles have been seen to increase efficiency and streamline services whilst maintaining quality and improving patient satisfaction in general practice (Oliver, 2017).

Investigations into the profession in recent years, such as the Department of Health (DoH, 2008) Work in Partnership Programme and Transforming Nursing for Community and Primary Care (HEE, 2015a), have sought to examine the general practice nursing workforce. The Primary Care Workforce commission (HEE, 2015b) highlighted the excellence, as well as the challenges, of general practice nursing and made recommendations which led to several policy changes to support the profession. Changes in nursing policy and education since the Shape of Caring Review (HEE, 2015c) have helped to transform general practice nursing with the introduction of a Health Education England Career Framework for general practice nursing, as well as opportunities for the Health Care Support Workforce to develop roles through apprentice routes and Nursing Associates through into Registered Nurse roles. The General Practice Nursing Workforce Development Plan (HEE, 2017) and the training hub networks developed by Health Education England in 2015 have seen a more coordinated approach to education and development for the profession, with the rapid expansion of placements for undergraduate nursing students in general practice and the development of mentorship for GPNs.

In 2016 the Chief Nursing Officer (CNO; the professional lead for nursing) for the NHS in England, Professor Jane Cummings, launched a 5-year nursing framework for nursing, midwifery and care staff (NHS England, 2017a) to support the delivery of the Five Year Forward View (NHS England, 2014b). In helping general practice to deliver this, NHS England launched the General Practice Forward View (NHS England, 2017b) with a dedicated action plan for general practice nursing. The General Practice Nursing Ten Point Plan (NHS England, 2017c) aimed to recruit, retain and return nurses to the profession by 2020. It suggested how GPNs can play their part in contributing to addressing challenges within the workforce and population health care by developing leadership skills and working more collaboratively. This direction of travel for general practice nursing is supported by the current CNO for NHS England, Ruth May, who strongly supports the development of nurses in general practice.

The NHS England General Practice Nursing Ten Point Plan programme of work has enabled leadership development for GPNs to become a priority in recent years. Opportunities to prioritise leadership development in addition to clinical development have provided GPNs with knowledge and skills to step up, take more responsibility and lead nursing teams within the practice or consider leadership positions in education within Clinical Commissioning Groups (CCGs) or PCNs. Some nurses have become clinical directors of PCNs, demonstrating for the very first time executive nursing leadership from within the general practice nursing profession.

Transformation of primary care

Primary health care and general practice in England have been undergoing dramatic transformation since the health reforms in 2012. Whereas much of this transformation has focused on the GP being the leader in the workplace, in recent years there has been a recognition that there are a vast number of untapped, high-quality leaders lying dormant within the general practice nursing and allied health professional population.

The NHS Long Term Plan (NHS, 2019) sets out a need and ambition for a team-based approach to deliver holistic, transformational change across the health care system to improve population health. In a system that has previously been developed and structured around top-down delivery approaches, shifting to a population-based local delivery model is complex. Since 2016 there has been a shift towards a new regional model, with the development of Sustainability and Transformation Partnerships (STPs) designed to address the ever-growing pressures on the health service. STPs are transforming into integrated care systems (ICSs) that cover all health care pathways across a geographical region, bringing with them wider-system working and more closely integrated working with other health care professionals.

The NHS Long Term Plan in 2019 and the GP contract review in 2020 saw the development of PCNs. PCNs involve general practices coming together to work across populations of approximately 30,000 to 50,000 individuals and aim to work together to focus on population health and preventive care. Working with other professionals in a multidisciplinary team is a key to the success of PCNs, and GPNs play a key role in enabling this success, bringing to PCNs their knowledge and experience of working closely with patients, communities, populations and wider multidisciplinary teams. The introduction of a wider multidisciplinary team in general practice, expanding the traditional structure of solely nurses and doctors, provides an opportunity to address workforce shortages. This will provide the opportunity to bring specialist multidisciplinary skills into primary care in the form of new roles such as pharmacists, paramedics and physiotherapists, and will enable care delivery to be shifted from hospitals into the community.

Nursing leadership in primary care networks

The development of PCNs provides opportunities for leadership and collaboration by encouraging GPNs, community nurses, public health nurses, hospital nurses and nurses in social care to work together for the benefit of patients, the public and communities. Nurses are vital to the forthcoming changes in the delivery of primary health care in England, as policy focuses on general practices working together in PCNs and involves nurses working more closely in larger, integrated teams. Recent proposals published by NHS England an NHS Improvement, Integrating care; the next steps to building strong and effective integrated care systems (ICSs) across England sets out legislative change to support ICSs. In April 2021 all areas of England had to become part of an integrated care system (ICS) which involved forming partnerships with health and social care working together to reduce health inequalities and to improve better outcomes for patients and populations. ICSs involve wider system collaboration and integration of services and professionals working together. Opportunities exist for GPNs to use their knowledge as holistic expert generalists in prevention, long term condition management and first contact care, to contribute to the and delivery of population health in an ICS working across organisational boundaries to deliver health care. The reforms in primary care make it clear that clinicians are in the driving seat, and that strong clinical leadership is needed. The recent focus on clinical leadership requires GPNs to become involved; however, as previously mentioned, it has now been recognised that historically there has been a distinct lack of nursing leadership within general practice because this area has had little support or focus in previous years. Despite this, there has been an emergence of nursing leadership within general practice nursing, and there are some nurses who are leading as Clinical Directors of PCNs and others who are leading on behalf of clinical specialities and workforce development within their PCNs. Opportunities for leadership positions that were previously absent from general practice nursing are emerging with the development of other new roles, such as becoming a Partner in the practice or taking on a Primary Care Lead Nurse role.

Barriers to leadership development

The unique employment conditions of nurses working in general practice mean that they are employed directly by GPs who are independent contractors that work on behalf of the NHS but are not considered to be part of the wider NHS workforce. GPNs do not benefit from the same terms and conditions of employment or career structure as other nurses who are NHS employees. Employment arrangements are widely variable, and this can mean that nurses are 'managed' by a GP or practice manager rather than by a nurse.

The nature of general practice work means that GPNs often work at a highly autonomous level. Physical and professional isolation are often experienced, and many GPNs have no recognised support structure. In general practice nursing there has historically been a lack of team working, integration and skills mix, as well as no effective workforce development. The challenge that this culture brings is that if nurses do try to initiate change and are not supported, they lose confidence and assertiveness and may feel disempowered. This may have a negative effect on them as they experience loss of self-esteem and dependence—causing workers to become disruptive, or to leave the organisation (Hyett, 2003).

It has been recognised that there is a wide variation nationally in access to education, training and development amongst GPNs. This variation has a direct impact on the level of skills and expertise amongst GPNs, and this has an impact on the quality of care delivered to patients. The lack of career development is another barrier, and the current perception is that the only way to progress a career for a GPN is through advanced clinical practice rather than advancement through any other alternative. The General Practice Nursing Ten Point Plan has included in its work an update to the Health Education England GPN career framework, which describes opportunities for creating portfolio careers that involve GPNs undertaking leadership roles in PCNs, research, mentorship and teaching to expand their clinical careers.

Despite these barriers, there are still some GPNs who have managed to take a leading role in their practice and have advanced their skills and competencies to become Independent Prescribers, Nurse Practitioners and even Partners in general practices; but generally these numbers remain low. The difference now is that these historical challenges have been recognised by the system and other professionals, and there is a willingness to address these issues to enable the sustainability of the general practice nursing workforce now and in the future. Opportunities for career and leadership development are emerging; however, as the system is changing there is a need for nurses to own and take control of their profession to engage and lead in these developments.

Understanding the theory of leadership

To be a successful leader, it is useful to understand something about the theory of leadership. Until most recently, leadership styles have been described as either 'transactional' or 'transformational'; however, new leadership theories are being introduced which bring a different approach and aim to transform health care.

Transactional leadership applies to older managerial styles. It involves the skills required in the effective day-to-day running of a team; for example, the autocratic style allows the leader to set an end goal without encouraging others to participate in the decision-making process, and often uses reward and punishment as a way of motivating people. A bureaucratic leadership style occurs when the leader is inflexible and adheres to policies, rules and regulations.

However, transformational leadership shows how an integrated team works together and encourages innovativeness. It focuses on having a vision, developing and empowering individuals and challenging traditional assumptions. Transformational leadership is about influencing others to do things and is connected to the process of addressing the needs of others so that the process of interaction increases their motivation and energy. It is commonly connected with clinical leadership and is a theory where the interdependence of followers and leaders is linked. Transformational leaders are often charismatic and inspirational, and they are more considerate towards others.

Becoming a transformational leader

New GPNs are in a unique position to model transformational leadership behaviours as they set out on this journey to become the primary care leaders of the future. When thinking about becoming a transformational leader, it is worth considering the work of Kouzes and Posner (2017), who offer five practices of exemplary leadership (Box 10.1).

Inspire a shared vision

Leaders are driven by a sense of the possible and what their team or the practice can become. Leaders can look to the future and see what is possible, imagining the opportunities that are in store and believing they can make a difference. However, leaders cannot be leaders without followers. They cannot command commitment from their followers; they have to inspire it, so that what was the

---

Box 10.1   Five practices of exemplary leadership

- Inspire a shared vision
- Model the way
- Challenge the process
- Encourage the heart
- Enable others to act

From Kouzes J. M., Posner B. Z. (2002). *The leadership challenge* (3rd ed.) Jossey-Bass.

leader's vision becomes everyone's vision. These leaders believe they can make a difference and inspire others to do the same, remaining positive and demonstrating the values that underpin and are at the core of nursing.

Model the way

The most important personal quality people look for and admire in a leader is credibility. People must believe in the leader to be able to believe his or her message. Leaders have strong beliefs and are willing to stand up for these beliefs. They set an example to others and 'walk the talk', doing what they say they will do. Their behaviours are what earn them their respect, setting an example through daily acts. They must be able to find their voice to be able to speak up against wrongs and share their values with others, expecting commitment without imposing their values on them. Leaders' belief and enthusiasm for their vision and excitement for the future are contagious. Leaders can uplift others, keep them motivated and instil hope.

Challenge the process

Leaders manage change well and look for ways of improving care and the culture of an organisation. Leaders understand that keeping things the way they have always been is not good. They challenge the process by searching for new opportunities, experimenting and taking risks but are willing to learn from their mistakes. Leaders are willing to change the status quo to improve conditions for themselves or others. Leaders remain open to new ideas and seize opportunities if they arise, such as a dramatic external event that impacts on an organisation or if a radical new way of working arises. Leaders are supporters and adopters of new ways of working and innovation, acknowledging that, if things do not work out, learning can come from this, rather than blame.

Encourage the heart

Leaders tend to be positive and optimistic and have a can-do attitude. They are aware that the road to achieving change can be a long one, and that there may be times when they themselves feel like giving up. Leaders overcome these obstacles to uplift the spirits of themselves and others and move people forward. Leaders encourage the heart by recognising the contributions of others and celebrating values and victories. They pay attention, offering encouragement and appreciation and maintaining a positive outlook. They show appreciation of others' contributions and look for ways to reward others for their performance, doing this with authenticity and building a strong sense of community spirit that can get their teams through difficult times.

Enable others to act

Leaders understand that they cannot do things alone, and that it is a team effort. They understand that teamwork, trust and empowerment are what will help to strengthen everyone's capacity to deliver on the vision and outcomes. They understand that collaboration is the skill that enables teams and partnerships to function effectively, and is at the core of enabling the project to work or making the change that is needed. Leaders make it possible for everyone to do extraordinary work by fostering trust and building confidence through relationships with others. Creating an environment where everyone contributes and can be involved enables followers to become leaders themselves. Empowering and enabling others to take ownership makes people feel strong, capable, informed and connected. Leaders do not reserve the power themselves; rather, they enable others to take informed risks and act, knowing that the leader has their back if things do not go to plan. Creating this positive culture enables everyone on the team to flourish, reach their potential and produce extraordinary results.

Reflection

What does leadership mean to you? Are you confident and comfortable calling yourself a leader? Do you think that only people at the top of an organisation or who have 'Leader' in their job title can be leaders?

Most people consider this to be true and might think that if they call themselves a leader then others might view them as being over-confident or big-headed. When we think of the word leadership, we might associate it with people who have accomplished amazing achievements, such as putting a man on the moon or conquering a mountain. If we only think of leadership in this context, we start to undervalue the everyday things that we all do that are, in fact, acts of leadership. These acts of everyday leadership involve the ability to influence others, something that General Practice Nurses do with their patients every day. If this ability to influence patients can be applied to others in the practice team or to other situations, this can be incredibly empowering and beneficial to the team.

Think about how you influence your work colleagues with your own behaviour. How do you persuade and influence others to follow you?

Styles of leadership

Peer leadership

There is recognition that people working in health and social care need to modernise services and harness the potential of new technologies. Peer leadership is currently being used and developed within the NHS. Peer leadership is, again, unlike the traditional leadership methods seen within health care, as it does not rely on positional authority alone (Douglas & Keep, 2012). It has a strong focus on health outcomes rather than organisational outcomes, is focused on output and encourages leaders to recognise that they do not have to achieve things through direct control, but rather by developing their ability to encourage others to work towards their vision. It allows individuals to develop the ability to influence others, whatever their role or position, as well as to challenge others' behaviour to get things done. The development of personal influence and authority comes through wisdom drawn from experience, as well as trusting relationships built from shared values.

Collective leadership

New theories around leadership are emerging to address the challenges that the health care profession is facing. Professor Michael West (West et al., 2014) suggests that collective leadership, a model in which everyone takes responsibility for the success of the organisation as a whole, and not just for their own jobs or area, is a preferred model of leadership. He goes on to suggest that, if leaders and managers create positive, supportive environments for staff, those staff members can then create caring, supportive environments for patients, delivering higher quality care. A culture of collective leadership means that all staff members are likely to intervene to solve problems, ensure quality of care and promote responsible, safe innovation (Fig. 10.1).

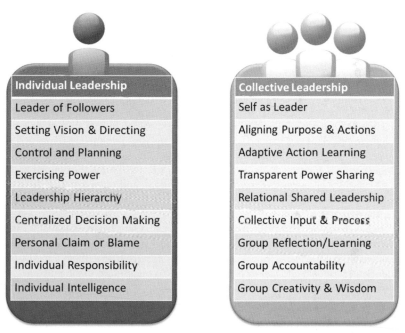

Individual Leadership	Collective Leadership
Leader of Followers	Self as Leader
Setting Vision & Directing	Aligning Purpose & Actions
Control and Planning	Adaptive Action Learning
Exercising Power	Transparent Power Sharing
Leadership Hierarchy	Relational Shared Leadership
Centralized Decision Making	Collective Input & Process
Personal Claim or Blame	Group Reflection/Learning
Individual Responsibility	Group Accountability
Individual Intelligence	Group Creativity & Wisdom

Fig. 10.1   Individual versus collective leadership. (From West, M., Eckert, R., Stewart, K., & Pasmore, B. (2014). *Developing collective leadership for health care.* https://www.kingsfund.org.uk/sites/default/files/field/field_publication_file/developing-collective-leadership-kingsfund-may14.pdf.)

Case study

In 2015 the author, as an employee of Health Education England, along with NHS Leadership Academy in the West Midlands, developed a primary care leadership programme. This included a model of interprofessional education known

Continued

as a 'Triumvirate'. The Triumvirate Leadership Programme was designed to bring three key professionals—General Practitioner, General Practice Nurse (GPN) and Practice Manager—from the same general practice together to attend a leadership programme together over a specific period of time. The programme provided protected time for the team to learn together and to develop shared leadership knowledge and skills.

GPNs in the Triumvirates reported that, as a result, the traditional hierarchical barriers that may have existed before participants entered the programme were challenged as the Triumvirate teams discovered that their colleagues possessed professional, technical and soft skills that could enhance the teams' working practices. Before the programme commenced, the organisations carried out a survey to see how participants felt about various aspects of their general practice. When this questioning was repeated at the end of the programme, improvements were demonstrated in all parameters, including shared leadership (+16%), communication (+24%), organisational culture (+29%) and strategic vision (+23%).

Several iterations of the programme have taken place, and some practices have developed the model further by inviting other allied health professionals to join the traditional Triumvirate, and clinical pharmacists, paramedics and other new roles have complemented the traditional team. This model is different from traditional leadership programmes, which aim to address individual development needs and usually involve the individual attending a development programme away from the practice. With traditional leadership programmes, the challenge then is for individuals to use what was learned on the programme and then put it into practice in the general practice environment on completion of the programme. This approach requires time, effort and the individual's influence or position in the general practice team, as well as persistence from the individual, and often results in little or no change being made.

The Triumvirate leaders reported that the impact of learning together in a classroom-based setting, away from the practice and with other Triumvirate teams, had not only brought about new learning, but had also strengthened the professional relationships of the team. They reported that this approach gave them added confidence and influence to make changes happen on their return to the practice.

What makes a good leader?

The NHS leadership academy has developed a leadership framework (available at https://www.leadershipacademy.nhs.uk/resources/healthcare-leadership-model/), which has been formed based on the principle of shared or collective leadership. It suggests that leadership is not limited to people who hold appointed leadership roles, and that the success of an organisation is a shared responsibility. It encourages all staff to contribute to leadership and to demonstrate appropriate leadership behaviours to empower the leadership capacity of colleagues. It acknowledges that not everyone is necessarily in a leadership role, but that everyone can contribute to the leadership process.

Mckeown (2014) suggests that we can all, any of us, lead at any time. We do not need to wait for permission to act, or to be the head of an organisation to be a leader. Myths exist that to be a leader you have to be heroic, or a certain type of person, or that you can only lead from in front, or that leadership is only visible in a time of crisis. It is now time to see leadership differently and to think of ourselves as everyday leaders.

Burns (2009) suggests that there are many views on what constitutes effective leadership. Leadership can be based on the leader's personal characteristics and the effect he or she has on the organisational function and culture, as well as leader and team behaviour. A good leader can be described as one who is confident and competent, who is aware of his or her own behaviours, strengths and areas for development, who works well with team members and is patient-focused, who is good at networking and who is politically aware.

Emotional intelligence

Good leadership starts with self; being able to manage ourselves, our responses and our relationships with others makes for good leadership. Having emotional intelligence (EI) is a valuable asset in leadership. Goleman (1998) describes EI as a person's ability to manage his or her feelings so that those feelings are expressed appropriately and effectively. He goes on to suggest that EI is the largest single predictor of success in the workplace. Good leadership requires individuals to have awareness of self, is one of the four dimensions of EI and demonstrates personal competence. EI includes how we manage ourselves and how we respond to situations and the acts of others, and this depends on our ability to manage and control our responses to these situations (Box 10.2).

Organisational culture

It is worth spending some time considering how the culture of the organisation affects leadership and how leadership can affect culture. The culture of the organisation refers to the working environment and, put simply, is how things get done in the organisation. Some cultures are stiff, formal, hierarchical and strictly business-like, whereas others are informal, creative, personable and less hierarchical. The way in which individuals communicate and relate to each other, organisational structure and transparency are all aspects of culture. The culture of an organisation can have an effect on the employee's development and potential, so getting the culture right in an organisation is crucial (Curtis, 2011).

The Care Quality Commission, in their inspection of general practice, focuses on the culture of the organisation and rates providers on a four-point scale of 'outstanding', 'good', 'requires improvement' or 'inadequate' for each of the five domains that it inspects. In order for a practice to obtain a 'good' or 'outstanding' rating, the Commission focuses on leadership and states that leadership at all levels within the organisation is key to the success

---

Box 10.2 The four dimensions of emotional intelligence

Personal Competence: These capabilities determine how we manage ourselves

Self-Awareness

- Emotional self-awareness: Reading one's own emotions and recognising their impact using 'gut sense' to guide decisions
- Accurate self-assessment: Knowing one's strengths and limits
- Self-confidence: A sound sense of one's self-worth and capabilities

Self-Management

- Emotional self-control: Keeping disruptive emotions and impulses under control
- Transparency: Displaying honesty and integrity; trustworthiness
- Adaptability: Flexibility in adapting to changing situations or overcoming obstacles
- Achievement: The drive to improve performance to meet inner standards of excellence
- Initiative: Readiness to act and seize opportunities
- Optimism: Seeing the upside in events
- Social competence: These capabilities determine how we manage relationships

Social Awareness

- Empathy: Sensing others' emotions, understanding their perspective and taking active interest in their concerns
- Organisational awareness: Reading the currents, decision networks and politics at the organisational level
- Service: Recognising and meeting follower, client or customer needs

Relationship Management

- Inspirational leadership: Guiding and motivating with a compelling vision
- Influence: Wielding a range of tactics for persuasion
- Developing others: Bolstering others' abilities through feedback and guidance
- Change catalyst: Initiating, managing and leading in a new direction
- Conflict management: Resolving disagreements
- Building bonds: Cultivating and maintaining a web of relationships
- Teamwork and collaboration: Cooperation and team building

From Goleman, D. (1998). *Working with emotional intelligence*. Clays.

---

with genuine engagement of staff. Good leadership is vital in creating and sustaining a culture in health care which understands that, if staff are to treat patients really well, then they themselves need to be really valued by their employers.

The unique organic structure of general practice means that in most cases the GP, as the employer, is considered the clinical leader of the practice team and the decision maker (McKenna, 2004). General practices in which the nurses are able to develop leadership skills are those that have good communication networks, value each others' professional opinions and have a culture where staff offer each other support and have a positive interest in performance. A healthy work environment is associated with job satisfaction, worker wellbeing and effective communication. Improving communication through clinical team meetings means that organisations can encourage innovation and creativity, which in turn will promote job enlargement and enrichment (Argyris, 1964). Clinical team meetings are crucial events in many work environments, and during team meetings many discussions take place on how to deal with practice issues, as well as clinical practice. GPNs should have input to the practice clinical team meeting, either directly or through a nursing team leader. Hughes et al. (2006) suggest that organisations that empower team members to lead in shared decision-making and shared leadership, encouraging a bottom-up approach that emphasises trust, ownership and change, where employees ask questions and make decisions, are more successful.

Structure leadership programmes

It has been recognised that GPNs' experience of leadership has previously been variable, depending on previous personal and professional experiences in secondary care or other settings. Action Two of the NHS General Practice Nursing Ten Point Plan has seen national investment in leadership programmes for GPNs to address this variation. Leadership programmes have been developed by NHS England nationally and regionally through the NHS Leadership Academy, CCGs and Training Hubs Programmes delivered by the NHS Leadership Academy. These programmes have included the Mary Seacole programme, the Edward Jenner programme and most recently the Rosalind Franklin leadership programme, which was developed specifically to meet the needs of GPNs.

Case study

As part of the NHS England and NHS Improvement General Practice Nursing Ten Point Plan programme of work, a structured bespoke leadership and resilience programme was developed to specifically meet the needs of General Practice Nurses (GPNs) during the COVID-19 pandemic. GPNs across the country benefited from CARE, which stands for connected, authentic, resilient, and empowered—the values and behaviours the programme promotes. It is a practical development programme that aimed to empower GPNs to drive innovation, strengthen relationships and develop a bottom-up, population health approach to health care. The programme supported GPNs to build their self-awareness and resilience, which in turn helped to unlock new and exciting innovation and system leadership, despite a time of heightened pressure.

The programme was developed in partnership with National Association of Primary Care, the General Practice Nursing Ten Point Plan team at NHS England and NHS Improvement (which commissioned the programme), the Bedfordshire, Luton

Continued

and Milton Keynes (BLMK) integrated care system (ICS) and specialist coaches ShinyMind. The programme offered practical and holistic learning through expert-led webinars, quality improvement project support and a dedicated community of support. Early success in BLMK has already led to innovation and joined-up working in the BLMK ICS, which piloted the approach. Janet Thornley, GPN Strategic Lead, BLMK ICS, said: 'CARE has been pivotal in helping the PCN Leads develop multi-professional relationships which have driven a bottom up, population health focussed approach to care. The programme has given the participants the tools to identify the needs as they are right now and actively participate with colleagues across the PCNs to improve patient health outcomes by connecting national and local strategy. The projects we are seeing emerge from CARE are exciting and innovative. Patients' lives will definitely be improved and joy at work has returned for the workforce. It really has exceeded our expectations.'

Leadership with patients

According to a Kings Fund (2018) report, public satisfaction with general practice has declined to the lowest level since the National Centre for Social Research's British Social Attitudes survey began. Satisfaction amongst those 65 years or older was previously much higher than that amongst other age groups; however, in 2017 satisfaction had fallen in all age groups. One of the top reasons was long waiting times for GP appointments. The national GP patient survey provides more insight and reports that patients are finding it harder to get through to their GP surgery on the phone and harder to see their GP of choice, and rate their overall experience in general practice more negatively.

To deal with complex health care and access demands, there are professionals in general practice who are looking at new ways of collaborating with patients that are moving away from the traditional consulting model to more innovative consulting models using technology and a concept of group consultations. GPNs in some areas of England have embraced these opportunities to lead on and develop group consultations.

Case study

General Practice Nurses (GPNs) in the north of England have been leading on a different way of consulting with patients. By changing the way clinicians consult, this approach shifts the balance of power, changes the clinical conversation, improves outcomes, creates time to care and improves both the patient and GPN experience.

Group consultations see 10–12 people consulting with a GPN at the same time. All patients in the group have been invited and given their consent to participate in the programme and share their information with others.

Supported by a facilitator (often a health care assistant), the GPN joins the consultation after 15–20 minutes once patients have looked at their results and thought of questions. The GPN consults one to one, with the other patients listening in and offering advice and support too. To understand the flow, go to: https://youtube /uZKVbKUvTfs.

Evaluation of GPN-led group consultation in the North West found that consulting with groups gave GPNs more time to explain and educate patients. GPNs got to know their patients better, repeated less, had more fun and found clinics more fulfilling and energising than one-to-one care. They also felt that group consultations shifted the power dynamic, with the consultation being more focused on the patients than on the clinician's Quality Outcomes Framework review.

Patients benefited from better clinical outcomes; for instance, in seven clinical trials, patients' HBA1c levels fell more than those of patients who received usual care. They also gained confidence and improved their knowledge of their condition. Satisfaction rates are very high, at over 97%.

Case study

As part of the North West General Practice Nurse (GPN) Group Consultations Practice Development Programme, in 2017, Premiere Health and West Gorton introduced group consultations for adults with diabetes.

West Gorton calculated 100% efficiency gains in clinician time and saw eight to nine patients in the time it would have taken to them to see four patients in regulated 4-minute-long one-to-one appointments.

Across these two practices, 31 patients, followed up after 3 months, achieved an average 10% reduction in HbA1c (65 to 59 mmol/mol). In Premiere Health, six patients achieved an average reduction in blood pressure (systolic by 12.5% and diastolic by 5%). In Premiere Health, the same six patients achieved an average weight reduction of 3.9%.

GPNs reported that group consultations shift the balance of power, are more person-centred and support peer connection, with friendships forming from the first session.

Patients report having high satisfaction rates and learning more compared with one-to-one consultations, even if their diabetes was already well controlled. Some found group care less intimidating than one-to-one reviews. Staff found introducing group consultations too time-consuming. Staff learnt a lot from patients. In addition, 93% of GPNs in this programme reported that group consultations were fulfilling. No GPNs reported that they felt stressed or burnt out by group consultations, and 57% of GPNs reported that group consultations energised them, compared with 19% describing one-to-one consultations as energising at baseline. Staff enjoyed consultations with less repetition. Group consultations accelerated skills development in health care assistants and student nurses, where they were involved.

Take a few moments to reflect on your consultations. What would it take to adopt group consultation into your practice?

General practice nurses leading through the COVID-19 pandemic

The COVID-19 pandemic placed a huge challenge on the health and social care system and on individuals themselves. Although primary care initially slowed down because patient footfall was reduced owing to patients being advised not to visit their general practices and to stay at home, GPs and GPNs recognised that they had to meet patients' needs in different ways.

Practical measures were put in place to allow minimal face-to-face contact with patients, and those who were to be seen were considered essential and high priority. In the main, patients were contacted through non–face-to-face methods (i.e., phone or video consultations). Extra resources were provided to primary care to allow for the expansion of digital technology. Many GPNs stepped up to demonstrate their leadership, rapidly learning how to consult with their patients through phone or video consultations. This rapid expansion of digital technology would have taken much longer to embed in normal circumstances, but happened out of need rather than desire.

GPNs learned to use digital technology and adapted their consultations with patients to use video for one-to-one consultations. Some considered video for group consultations using the same principles as those used for face-to-face group consultations, but managing the group through a virtual meeting using Zoom or Microsoft Teams. GPNs who adopted these ways of working demonstrated the ability to adapt to change, one of the key principles of good leadership, and an important EI competency.

GPNs in some parts of England started to look at how essential face-to-face care could be delivered in alternative, innovative ways whilst maintaining social distancing. Drive-through childhood vaccination clinics were set up following a thorough risk assessment and a 'Plan Do Study Act' cycle. This creative ability to lead services in different, adaptable ways was a great demonstration of leadership by GPNs. These clinics were set up by GPNs, GPs and other practice staff working together collaboratively, demonstrating inclusive and distributive leadership, doing things for the first time and learning as they went along to respond to the crisis.

The COVID-19 pandemic brought about the ability for rapid and adaptable change that transformed primary care delivery and introduced new ways of working, and GPNs contributed to this transformation. What is needed as we move forward is for GPNs to continue to lead and to lock in these new ways of working as the 'new normal'.

Conclusion

The nursing role in general practice is an important and valuable contributor to the delivery of patient care. GPNs in this role have now become a highly skilled, accomplished and essential asset to the general practice team. GPNs, as leaders and enablers in the system, require investment and support from GPs (as their employers) to promote their wider recognition as highly competent members of the interdisciplinary team. Leadership that is shared and involves all members of the practice is integral to creating a motivated team. Distributive, inclusive, shared leadership with the general practice culture is essential if nurses are to be supported to develop their leadership skills. The COVID-19 pandemic provided an opportunity for GPNs to step up and lead alternative ways of care delivery to their patients. Ensuring that these new ways of working are locked in and used to transform general practice nursing in the future is essential. GPNs who are able to own their space in the leadership arena, develop themselves and influence and deliver excellent care to patients must be a priority for general practice teams now and in the future.

> A leader is best
> When people barely know he exists
> Of a good leader, who talks little,
> When his work is done, his aim fulfilled,
> They will say, 'We did this ourselves'.
> *Lao Tzu, Tao Te Ching*

References

Argyris, C. (1964). *Integrating the individual and the organization.* Wiley.

Burns, D. (2009). Clinical leadership for general practice nurses, part 1: Perceived needs. *Practice Nursing, 20*(10), 519–523.

Douglas, R. & Keep, J. (2012). *Why collaborative leadership is the new tool of effective peer leadership.* http://www.hsj.co.uk/resourcecentre/leadership/why-collaboration-is-the-new-tool-of-effective-peerleadership/5043520.article.

Goleman, D. (1998). *Working with Emotional Intelligence.* Clays London.

Gordon, G. & Buresh, B. (2013). *From silence to voice: What nurses know and must communicate to the public.* Cornell.

Health Education England. (2015a). Transforming nursing for community and primary care. https://www.hee.nhs.uk/our-work/transforming-nursing-community-primary-care.

Health Education England. (2015b). *The future of primary care: Creating teams for tomorrow.* http://hee.nhs.uk/wp-content/blogs.dir/321/files/2015/07/The-future-of-primary-care.pdf.

Health Education England. (2015c). Shape of caring review. https://www.hee.nhs.uk/our-work/shape-caring-review.

Health Education England. (2017). *The general practice nursing workforce development plan.* https://www.hee.nhs.uk/.../The%20general%20practice%20nursing%20workforce%20.

Howie, K. (2006). Management skills in the primary care team. *Practice Nurse, 31*(4), 505. 4.

Hughes, A., Elson, P., & Govier, J. (2006). Developing practice nurses leadership skills. *Practice Nursing, 17*(8), 376–378.

Hyett, E. (2003). What blocks Health Visitors from taking on a leadership role. *Journal of Nursing Management, 11*(4), 229–233.

Kouzes, J. M. & Posner, B. Z. (2017). *The leadership challenge: How to make extraordinary things happen in organisations,* (6th ed.). John Wiley & Sons, Hoboken, New Jersey.

Laurant, M., van der Biezen, M., Wijers, N., Watananirun, K., Kontopantelis, E., & van Vught, A. (2018). Nurses as substitutes for doctors in primary care. *The Cochrane Database of Systematic Reviews, 7*, CD001271.

McKeown, G. (2014). Essentialism: *The Disciplined Pursuit of Less:* Random House ISBN 0753550288, 9780753550281

NHS England. (2015). *Five year forward view.* https://www.cngland.nhs.uk/five-year-forward -view/.

NHS England. (2017a). *Leading change adding value – a framework for nursing, midwifery and care staff.* https://www.england.nhs.uk/wp-content/uploads/2016/05/nursing-framework.pdf.

NHS England. (2017b). *General practice forward view (GPFV).* https://www.england.nhs.uk /publication/general-practice-forward-view-gpfv/.

NHS England. (2017c). *General practice – developing confidence, capability and capacity. A ten-point action plan for general practice nursing.* https://www.england.nhs.uk/publication/general -practice-developing-confidence-capability-and-capacity/.

NHS England. (2019). *The NHS long term plan.* https://www.longtermplan.nhs.uk/.

Queen's Nursing Institute. (2016). *General practice nursing in the 21st century: A time of opportunity.* https://www.qni.org.uk/wp-content/uploads/2016/09/gpn_c21_report.pdf.

Scott, G. (2016). *Nurses' voices must be heard by those in power.* https://rcni.com/nursing-standard /opinion/editorial/nurses-voices-must-be-heard-those-power-64796.

Sfantou, D., Laliotis, A., Patelarou, A., Sifaki-Pistolla, D., Matalliotakis, M., & Patelarou, E. (2017). Importance of Leadership style towards quality of care measures in healthcare settings: A systematic review. *Healthcare (Basel), 5*(4), 73.

Thyer, G. L. (2003). Dare to be different: Transformational leadership may hold the key to reducing the nursing shortage. *Journal of Nursing Management, 11*, 73–79.

West, M., Eckert, R., Stewart, K., & Pasmore, B. (2014). *Developing collective leadership for health care.* https://www.kingsfund.org.uk/sites/default/files/field/field_publication_file /developing-collective-leadership-kingsfund-may14.pdf.

While, A. & Webley-Brown, C. (2016). General practice nursing: Who is cherishing this workforce? *London Journal of Primary Care, 9*(1), 10–13.

Chapter 11

Quality and safety

Rhian Last

Learning outcomes

After reading this chapter you should be able to:

1. Introduce improvement theories for managing change
2. Explore effective collaborative team working and multidisciplinary team working
3. Emphasise the imperative for improving patient safety, experience and outcomes

Introduction

The National Health Service (NHS) is continuously changing, and this can be both exciting and challenging. The current emphasis on personalised care, the need for improved efficiency and effectiveness and a commitment to collaborative working is necessitating the redesign of services (NHS England, 2019). Front-line staff members in primary care, including General Practice Nurses (GPNs), are becoming involved in developing or redesigning systems and processes within their working area to meet the demand for user-friendly, efficient and convenient services which provide high-quality outcomes for patients, their family and carers.

It is often at the front line of working that some of the best ideas for making improvements can arise. Knowing how to put a good idea into practice is the fundamental next step. As a nurse new to general practice, you may have an opportunity as part of the nursing team to contribute to change in delivery of services in the practice, and certainly with individual patients in your care. Discussing this through regular clinical supervision and allowing time to reflect on clinical practice with your mentor and others will enable a culture of continuous reflective learning to improve the quality of care delivered to patients in the practice population.

Improvement science theory and methods

Improvement science is a concept that is rapidly gaining momentum and is used to address challenges and drive a culture change of continuous learning and improvement. There are many tools and models for improvement, and some of the key ones are explored in the next sections of this chapter.

Theory of profound knowledge

William Edwards Deming, an American statistician, suggested that quality can be improved, at reduced cost, by the practice of continual improvement and by thinking of the work of an organisation as a system, not as disparate 'bits and pieces' (Deming, 1986). What this means for GPNs is that, when seeking to improve, it is important to consider the 'whole picture' from our patients' perspective; and in order to achieve quality and improvement that are continuous and sustainable, we need to understand processes and systems. Many of the problems that NHS organisations, including general practice, have in serving their patients and populations are caused by the systems and processes in place. Discrepancies, or gaps in processes, can lead to unacceptable delays, steps not being performed correctly, important steps being omitted and myriad other difficulties that result in inefficient and costly services and disgruntled customers. There is a need for an understanding of the complexity of, and relations between, organisations within health and social care overall and within general practice. This is because there is so often a breakdown of communication or a lack of understanding of who does what, when and where. It can lead to confusion, duplication and a general driving up of costs and, importantly, can impact negatively on patient safety, outcomes and experience.

Each part of an organisation impacts on the functioning of other parts. According to Deming's theory, to effect meaningful and impactful change we need profound knowledge of:

- The systems and processes of the organisation.
- The natural variation that occurs within those processes, so that overreaction to normal variation is avoided (we will discuss variation in more detail later when we look at statistical process control [SPC]). A simple example in a General Practitioner (GP) surgery will be that Monday mornings tend to be busier than other times of the week (this would be deemed a natural variation). To assist with this, the practice manager may arrange extra staff cover on a Monday morning. If the practice manager judged every day on the basis of how busy a Monday morning is and arranged extra staff to cover throughout the week on this basis, this would be an overreaction to normal variation.
- Knowledge of how the various systems and processes interrelate. This is important both within the GP surgery and also within the wider health and social care teams that we refer to and liaise with on behalf of our patients. Change in one part of a system will have a wider impact. To be able to effectively factor this in during the planning stage of any proposed change, it is important to have a good knowledge of systems and processes.
- Psychology, an understanding of how change impacts on individuals and the importance of building trust within the workforce and with customers. Change is hard for everyone, and it is always important to give this full consideration when planning new ways of working.

Reflection

- Think about a change that you have made or been involved with.
- It may have been a lifestyle change, perhaps losing weight or taking up exercise, or maybe moving to a new house, perhaps to a completely new area. What impact did it have on you? How were you feeling about this change?
- You may have been involved in changes at work.
- What were the challenges? Were they overcome? If so, what helped to make this happen?

In addition, for optimal functioning, everyone in an organisation must share a clear understanding of and commitment to the organisation's aim or purpose. This is the nub of successful collaborative working. Among the critical success factors for organisational change identified by Deming are:

- Constancy of purpose
- Building quality into the process, rather than relying on constant checking that quality is being achieved
- Ceasing to judge success based on cost alone
- Striving for continuous improvement
- Learning by experience and discovering better ways of doing things
- Having leaders who support people to do a better job. Management by fear stifles innovation and collaboration
- Removal of barriers between different departments and agencies. Change requires a team approach
- Elimination of management by targets and numbers. Performance reviews based on these factors alone, particularly when the means of reaching an objective are unclear or unstated, are demotivating and demoralising
- Giving people the means to take pride in their work
- Instituting educational and self-improvement initiatives
- Engaging everyone in the change process (Deming, 1986)

'Plan Do Study Act' cycles

'Plan Do Study Act' (PDSA) cycles are a way of testing an idea by trialling a change on a small scale, assessing its impact and learning from previous cycles before blanket implementation (NHS, 2018).

The Model for Improvement (Langley et al., 1996) is a method often used for continuous quality improvement initiatives (Fig. 11.1). Based on improvement science theories, the Improvement Model is logical, uncomplicated and based on three fundamental questions:

What are we trying to accomplish?

It is very important here not to jump into unconsidered, knee-jerk reactions. Time must be taken to examine and consider the whole picture and determine

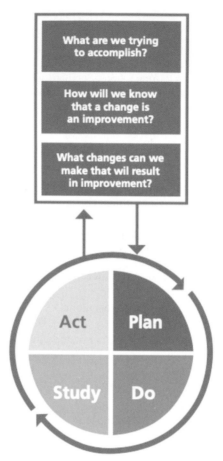

Fig. 11.1 The model for improvement. *Source: NHSE / NHSI Quality, Service Improvement and Redesign (QSIR) Tools.* https://www.england.nhs.uk/wp-content/uploads/2021/03/qsir-plan-do-study-act.pdf.

what exactly you are aiming to achieve. This will help to ensure that any action taken will lead to improvement that is meaningful and sustainable.

How will we know that a change is an improvement?

This will require an appropriate process and method for capturing and measuring data. This will help everyone to understand where you are and where you are going.

What changes can we make that will result in improvement?

This is where the PDSA cycles come into play. By trying out small incremental changes it will be possible to monitor what is working well and not so well so that long-term changes will lead to sustainable improvement. It is important to keep things simple and specific. This will also help to keep things manageable.

The PDSA cycle is initially undertaken on a small scale over a short time frame, and data are collected. If the results of the small-scale trial look promising, the initiative is then rolled out to a slightly larger group. If things continue to look promising, a further step change is then undertaken, and so on. The progressive steps of the PDSA cycle allow us to learn what works and what does not (at little cost if things go wrong), and to continuously improve the process with each step change. The PDSA cycle used in this way is an effective method of 'rapid cycle testing', a practice recommended by Deming. It should be a dynamic, fluid and continuously rolling process of incremental change.

Lean production

Lean production, also referred to simply as 'lean', refers to systems or processes that are not wasteful of resources, materials or humans. The principles of lean originated in Japanese manufacturing, and its basic philosophy is centred on preserving value with less work – working smarter, rather than only working harder (Holweg, 2006). Lean aims to:

- Improve quality: Understand the customer's (or in this case patient's) needs and design processes that meet their expectations and requirements
- Eliminate waste: Any activity that consumes time or resources that does not add value
- Reduce the time an activity takes: This is one of the most effective ways of eliminating waste and lowering cost
- Reduce overall cost: By only producing enough to meet demand

Although lean originated in industry, some of its principles and methods may be applied to the settings of health care and general practice:

- Designing and using a system that is simple and eliminates steps in the process that do not directly contribute to the end goal of improved patient care
- Recognition that there is always room for improvement and continuously improving the system for improved efficiency and less waste

Statistical process control

To identify improvement, data need to be collected. However, as discussed earlier in this chapter, there will be some degree of natural variation in every process, e.g., waiting time in a particular clinic, patient satisfaction data and serial blood pressure measurement. Variation comes from two main sources:

- Common: Also known as normal, random, chance or unknown
- Special: Assignable (Shewhart, 1931)

Common variation is natural and causes a stable, repeating pattern of variation. Special causes of variation are unpredictable. For example, we would expect to have some snow in winter (common variation), for which we can plan (gritting). We may also experience extremes of weather, such as flash flooding or unusually heavy snow fall, examples of special variation, which is less easy to plan for.

Improvement initiatives aim to reduce (or eliminate) special sources of variation and may also seek to reduce the degree of common variation. To determine whether variations in the data collected are attributed to common or special variation, and whether any initiative to reduce variation is effective, requires repeated measurement over a long period of time.

SPC is a statistical method developed in the 1920s by Shewhart and popularised by Deming (Shewhart, 1931; Deming, 1986). SPC is a good technique to use when implementing change, as it enables an understanding of whether changes underway are resulting in improvement – a key component of the Model for Improvement. SPC is widely used in the NHS to understand whether change results in improvement. The tool provides an easy way for people to track the impact of improvement projects. The results of SPC analysis are presented graphically in a 'control chart'. This is a powerful and user-friendly method of helping managers and practitioners understand variation and make appropriate decisions. More information on the application of SPC can be found here: https://improvement.nhs.uk/resources/statistical-process-control-tool/.

Working in a multidisciplinary team for effective quality improvement

GPNs work regularly with people with long-term conditions, especially those with comorbidities, and these patients pose challenges, as their needs often cut across health and social care boundaries, as well as across various medical disciplines. Primary Care Networks (PCNs) require individuals to deliver effective multiagency and multidisciplinary working if they are to deliver seamless, cost-effective care. The establishment of this way of working requires changes to the way health and social care services have traditionally been organised.

We know that a multidisciplinary team (MDT) approach to long-term conditions can produce improved outcomes for patients with a number of conditions. In heart failure, for example, a multidisciplinary approach can reduce both hospital admissions and overall mortality (McAlister, 2004). Weekly MDT meetings and the use of clinical protocols were found in another study (Jackson et al., 2005) to result in better glycaemic control in a large number of diabetic patients.

There are several benefits from MDT working in primary care:

- A more responsive service
- Greater patient centredness
- A more clinically and/or cost-effective service
- More job satisfaction and improved career paths for health care professionals

Multidisciplinary working, however, is not always easy, and is a relatively new concept for general practice. The introduction of a variety of new roles into the general practice team will mean that the traditional roles of doctors and nurses will change, allowing for the professional with the most appropriate skills and expertise to deliver care to patients. As discussed in other chapters, the tradition in the United Kingdom has been for different health care disciplines to train, learn and practise separately. Health care professionals have also, until relatively recently, tended not to involve themselves in 'management'. 'Management' has been viewed as something that is 'imposed' and has to be 'tolerated', rather than as something that clinicians need to be actively involved in.

Lack of mutual trust between different health care disciplines can be a major barrier to effective multidisciplinary working. Joint training and team-building exercises can foster confidence in fitness to practise and keeping up to date. Continuing professional development is essential, and learning together is one way of understanding each others' roles, building trust and working more closely. PCNs have an invigorated focus on MDT working, and this is creating an imperative for practice teams to consider working in this way. Future systems will involve introducing these new allied health care professional roles to the practice. This will widen knowledge, increase skills and introduce new ways of working that can complement nursing.

Building multidisciplinary teams to improve quality

Initiatives such as NHS England's 'Time For Care' programme have been designed to help practice teams manage their workload, adopt and spread innovations that free up clinical time for care and develop the skills and confidence to lead local improvement.

The case studies provided at the following link demonstrate some positive examples of the NHS delivering improved high-quality care in a number of different settings across the country: https://www.england.nhs.uk/gp/case-studies/. They provide some context and background to the challenges being faced by the NHS and the solutions developed to ensure better, cost-effective outcomes for patients and the public. Many involve multidisciplinary approaches and are good examples of effective collaborative working in practice.

Team working does not automatically happen when people work alongside each other, even when they share the same office. Many structural, historical and attitudinal barriers can, and do, cause difficulties. There may be competing demands, diverse lines of management and funding, poor communication and personality clashes, as well as problems generated by the differing status and gender of team members.

The role of GPNs is often isolating, and the chance to come together as a team during the working day is important to build relationships and team cohesion. This can be easier said than done, but having awareness of self and how other people interact and function can help GPNs understand not just what needs to be improved, but also what methods of approach will support quality improvement. A simple tool that GPNs can be aware of is the Johari window, a cognitive psychological tool that can be used to increase self-awareness and understanding between individuals within an MDT. This can lead to more efficient teams that make the best use of the talents of each individual member. The Johari window exercise was developed by American psychologists Joseph Luft and Harry Ingham (Luft & Ingham, 1955). The name, Johari, is derived from the authors' first names, Joseph and Harry.

The Johari window

As demonstrated in Figure 11.2, the Johari window has four panes:

● What is known by the individual about himself/herself and is also known by others: the 'open pane' or 'arena'
● What is not known by the individual, but is known by others: the 'blind pane' or 'blind spot'
● What the individual knows about himself/herself, but is not known by others: the 'hidden pane' or 'façade'
● What is not known by the individual about himself/herself and is also unknown by others: the 'unknown pane'.

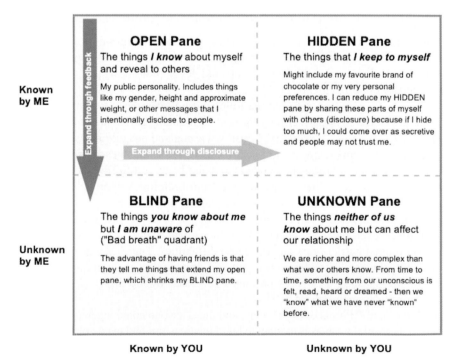

Fig. 11.2   The Johari window. (From The Johari Window 2020: https://www.nwacademy.nhs.uk /discover/toolkits-documents/johari-window-2020.)

The aim of the model is to consider how to increase the size of the open pane for every individual in the team because this is where we are at our most productive and effective. People who are already working in established teams will have larger open panes than people who have just joined. New members will not know their colleagues well and will have had little opportunity to share information. A person's open pane can be expanded horizontally, reducing the blind pane, by seeking and actively listening to feedback from other members of the group. Where feedback is sought or given, however, it is vital that this is conducted sensitively. Ensuring that this happens is a key role of the facilitator of the exercise. Feedback must never be allowed to become character assassination!

The open pane can also be enlarged by the individual disclosing information about himself/herself to the team. In this situation the open pane expands vertically into the hidden pane.

The issues in the fourth Johari window, the unknown pane, can take a variety of forms: feelings, behaviours, attitudes and capabilities. These can be close to the surface, positive and useful, and can also be deeply engrained aspects of an individual's personality, affecting his or her behaviour to various degrees. Some examples of issues in the unknown area include:

- An ability or skill that is underestimated or untried, through lack of opportunity, confidence, encouragement or training
- A natural talent that the individual is unaware that he or she possesses
- Fears that individuals do not know they have
- Repressed or unconscious feelings
- Conditioned behaviours and attitudes

Some of these issues, particularly the first two, can benefit the team as a whole if they can be brought into the open pane.

The size of the unknown pane can be reduced in a variety of ways. The observation of others will reduce the unknown area by increasing the blind pane. Self-discovery can reduce it by increasing the hidden pane. Mutual enlightenment, such as may happen during a group development experience, can expand the open pane into the other three windows.

Case study

A newly qualified nurse (NQN) had recently started at the surgery and was very keen to learn and get involved. Consequently, the NQN was asking the lead General Practice Nurse (GPN) lots of questions about systems, processes and procedures. The GPN found this intrusive and perceived the NQN as critical and pushy. The GPN was also worried that the NQN might get involved in work that was outside of his scope of professional practice without the necessary further training and education that might be needed for certain tasks, so lots of the questions were deferred.

Continued

The NQN perceived the GPN's attitude as dismissive and unfriendly, and there was some friction which was impacting on the wider surgery team.

The practice manager arranged some protected time for the lead GPN and the NQN to get together. Through some deeper asking and careful listening the GPN was able to establish that the NQN was simply keen to learn and was equally concerned that his professional practice was safe and within scope. The GPN was also able to tell the NQN that their journeys were similar, and that there was much that the GPN had had to learn when she first started in general practice. They set about planning a programme for learning and development together.

Through asking, listening and sharing together they were able to create a more open environment and foster a bond of trust between them in which their professional relationship could flourish and the wider surgery team would benefit as a result.

Implementing organisational change

GPNs have an important part to play in supporting and realising change that will lead to improved, safer and more cost-effective care. Threaded throughout this book is the belief that GPNs are involved in care from preconception right through to end of life and are the linchpins of general practice. GPNs are rooted in their communities and committed to best practice. In their day-to-day practice they have the opportunity to identify areas requiring improvement. A growing number of GPNs are developing their leadership skills and expertise and taking up the baton as PCN clinical directors and deputy clinical directors. They are ensuring that GPNs will influence the design and delivery of organisational change that will lead to improvement.

Improvement requires change, but not all changes result in improvement (Berwick, 1996). Organisational change within the NHS is about improving the safety, experience and outcomes for our patients and their families and carers. Solving problems and implementing change in primary care and general practice is the same as solving any other problem or making any change.

You will need to:

- Define what the problem is/what change you want to make
- Generate solutions/decide how you are going to make the change
- Implement the solutions/changes
- Evaluate the effect...
- ...and repeat these four steps until the problem is solved or the change is made

This seems straightforward, but you will doubtless know from experience that achieving a sustainable change is usually not that simple.

Before embarking on organisational change, some key questions need to be asked:

- What current or future issues is this change going to address, and are these important? If you are unable to answer this question, then either the change is not worthwhile or you have not yet grasped the key issue.
- What are the consequences of not making the change?
- Do you have the right leader to take change forward? An effective leader and change agent is of fundamental importance to the success of any organisational change, large or small.
- Do you have wholehearted 'buy-in' from everyone involved?
- Who are the key people needed to take this change forward? Who do you really need to sell the idea to?
- Who is likely to feel threatened by the change, and how will you address those fears?
- Have you fully explored the implications of change and the barriers to its successful implementation?
- What are the processes that you will need to change, or what new processes will you need to introduce?
- How will you measure success? How will you change people's behaviour?

Change needs to be carefully planned and led if it is to be successful. This is particularly relevant to current primary care and the development of Integrated Care Systems and the embedding of PCNs, where we have new, larger and more diverse teams creating new ways of working. GPNs need to get involved and bring the added value of their rich expertise to the table. There is certainly scope and opportunity for GPNs to take a lead.

Change will require people to think and behave in different ways. This may have implications for training, and a first step may be to conduct a training needs assessment. A team leader needs to be able to explain why the change is necessary, but also to enthuse and excite the rest of the team and those whom the change will affect. A plan (usually known as a project management plan) needs to be set out, including a schedule with appropriate milestones (who will do what by when). Regular meetings with a clear agenda will help keep the process on track. It is helpful to identify key 'tipping points'. Meetings with key team members can be scheduled before these points to ensure that the necessary preparations are in place. Within general practice, team meetings may involve all members of staff, but this is not always the way in all practices.

Reflection

How are meetings organised at your place of work? Are all staff involved? Are staff involved in some meetings but perhaps not in others? Are they never involved? If that is the case, how is everyone kept informed?

Consider how you can become involved in team meetings and what you can bring to the meeting.

Consider what makes a highly effective team.

This chapter has already stressed the need to measure the effect of any change. Monitoring needs to continue throughout the change process to ensure that milestones are met and that the project remains on schedule overall. Ongoing progress reports will enable refinements and adjustments to be made as you go.

It is also important to maintain momentum and motivation. People's achievements in reaching milestones and targets need to be recognised and rewarded. Momentum and motivation are also kept alive by keeping the team informed. There is a practice based in greater London which regularly organises team 'huddles', informal meetings where everyone is kept updated, can raise any issues for discussion, etc. This helps to ensure that people feel involved and have an opportunity for their voice to be heard. (This relates well with the 'open pane' of the Johari window, which was covered earlier in this chapter). Involving people and acknowledging their input also helps to engage those resisting change. It is important to listen to concerns and comments. There may be some valid points made. If you listen to people's concerns, they will be more likely to remain open to persuasion. Once feedback has been obtained and analysed, it is time to start planning a way forward that will lead to an improved service.

Working well in collaboration can reap many rewards and build a culture of sharing which provides consistency and continuity and reaps many rewards. People also benefit from wider networks, finding out about and adopting what is working well elsewhere (Fraser, 2007).

Collaboration will work well when strong bonds of trust are formed and where there is a mutual trust for everyone's contributions. This trust empowers all members. There needs to be good communication flow and a clear understanding of what everyone contributes to the team. A collaborative culture is one of sharing. Think of it as a jigsaw: it will only work well when all the pieces are in place and connected. Regular communication that is honest, respectful and purposeful is the key to collaborative working.

Reflection

Who is the leader of change in your place of work? It could be that this is the remit of one person (top-down leadership), or perhaps the leader will change according to the type of change (distributed leadership). Consider how this impacts on whether people feel involved or whether they feel that change is being done 'to' them rather than 'with' them.

Reflection

Do you currently work in a collaborative team? What do you think makes it work well? If you are yet not part of a collaborative team, think about the other health care workers involved in the care of your patients. How might you find out some more about the work they are doing, and how might that link in with you?

Case study

This concerns an inner-city general practitioner (GP) surgery which needed to develop a more robust system for reviewing patients with multiple long-term conditions.

Challenges
- Initially, patients were being called in for reviews of each individual long-term condition.
- This was inconvenient for patients and resulted in a great deal of duplication of tests, repetition, etc. Data capture was also incohesive and inconsistent.
- Because of this, time spent with the patients was not being used to their best advantage.

What did the general practice nurse do?
- As the person who was responsible for running review clinics, the General Practice Nurse (GPN) was aware of the issues and came up with a possible solution.
- At that time, the GPN had taken the initiative to enrol in a Leadership Programme which afforded the knowledge, skills and confidence to push forward.
- The GPN devised and presented a plan to the GP partners and the practice manager to set up specific clinics for patents with multiple long-term conditions, with longer appointment times where they could have a complete holistic review.
- The plan was agreed on the basis that this would be started on a small scale (for one week, initially), applying Plan Do Study Act (PDSA) cycles to understand what was working and what needed to improve. This would be extended for a longer period if the findings indicated that the method was working.
- All staff were informed and engaged.
- Processes for improved data capture were put into place.
- A letter was devised to inform patients about the changes to their review appointment so that they knew what to expect.
- The process was mapped, involving all staff, to understand the wider implications this service might bring to the day-to-day running of the surgery and to provide robust safety netting (for example, taking into consideration the current system for call and recall of patients and what would happen next following the review).

This was a GPN-led initiative that involved all practice staff. This system proved successful, and the practice won a national quality improvement award. That was in 2005. The really important factor here is that the surgery still uses this system for reviewing patients with multiple long-term conditions, so this is a change that has proved sustainable. The surgery is continually applying PDSA cycles to understand what is working well and to make any necessary improvements. This is also a method of review that has now been adopted by many other GP surgeries around the country, so there has been adoption and spread of good practice.

Case study

This concerns an inner-city practice in South Yorkshire that cares for more than 8000 patients, 80% of whom are migrants. As part of the routine health check for new patients, routine screening for bloodborne viruses including hepatitis B virus is offered. With opening boarders and European Union migration, increasing numbers of Slovak Roma registered and were offered screening.

Following identification of a previously unknown high level of active hepatitis b infection within this population, the practice was able to put a business case to the Clinical Commissioning Group (CCG) to enable a city-wide screening and vaccination programme of approximately 3000 members of the Slovak Roma community.

Challenges
- A population that has historically not seen health as a priority. To address low health-seeking behaviour the introduction of a nurse-led clinic dedicated to the needs of Slovak Roma patients, with provision of interpreters was established.
- The screening, vaccination and possible treatment of a transient and non-English-speaking population.
- Initially having to manage this without external support, until the Locally Enhanced Service (LES) was in place.

What did the general practice nurse do?
- Based on an interest in hepatitis b, became an expert in the processing, interpretation and recording of patients' results, thus gaining the evidence required for the LES.
- Liaised with secondary care experts in infectious diseases on management of patients and worked with these colleagues to produce detailed information in video and written form in the patient's own language.
- Counselled and referred newly diagnosed patients to secondary care colleagues.
- Developed and delivered a programme of education for General Practice Nurses explaining the LES, as well as detailed guidance for all staff on management of patients on the CCG education portal website.
- Published research in a national journal and subsequently spoke at national conferences about this work.

Patient safety

The NHS Patient Safety Strategy (Improvement.nhs.uk, 2020) informs us that 'patient safety is about maximising the things that go right and minimising the things that go wrong' for people using health care services. Patient safety is integral to the NHS's definition of quality in health care, alongside effectiveness and patient experience. This strategy describes how the NHS will continuously improve patient safety over the next 5 to 10 years.

The strategy was designed to complement the NHS Long-Term Plan (NHS England, 2019), the vision is for the NHS to continuously improve patient safety. More information about the NHS Patient Safety Strategy can be found here: https://improvement.nhs.uk/resources/patient-safety-strategy/.

Patient safety is also a core component of the governance of health and social care standards, as discussed in Chapter 2, and is an intrinsic constituent of clinical and nursing governance.

Reflection

Have a look through the links below to remind yourself of the key drivers which support governance and best practice:

Nursing and Midwifery Code of Conduct:
> https://www.nmc.org.uk/standards/code/

Royal College of Nursing, Clinical Governance:
> https://www.rcn.org.uk/clinical-topics/clinical-governance

Care Quality Commission:
> http://www.cqc.org.uk

When things go wrong

Despite appropriate training and experience, and irrespective of the motivation to get things right, mistakes will be made. James Reason describes different types of error (Reason, 1990). Unsafe acts can generally be broken down into intended actions and unintended actions. Intended actions can be further broken down into violations and mistakes. Violations can occur from what is routine (how we have always done it), reasoned (where even with careful thought a mistake is made), reckless (where little or no thought is given) or malicious (that is, with bad intent) – thankfully, malicious violations are rare. Mistakes, on the other hand, will be rule- and knowledge-based errors. An example would be a prescriber missing a decimal point in a dose that should be 2.5 mg and issuing 25 mg in error.

Unintended actions consist of slips and lapses and will be caused by skill-based errors such as memory lapse or attention failure. An example would be a practitioner prescribing a standard dose of morphine to a petite, frail patient with chronic renal failure, having failed to take into consideration the compromising factors relevant to that specific patient.

Research findings inform us that, in general practice, 4.9% of prescription items have at least one prescribing and/or monitoring error, with a small number of prescriptions containing more than one error (Avery et al., 2013). However, it is one of many areas open to the possibility of error; for example, errors can occur during a patient consultation, in wider communication flows such as poor record keeping, during handovers, attributed to technology malfunctions, involving inappropriate treatment, and more (the list is not exhaustive).

Ensuring patient safety

To minimise the likelihood of human error we need to carry out risk assessments and then identify and instigate appropriate actions to avert or reduce the risk of mistakes. This is always important and particularly so when undertaking new ways of working. Acknowledging when something has gone or is going wrong can be challenging for both the individuals concerned and their organisation. It is very important that we develop the personal integrity to be able to speak up and acknowledge a mistake.

How we consequently respond to mistakes will have an impact on what happens next. It is far easier for someone to speak up in an organisation with a culture that is open and nonblaming, where everyone can learn and grow from mistakes to ensure there is no recurrence. This type of organisational culture will help to avoid crisis situations such as occurred in Mid Staffordshire, where a catalogue of events led to patients suffering and unacceptable deaths.

Reflection

What is the process for reporting an adverse event at your place of work? How is an adverse event managed and processed?

Involving patients, carers and service users

Involving patients, carers and service users can have a beneficial effect on how services are planned, organised, delivered and, importantly, used. This involvement can, in turn, have a positive effect on care outcomes. Through involvement they will learn more about health conditions and treatments. This can improve confidence in services and can make services more responsive to their needs. Feedback can be particularly valuable when practices are considering what is working well and what might be improved.

Obtaining and learning from patient feedback

Feedback can be obtained in several ways: individually or in a group, at the time or retrospectively and anonymously or named. Some people will prefer to give their feedback as individuals, whereas others may prefer a collective approach. Very often people will feel more comfortable with being open and frank if the feedback they give can be anonymous. Anonymous feedback, however, does mean that you and your team will not be able to reply directly to individual comments.

'Patient stories' are, essentially, the narrative of an individual's health care experience. This could be positive, negative or both, and might be told by patients themselves or someone close to them, such as a family member or carer. Once a story has been captured, an individual response or action might be required. When a number of stories have been collected, however, it becomes possible to search for any emerging themes or trends which might benefit from attention and improvement.

Some people will prefer to be asked retrospectively for their views on their experience of care, as this can be less intrusive and allows time for reflection. Others are happy to be asked at the point of care, when their experience is fresh in their minds. These are all options that need to be considered. Interviews can be conducted face to face or by telephone. Other methods of collecting feedback include paper-based or online questionnaires. All these options for gathering feedback need to be considered.

There are different ways of capturing stories; for example, visual narratives, which involve drawing out information utilising pictures and/or photographs. This has been usefully implemented for children with asthma (Rich et al., 1999) and wider groups of young people (Drew et al., 2010). The important thing with all feedback is to ensure that someone collates the information and that there is some sort of process in place to follow this up and address any issues. It is always useful to learn from what we might do better, as well as what went well.

Reflection

Find out the principles and processes for obtaining patient feedback that are applied within your place of work. You can ask your practice manager about this:

- Who is responsible for collecting feedback from patients/service users in your General Practitioner (GP) surgery?
- Who collates this information, analyses and disseminates it and then ensures appropriate actions are taken?
- Ask your practice manager if they can think of an occasion when the GP surgery has been able to make an improvement based on patient/service user feedback.
- Are there any other ways that patients have been involved in making improvements?

Useful resources

The NHS Change Model is a framework for any project or programme that is seeking to achieve transformational, sustainable change. The model, originally developed in 2012, provides a useful organising framework for sustainable change and transformation that delivers real benefits for patients and the public. It was created to support health and care to adopt a shared approach to leading change and transformation.

The model has eight components, all of which should be considered when implementing change. The components act as a guide to ensure all elements of change are considered and implemented effectively, creating an environment where change programmes deliver transformational, sustainable change.

You can find more information and valuable resources on the link here: https://www.england.nhs.uk/sustainableimprovement/change-model/.

In April 2021 The Health Foundation published: Quality Improvement Made Simple. This updated guide to quality improvement is informed by latest research and can be accessed here: https://www.health.org.uk/publications /quality-improvement-made-simple.

Next steps for personal development

It is important to be proactive in seeking out opportunities for personal development that will support improved and safer care delivery. Some inspiring examples are listed below. As highlighted earlier, the NHS 'Time For Care' Programme aims to help practice teams manage their workload, adopt and spread innovations that free up clinical time for care and develop the skills and confidence to lead local improvement. In 2019 the programme grew to offer bespoke support to PCNs. Importantly, they set up a quality improvement programme for GPNs. Have a look at the Time to Care website of Integrated Care Systems to find out further information: https://www.england.nhs.uk/gp/gpfv/redesign/gpdp /releasing-time/.

Further opportunity for personal development became available through CARE, a learning and development programme to empower general practice nurses and other primary care professionals to play a key role in their primary care network, to shape services based on population health needs and to strengthen their leadership. Focussing on wellbeing and building and harnessing resilience, the programme uses digital technology to connect primary care professionals and to support joined-up, multi-professional working. More information is available here: https://napc.co.uk/gpncare/.

NHS England / NHS Improvement offer a range of online learning resources to facilitate change that will lead to improvement. More information is available here: https://www.england.nhs.uk/sustainableimprovement/improvement-fundamentals/.

COVID-19

At the time of writing this chapter the COVID-19 pandemic erupted and entailed rapid change and adaptation of service delivery in primary care to facilitate safe environments and channels of communication that would minimise the spread of infection.

Primary care saw a rapid escalation of the adoption of digital consultations via telephone, email and video consultation. For those patients who did need to be seen face to face (with or without COVID-19 symptoms), general practices worked speedily within their own practices and in collaboration with other local practices and local councils to arrange safe ways of working and appropriate environments; some examples were developing areas such as 'hot hubs', where high risk patients could be assessed, and the use of marquees and open-air facilities where patients could be seen in their cars (The King's Fund, 2020).

In conjunction with the immediate and fast responses required to cope with a pandemic, quality improvement and patient safety principles using PDSA cycles were applied to understand what is working well and what might be improved (Staines et al., 2020). Indeed, findings were published rapidly, which indicated that the application of PDSA cycles proved essential to overcoming barriers when implementing virtual consultations for an orthopaedic outpatient service in response to COVID-19 (Gilbert et al., 2020).

Conclusion

In all the work that we undertake in day-to-day general practice there is always room for improvement. Some of the best ideas for making changes that will lead to improvement will come from GPNs, with their firsthand experience of working at the front line of primary care. Improvement theories and tools are valuable to apply when making changes to the way we work, to understand what is working well and what might be improved. In this continuing evolvement of primary care, there is a need to engage and work well in collaboration with others. Fostering good relationships within MDTs can support best practice, improve staff experience and maintain the imperative for improving the safety, experience and outcomes of patients through sharing and learning together.

At this time of significant change in primary care, with the introduction and embedding of PCNs and the added challenge of a pandemic, there is huge opportunity for GPNs to take up the baton and develop their knowledge and skills in quality improvement methodology and patient safety initiatives that will lead to improved, safer, more efficient and sustainable care delivery.

References

Avery, A., Ghaleb, M., Barber, N., et al. (2013). The prevalence and nature of prescribing and monitoring errors in English general practice: A retrospective case note review. *British Journal of General Practice, 63*(613), e543–e553.

Berwick, D. (1996). Harvesting knowledge from improvement. *JAMA: The Journal of the American Medical Association, 275*(11), 877–878.

Deming, W. (1986). *Out of the crisis*. Institute of Technology Center for Advanced Engineering Studies.

Drew, S., Duncan, R., & Sawyer, S. (2010). Visual storytelling: A beneficial but challenging method for health research with young people. *Qualitative Health Research, 20*(12), 1677–1688.

Fraser, S. (2007). *Undressing the Elephant: Why good practice doesn't spread in healthcare*. Lulu.

Gilbert, A., Billany, J., Adam, R., et al. (2020). Rapid implementation of virtual clinics due to COVID-19: Report and early evaluation of a quality improvement initiative. *BMJ Open Quality, 9*(2), e000985.

Holweg, M. (2006). The genealogy of lean production. *Journal of Operations Management, 25*(2), 420–437.

Improvement.nhs.uk. (2020). https://improvement.nhs.uk/documents/5472/190708_Patient_Safety _Strategy_for_website_v4.pdf.

Jackson, G. L., Yano, E. M., Edelman, D., et al. (2005). Veterans Affairs primary care organizational characteristics associated with better diabetes control. *Am J Manag Care, 11*(4),225–237. PMID: 15839183.

Langley, J., Nolan, K., Nolan, T., et al. (1996). *The improvement guide: A practical approach to enhancing organizational performance*. Jossey-Bass.

Luft, J. & Ingham, H. (1955). The Johari window, a graphic model of interpersonal awareness, *Proceedings of the Western Training Laboratory in Group Development*. Los Angeles: UCLA.

McAlister, F., Stewart, S., Ferrua, S., & McMurray, J. (2004). Multidisciplinary strategies for the management of heart failure patients at high risk for admission. *Journal of the American College of Cardiology, 44*(4), 810–819.

NHS England. (2019). NHS Long Term Plan.

Reason, J. (1990). *Human error*. Cambridge University Press.

Rich, M. & Chalfen, R. (1999). Showing and telling asthma: Children teaching physicians with visual narrative. *Visual Sociology, 14*(1), 51–71.

Shewhart, W. (1931). *The economic control of quality manufactured product*. D Van Nostrand.

Staines, A., Amalberti, R., Berwick, D., Braithwaite, J., Lachman, P., & Vincent, C. (2020). COVID-19: Patient safety and quality improvement skills to deploy during the surge. *International Journal for Quality in Health Care*.

Staines, A., Amalberti, R., Berwick, D. M., et al. (2021). COVID-19: patient safety and quality improvement skills to deploy during the surge. *Int J Qual Health Care, 33*(1):mzaa050. doi: 10.1093/intqhc/mzaa050. PMID: 32400870; PMCID: PMC7239133.

The King's Fund. (2020). *How has general practice responded to the Covid-19 (Coronavirus) outbreak?* https://www.kingsfund.org.uk/blog/2020/04/covid-19-general-practice.

Chapter 12

Primary care networks and multidisciplinary team-based working

Clare Simpson

Learning Outcomes

After reading this chapter you should be able to:

1. Define a Primary Care Network
2. Describe the critical role of General Practice Nurses in Primary Care Networks
3. Understand multidisciplinary team-based working in a Primary Care Network

Introduction

As a nurse, your priority will always be your patients. This chapter aims to show you the importance of the role of General Practice Nurse (GPN) in shaping and delivering local and national strategies to continuously improve the health and well-being of your patients. Although many GPNs might not think of themselves as leaders now or in the future, ongoing assessments and reviews of their day-to-day clinical work greatly contribute significantly to system change.

What is a primary care network?

The health and well-being needs of the population are becoming increasingly complex and require health and care policy makers and providers to take into account more of the things that contribute to people's health and well-being alongside healthcare. This includes things like lifestyle, employment, housing, education and adequate personal finance.

As a consequence, the National Health Service (NHS) Long Term Plan (NHS England, 2019) sets out a new approach for General Practice called a population health management approach. This includes a more pro-active assessment of an individual's health and well-being needs to inform more personally tailored and holistic care. For example, the 2020 acute population health need related to the COVID-19 pandemic includes clear physical and mental health needs along with risks associated with where and how people live and work.

Primary Care Networks are being established to connect General Practice staff, including GPN with each other, their system and their communities to work in partnership to respond to both the COVID-19 pandemic and help shape future services for the better.

NHS England describes Primary Care Networks (PCNs) as consisting 'of groups of general practices working together with a range of local providers, including across primary care, community services, social care and the voluntary sector, to offer more personalised, coordinated health and social care to their local populations' (NHS England, 2020a). PCNs are designed to focus on population health management (PHM), which is an emerging method for local health and care partnerships to use data to design new models of proactive care and deliver improvements in community health and well-being that make the best use of resources. It aims to improve physical and mental health outcomes, promote well-being and reduce health inequalities across an entire population. It involves focusing on the wider determinants of health, which have a significant impact, as only 20% of a person's health outcomes are attributed to the ability to access good quality health care. GPNs are integral to PHM approaches, as they are well used to meeting patients' individual holistic needs. Fig. 12.1 illustrates the system transformation PCNs have been established to create (NAPC, 2016a).

Current state

Current state refers to the traditional general practice operating model that uses a siloed disease- and service-based referral system for all primary care needs. Organisations and teams are financed and work independently from one another, often competing around resourcing and service delivery, rather than working together for the good of their shared population. This approach is not only confusing for patients and their carers, but has become increasingly inefficient and less impactful, particularly involving prevention and sustainable health outcomes.

For example, Kings College Hospital, NHS Foundation Trust in London has some of the best stroke outcomes in the world but is also located in one of the highest stroke risk areas in England. You might ask yourself this: 'Would I rather have access to the best stroke treatment, or avoid having a stroke at all?' In response, NHS England and NHS Improvement has recognised the need for a more population health–focused policy and funding model: 'We believe… that NHS bodies should have shared responsibility for wider objectives

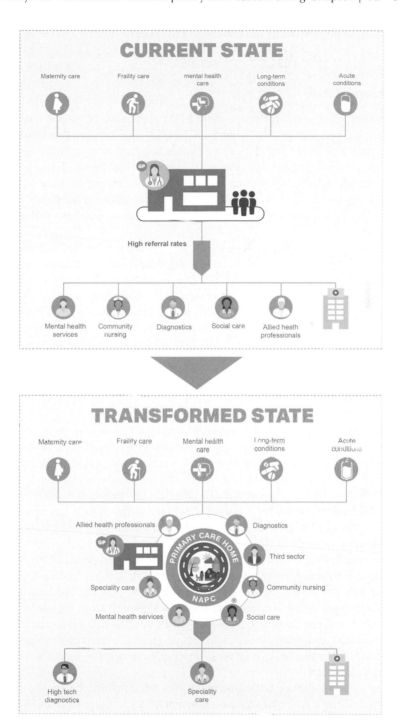

Fig. 12.1   The system transformation primary care networks have been established to create. (From NAPC [2016a]. *Illustration of system transformation* [*Primary Care Home*].)

in relation to population health and the use of NHS resources' (NHS England, 2019a).

Transformed state

The 'transformed state' reflects a more PHM approach. PCNs are redesigning existing services around groups of people with similar characteristics across their registered populations to enable targeted interventions for both those population groups and the individuals within them. They look at health management not just from the perspective of trying to make existing services more efficient and effective, but also considering the needs of the population as a whole and being prepared to organise services differently around them.

To support the development of the PCNs and deliver the NHS Long-Term Plan, a £4.5 billion increase in funding for primary and community care was announced by NHS England and NHS Improvement in 2019, along with the introduction of new PCN contracts to extend the scope of primary and community services. The original General Medical Services Contracts have been supplemented by these network contracts as part of the Directed Enhanced Service element (NHS England, 2020b).

The critical role of General Practice Nurses in primary care networks

As a nurse, you might well have been attracted to work in general practice because of the opportunity it gives to work in a small and reasonably autonomous team and develop long-term relationships with the individuals and families you provide care for. There is considerable evidence to show the significant benefits to individuals' health and well-being from regular social interaction and strong personal relationships, which has made the role and function of general practice critical to the health and care system as a whole.

This is reflected in the NHS Long Term Plan (NHS England, 2019), which puts General Practice at the centre of every network. Understanding and connecting with the people the NHS provides care for is clearly fundamental to the effectiveness of the services it delivers. Designed to serve registered populations of between 30,000 to 50,000, each PCN aims to harness the closer, more personal and established relationships general practices develop with their patients. In this way, it is clear that GPNs must play a central role in PCN development.

The unique role the GPN plays and the relationships he or she forms with patients as a result of this role fundamentally underpin the PCN PHM approach.

Case study

The National Association of Primary Care (NAPC) was commissioned by NHS England as part of the General Practice Nursing (GPN) Ten Point Plan commission to work with the Bedfordshire, Luton and Milton Keynes (BLMK) Integrated Care System to codesign an approach for reaching, engaging and developing a talent pipeline of future GPN leaders (BLMK, NAPC, 2018). NAPC was already working with BLMK to support Primary Care Network (PCN) development, and the idea was to build on these relationships and use the NHS Long Term Plan to demonstrate the value of GPNs across the locality.

PCNs are about local communities working together and building a strong sense of belonging that are relationship- and person-centred and build on one-to-one interactions with people. When PCNs were described in this way, people across the system immediately started to understand the critical role GPNs played in their success. GPNs and others realised that GPNs were able to support PCN development because of their experience of working in the community, and their inherent person-centred, holistic approach.

As a result of the work to date, BLMK has identified and energised a group of nurses across the patch, and particularly in Milton Keynes (MK), where the Primary Care Nursing Lead in the Clinical Commissioning Group (CCG) is herself a registered nurse. Working with the MK Federation, the CCG has established a strong GPN network with nurses across the local area. Initially PCNs were heavily focused on effecting operational changes to improve service provision and were not really understanding what population health management and multidisciplinary team-based working really meant in practice. Now GPNs across MK are asking to be involved in PCN development and challenging existing ways of working in general practice. This work has not only raised the profile of BLMK – Ruth May, Chief Nursing Officer, NHS England, visited in May 2019 and presented silver awards to two outstanding GPNs there – it has changed the way they are developing their PCNs. One GPN put herself forward to become a Clinical Director (CD) and, supported by the CCG, Federation and NAPC, she was appointed as a deputy CD. The CCG has invited all PCNs to nominate and appoint nurse deputies throughout the vicinity.

PCNs are not all about general practice or about a single profession; they are designed to be small enough to provide patients and staff alike with personalised care in a community-based setting and large enough to impact the health and care of the nation. They are designed to deliver economies of scale through better joined-up working and to bring together a range of health and social care professionals to work together as a complete care community. The workforce of each PCN is drawn from general practice surgeries, community, mental health and acute trusts, social care, local councils, police and fire services, youth clubs, schools and the voluntary sector, whose collective focus is on local population needs and providing care closer to patients' homes.

PCNs have been described as the 'building blocks' for system change; they aim to enable better and more sustainable services for local populations. NHS

England describes PCNs as networks that build on the core of current primary care services and enable greater provision of proactive, personalised, coordinated and more integrated health and social care (NHS England, 2019c).

Case study

The Beacon Medical Group is a partnership combining three practices in the Plymouth and South Hams Area: Ivybridge Medical Practice, Plym River Practice and The Ridgeway Practice. As a partnership they formally merged on 1st April 2014 and provide general practice services to approximately 33,000 patients.

Working together as a Primary Care Network, they cut the average waiting time to see a General Practitioner (GP) by 6 days by redesigning the Urgent Care Team, and extended the practice to include another 7000 patients. The team has an additional two nurse practitioners and a paramedic, as well as GPs and pharmacists. The group ensures that people seeking an urgent appointment are seen quickly by one of their specialist staff, rather than having to wait to see a doctor. Over 6 months, the average waiting time for a GP appointment fell from 14 to 8 days.

The group also worked with its local community pharmacists to help improve local flu vaccination rates. Instead of competing for patients, surgeries and pharmacies worked together, taking advantage of all opportunities to promote the vaccine and recommend the easiest, most appropriate setting for each individual patient. The joint working led to an increase in the number of people taking up the vaccine, including those with respiratory conditions, where the rate increased from 39% to 52%.

NAPC

Reflection

Take time to find out which Primary Care Network (PCN) your practice is connected to and who is in your PCN.

How do you, as a General Practice Nurse (GPN), work with other GPNs in the PCN?

What is multidisciplinary team-based working?

The ethos of PCNs is to foster and grow multidisciplinary team-based (MDT-based) working. There are a number of different definitions and approaches around MDT-based working in health, but in relation to the PCNs and its Primary Care Home model, the National Association of Primary Care (NAPC) defines it as bringing 'together a range of health and social care professionals to provide enhanced personalised and preventative care for their local community. Staff come together as a complete care community – drawn from GP surgeries, community, mental health and acute trusts, social care and the voluntary sector – to focus on local population needs and provide care closer to patients' homes' (NAPC, 2019a).

Thanet Health Community Interest Company provides a good illustration of what effective MDT-based working might look like in practice.

Case study

Thanet recognised an urgent need to pool its collective health and care resources across the locality on a voluntary basis to start building an integrated approach to improve care for frail elderly people and reduce demand. It started by introducing an integrated nursing team to provide an enhanced frailty pathway and an acute response team to provide a range of treatment and personal care support to keep people out of hospital. The team comprises a General Practitioner, nurses, health care assistants, a physiotherapist, an occupational therapist, voluntary care and a care agency working closely with social services. The team assesses patients and puts a package of care in place to enable patients to remain at home or be discharged. Health and social care coordinators have been brought into general practice to provide nonclinical support to patients, and surgery hours have been extended to include weekends and bank holidays.

NAPC (2018b)

Working with local systems, the NAPC has identified a number of emerging care models based on population need and involving MDT-based workforce solutions. These are illustrated in Fig. 12.2. Critically, its approach focuses on wrapping teams of multiprofessional people from multiple employing and voluntary local organisations across the PCN around population cohorts and the individuals within them, rather than around diseases such as cancer or diabetes. This approach has identified a particular need for a MDT-based approach for managing complex long-term conditions and/or disability (Fig. 12.2).

New roles in the multidisciplinary team

As a result of the establishment of PCNs and incentives, an approach to integrating care across different provider organisations and professions, there are a number of new roles emerging. These new roles include social prescribers. NHS England describes social prescribing as a way for local agencies to refer people to a link worker who will then connect people to support them in their health and well-being. The concept has gained support in NHS organisations to address social isolation. Link workers give people time, focusing on what matters to them as individuals and taking a holistic approach to their health and well-being. They play a significant role in connecting people to the most appropriate and relevant professions and support, including community groups and statutory services for practical and emotional support (NHS England, 2019d).

Other roles general practices are being encouraged to recruit and share across their network are being introduced to the MDT as plans for PCNs develop, with the aim of creating an MDT structure that is similar to that of teams traditionally associated with hospitals and community trusts.

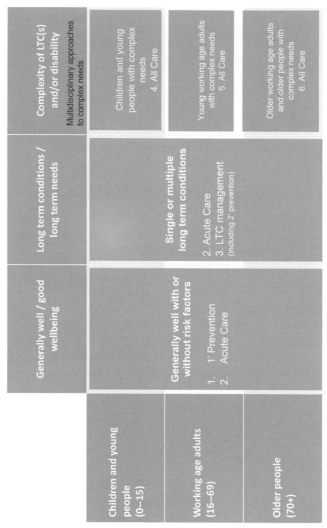

Fig. 12.2 *LTC*, Long-term condition. (From NAPC, 2016 and NAPC BLMK ICS, 2018.)

New roles include:

- Clinical pharmacists who help to alleviate the pressure of work relating to prescriptions and medication reviews, to help support General Practitioners (GPs) and Independent Nurse Prescribers.
- Paramedics who are undertaking home visits and same-day urgent care appointments, work that is traditionally performed by GPs.
- An enhanced Acute Response Team (ART), such as that set up by Thanet Primary Care Home, which involved a GP and a paramedic based in Accident and Emergency (A&E). This team cared for patients with conditions varying from normal primary care–type problems to more challenging conditions such

as chest or acute abdominal pain. The latter could often be managed by primary care clinicians with access to basic investigations, without necessarily needing the expertise of the A&E team and more complex diagnostics (NAPC, 2018c). Thanet Primary Care Home also runs a complex care ART consisting of a GP, an integrated nursing team, a health care assistant, an occupational therapist, physiotherapists, volunteer care workers and care agency staff.

There are significant benefits to being part of an integrated MDT for both patients and staff. For example, patients who are unable to leave their homes because of heart failure can receive care from a GPN specialist, or patients living at home or in care homes can receive their flu jabs from the District Nursing teams. Another theme around roles and functions is the emergence of integrated nursing teams that bring nurses from primary, community and secondary care together to break down silos and provide joined-up care for patients with multiple comorbidities and complex care needs.

Critical factors for successful primary care networks

Learning from the NAPC's community of practice shows that at the heart of any effective health and care system is an engaged and capable workforce (NAPC, 2019b). Involving the whole workforce, including patients and carers, in the service redesign process improves the quality and experience of providing and receiving care. This inclusive approach to managing change is proving critical to the effectiveness and sustainability of local system change. The will of the workforce to make the networks work is at the heart of their success.

A paper delivered at the Economic and Social Research Council Research Seminar Series (University of Birmingham, 2010) described the human factors relating to effective collaboration and cross-boundary working. It stated that 'the evidence is that joined up delivery has occurred extensively but in an ad hoc, almost accidental manner is dependent on the energy and imagination of individuals' (Savoie, 2009). A later paper stated: 'The thing that makes it work in any type of structure is the commitment of the person – structures can be enabling or difficult' (NLIAH, 2009). The paper also points to the development of trust as central to the maintenance of effective interpersonal relationships, which is best developed through individuals ('boundary spanners') freed from the 'rigid rules and requirements of their own organisations' but with the endorsement and authority of these organisations to act on their behalf.

Reflection

Caroline Rollings, RN, MBA, a previous managing partner at the Newport Pagnell Medical Centre practice and a National Association of Primary Care Faculty member, shows how a change in working practices can benefit the working of a whole system and asks nurses to consider the following: 'This is completely our experience. Going from "how can I not take up this referral into our organisation?" to '"how can I help my colleague with this patient?"'.

Case study

Further success factors have emerged in some of the local systems that the National Association of Primary Care has been working with. These include:

1. Aligned leadership strategies (purpose), messaging and focus: in the face of ever-increasing demand on existing services, leaders and teams tasked with delivering effective and sustainable system change are responding faster and better to a clearly articulated and simple description of their shared purpose. Involve General Practice Nurses in the strategic planning of the organisation.

    NOTE: The 2020 COVID-19 pandemic provides an excellent example of how a shared national and local purpose with messages such as, "Stay at home, protect the NHS, save lives", has served to speed up system integration by bringing communities and healthcare teams together as one; united by a common cause.

2. Starting where the system is at, not where you think it should be.

    a. Let networks develop at their own pace by enabling easy access to expertise, good practice solutions and shared learning (and pain!).

    b. Develop network leaders on the proviso that they develop the next cohort of leaders, and so on.

    c. Take development to the networks – make it real and practical and focused on helping individuals develop their own networks in their own way, using their own style, skills and capacity.

3. Relationships/networks:

    a. Connecting people to enable peer-to-peer influence to engage and involve people at all levels and across all professions is critical. *These connections have provided significant support to GPNs during the COVID-19 pandemic, and played a critical role in providing much needed workforce resilience.*

    b. Recognising that interactions with and the influence of other organisations/stakeholders impacts the pace and scope of the work. Some networks have needed to reframe their relationships with key stakeholders to move forwards.

4. Leadership: where primary care network development is working well, there is a balance of clinical and operational leadership. The need to build strong, effective and sustainable patient and public leadership has also been recognised across the Bedfordshire, Luton and Milton Keynes Integrated Care System (NAPC/NHS England, 2019).

What does all this mean for General Practice Nurses?

Throughout this chapter, we have highlighted the critical role of GPNs in shaping and delivering national and local strategy to improve patient health and well-being.

Changing entrenched organisational cultural norms and independent decision-making across general practice is no easy task, and general practice clinicians, including GPNs, will play a critical role over the next decade in helping shape and embed new ways of working across many of the emerging local health and care systems.

Reflection
___

Coming into an ever-changing system, there are some things nurses new to general practice might want to consider:

1. General Practice Nurses (GPNs) are responsible for providing the best possible care for their patients. As part of a Primary Care Network, this responsibility extends beyond doing a good job individually with and for patients to requiring an active contribution to the services delivered across the whole network; for example, the role of a shared diabetes nurse specialist working across a Primary Care Network (PCN).

2. As one of the largest representative groups across the general practice workforce, it has often been remarked that the voice of GPNs could be a lot louder.

    a. Understand your own value as a GPN. GPNs are 'super connectors' of the whole primary care workforce and as such are the catalysts for primary care transformation – reducing demand and improving patient health and well-being.

        i. looking at 265 population health improvement initiatives, covering over 10% of primary care, GPNs have a disproportionately high representation in starting, leading and delivering these initiatives.

        ii. Patients who had one or more contacts with a GPN saw their GP demand fall by 1.6 appointments, compared with patients with no contact with a GPN who saw their GP demand grow by 0.5 appointments. (CARE Programme, NHS England and NHS Improvement, 2021).

    b. Recognise your 'strength in numbers'. Get involved in established nurse forums, or start your own. Find your voice by connecting with like-minded colleagues across your locality to ensure practice nurses play an equal part with other clinical groups in any multidisciplinary team-based approach.

    c. Make it your mission to ensure that it becomes an automatic consideration to include practice nurse leaders in any primary care change initiative. Actively seek opportunities to get involved in your PCN, or any other planned changes or improvement initiatives in your locality.

3. PCNs require distributed, connected leadership across multiple professions and organisations. To enable a balance of clinical input and leadership, be bold and actively seek opportunities to develop your leadership and management capabilities as much as you do for your clinical expertise. Encourage others around you to have ambitions around leadership and career progression.

In February 2019, Ruth May, Chief Nursing Officer for England, NHS England and NHS Improvement, set out her priorities for the future of nursing and stated that boosting pride in nursing and midwifery was her 'first priority' and a key focus during her tenure. The World Health Organisation named 2020 the International Year of the Nurse, and in England this was extended to the Year of the Nurse and Midwife. Nurses representing all disciplines are encouraged to promote their roles and the contribution of nursing. GPNs have been supported by the NHS England General Practice Nursing Ten Point Plan, and this has raised the profile of nurses working in general practice, as well as encouraging new nurses into the profession.

Insights from people working directly with patients and who have unique understanding of the needs and wants of their local population, including GPNs, are critical for informing national policy. As a GPN, always remember your value in the system. National bodies are bound to want and need to continue working in partnership with local systems and nursing colleagues to address cultural issues in general practice (e.g., greater alignment and equity around nurse pay and terms and conditions, improved access to training and leadership development and better and more consistent use of data to report successes). GPNs often find themselves working in isolation, and networks are a great way of reducing isolation. Many more GPN forums and networks are being set up in primary care, and it is essential that GPNs find the key influencers in their areas.

Forums and network groups are also effective ways of sharing good practice, learning and having an opportunity to share experiences and skills, as well as keeping up to date with the policy changes effecting general practice.

Case study

The Bridge Primary Care Network in Newport Pagnell has established a Legs 11 club, which is a leg ulcer clinic run jointly by the District Nursing and General Practice Nurse teams. The multidisciplinary team consists of specialised nurses who have an interest in leg management, three volunteers who register clients, make the tea and stock up the biscuits and a Red Cross driver who brings housebound patients to the clinic. The team manages leg ulcers, wound care, varicose veins, varicose eczema, compression therapy including hosiery and bandaging and Dopplers...to name just a few tasks.

The team takes a holistic approach to all of its clients, assessing the person and not just his or her legs. The team assess patients' mental health needs and the impact their condition has on their day-to-day living and ability to maintain a good quality of life. Treating multiple patients at the same time makes them aware that they are not alone, and lets them see that there are others who are worse off but can still heal. They ask each other about their treatments and even compare their wounds when dressings are removed.

This clinic is healing approximately 80% of patients' leg ulcers and all wounds within 4 months. After healing, recurrence is prevented by following up with regular assessment and Dopplers and by supplying compression hosiery. The team offers advice at any time, as prevention is better than cure. Clients drop in for a coffee and to be offered reassurance once healed.

The emphasis of the Leg Clinic is to empower members to participate in their care, in a social environment that eases loneliness by providing congenial surroundings where old friends can meet and new friendships be formed.

Noncompliance with treatment has been virtually eliminated, and evidence of greater healing rates has been illustrated through many patients whose longstanding ulcers have healed or greatly improved as a direct result of this change in approach.

Patients' willingness to attend for systematic 'well leg' checks and ongoing health education has dramatically reduced the incidence of recurrence.

Conclusion

As a nurse, your priority will always be your patients. As a GPN, you have a unique and critical role to play in shaping and delivering local and national strategies to continuously improve the health and well-being of patients as part of a PCN. PCNs have been described as the 'building blocks' for system change; a central part of the NHS Long Term Plan, they aim to enable better and more sustainable services for local populations using a PHM approach which takes into account more of the things that contribute to people's health and well-being alongside healthcare. This includes things like lifestyle, employment, housing, education and adequate personal finance.

Primary Care Networks have been central to the nation's response to the COVID-19 pandemic which represents an acute population health need and have served to connect General Practice staff, including GPNs with each other, their system and their communities to work in partnership to respond to both the current COVID-19 pandemic and help shape future services for the better. PCNs are not all about general practice, nor are they about a single profession. Nationally, there are new funding and new contracting models to extend the scope of primary and community services, and the NHS Long Term Plan places a significant focus on MDT-based working to enable effective and sustainable change to patient care in a primary care setting.

PCNs bring together a range of health and social care professionals to work together as a complete care community. A number of emerging care models that are based on population need and involve MDT-based workforce solutions are emerging. New roles are also being created as a result of this approach to integrating care across different provider organisations and professions. Learning from models and approaches from the NAPC's community of practice shows that involving the whole workforce, including patients and carers, in the service redesign process improves the quality and experience of providing and receiving care. Changing entrenched organisational cultural norms and independent decision-making across general practice is no easy task. GPNs should always remember their value in and to the system. The recent changes in primary care can only be achieved if there is partnership working with local systems, professional and nursing colleagues to address cultural issues in general practice.

References

NAPC. (2016). *Illustration of system transformation (Primary Care Home)*.

NAPC. (2018a). *Primary Care Home, Case study*. https://napc.co.uk/wp-content/uploads/2017/08/NAPC-case-study-Beacon-Medical.pdf.

NAPC. (2018b). *Primary Care Home, Case study*, Thanet.

NAPC. (2018c). *Population health–based workforce redesign, Booklet*.

NAPC. (2019a). *Primary Care Home, Definition of multidisciplinary working*.

NAPC. (2019b). *Primary Care Home, How to develop an enhanced acute response team*.

NAPC and BLMK ICS. (2018). *New service model design.*

NAPC/NHS England. (2019). *Engaging general practice nurses in leading service change, draft report.*

National Leadership and Innovation Agency for Healthcare. (2009). *Getting collaboration to work in Wales: lessons from the NHS and partners.* Cardiff: NLIAH.

NHS England. (2019a). *Implementing the NHS Long-Term Plan Proposals for possible changes to legislation.* https://www.longtermplan.nhs.uk/wp-content/uploads/2019/02/nhs-legislation -engagement-document.pdf.

NHS England. (2019b). *NHS Long-Term Plan.* https://www.longtermplan.nhs.uk.

NHS England. (2019c). *Integrated care, The building blocks of integrated care.* https://www .england.nhs.uk/gp/case-studies/primary-care-networks-the-building-blocks-of-an-ics/.

NHS England. (2019d). *Personalised Care, Social prescribing.* https://www.longtermplan.nhs.uk /areas-of-work/personalised-care/.

NHS England. (2020a). *Primary Care Networks, Frequently asked questions.* https://www .england.nhs.uk/primary-care/primary-care-networks/resources/pcn-faqs/.

NHS England. (2020b). *Network Contract Directed Enhanced Service (DES) specification.*

NHS England and NHS Improvement/NAPC. (2021). CARE Programme: *Connected, Resilient, Authentic and Empowered.*

Savoie, D. (2009). *National Leadership and Innovation Agency for Healthcare*: NLIAH. Court Government and the Collapse of Accountability in Canada and the United Kingdom.

University of Birmingham. (February 2010). 'Collaborative Futures: New Insights from Intra and Inter-Sectoral Collaborations', entitled, "Special Agents: The Nature and Role of Boundary Spanners".

Chapter 13

Digital health management

Rachel Hatfield, Ann Hughes, Ruth Chambers

Learning outcomes

After reading this chapter you should be able to:

1. Understand how digital technology/technology-enabled care can help to achieve prompt individualised care
2. Describe how technology-enabled care services (TECSs) are supporting productive delivery of health and social care at the front line and across organisational boundaries
3. Understand how TECSs can assist General Practice Nurses, the patient and the clinician efficiently to provide safer ways of working together to manage health and long-term conditions

Introduction

The National Health Service (NHS) is evolving, and to deliver the care that patients deserve the NHS needs to be forward-thinking. To ensure the sustainability of the NHS, more emphasis is needed on self-care; this can be achieved with the help of digital technology/technology-enabled care (TEC), empowering patients to take more responsibility for their self-care and management of their long-term health condition(s) or adverse lifestyle habit(s), preventing further deterioration and increasing medicine adherence as required. Access to digital technologies can enable patients to understand and learn more about their condition(s). However, adoption of technology-enabled care services (TECSs) in primary care is often still seen as a complex process, with only a minority of frontline health care teams embedding technology into their everyday processes, resulting in vast numbers of practitioners and patients being left behind. There is a need to change this perception and embrace the possibilities of using digital technology alongside or in place of more traditional methods to realise its true potential. The expectations of the workforce and the population are changing, and digital health care technology should be used to address the health care challenges of the 21st century to enhance patient care and allow clinicians more time to improve outcomes and empower patients to take more responsibility for their own health condition(s) and care (Health Education England, 2019).

There have been huge advancements in the use of technology across all other industries, and to ensure the sustainability of the NHS it is vital that these digital technologies are used effectively and efficiently in frontline health and care settings. The introduction of simple technological and digital tools can have a dramatic and positive impact on the way that frontline clinicians practise, as well have having cost, clinical and quality benefits for both clinicians and patients.

A substantive contribution can be made to creating a sustainable NHS, and general practice in particular, by embedding a range of digital tools as part of usual service delivery, resulting in more efficient, effective and productive working across the whole general practice team. General Practice Nurses (GPNs), as the frontline staff members with substantive direct interaction with patients in relation to their health conditions, are key to this successful implementation and the future of the NHS. Introducing digital tools welcomed by clinicians and patients (and their carers) can encourage and enhance patient engagement, increase patient adherence to treatment, prevent deterioration of health condition(s) and encourage patients to positively change their behaviour and actively redress their adverse lifestyle habit(s).

Evolution of the digital General Practice Nurse

Health care delivery has evolved drastically over the years, and arguably nowhere more so than in the primary care setting. Maybe that is because the role of GPNs, who in the 1980s were seen as the General Practitioner's (GP's) 'hand maidens', has evolved tremendously as their responsibilities have developed and expanded.

Primary care now offers a whole new career pathway for the enthusiastic registered nurse to play an integral role in the primary care team. GPNs are often the first port of call for management of both long-term conditions (LTCs) and minor ailments, with nurse-led clinics now commonplace in general practice.

Outdated practices such as manual blood pressure checks with a sphygmomanometer have been replaced by evaluation with an array of devices that provide additional speed, accuracy and convenience. One recent example is the drive to reintroduce the practice of manual pulse checking to identify patients who have atrial fibrillation, alongside development of devices like AliveCor to support diagnosis. These devices are in use across the primary care team, with growing public health and system efficiency benefits stemming from early intervention, thus triggering anticoagulation at an earlier stage.

Many GPNs probably remember using physical lifting and handling techniques such as the 'Australian' or shoulder lift in the past, well before the advent of a shift to manual handling guidelines and present-day policy, with the many aids available such as slide sheets or mechanical hoists. At that time this was just accepted as part of the role, but as time and machinery have advanced, the need for a nurse to undertake this type of task has thankfully disappeared.

Everyone can appreciate that the introduction of new ways of agile working have had a dramatic impact on the health and safety of both the patient and the nurse, and probably helped to reduce workplace injury to the nurse dramatically! Advancements like this, which at the time may have been viewed warily and with distrust, have now become the usual way of working.

The last task of a GPN's day used to be thorough cleaning and sterilisation of any instruments used over their clinical session, using an expensive autoclave machine maintained by each practice; whereas today there is widespread use of single-use instruments to prevent infection. The advancement of knowledge and technology to produce single-use instruments has had a significant impact on the infection prevention agenda and a positive impact on patients well-being, as well as releasing nurses' time for other tasks.

In primary care one of most significant technological changes has been the introduction of electronic patient records. Gone are the days of endless freehand documentation in 'Lloyd George' notes, and now it is much easier to document, retrieve and share relevant patient information via the electronic records system.

GPNs have always been adaptable and able to embrace change and new ways of working that benefit patients. The introduction of digital technology and digital tools should also be seen as an advancement in this patient-centred agenda, allowing the patient and the clinician a better, more efficient and safer way of working together to manage health and LTCs. The use of digital tools and TECSs can improve medication adherence through better interactive communication, increase shared care with enhanced patient empowerment and encourage patients to take more responsibility for their own health and well-being by boosting the digital inclusion of patients in delivery of their care. The use of digital technology in people's everyday lives has escalated over the last decade. Most of the UK population now uses, or has access to, the internet, and over 80% of adults access the internet via a mobile phone, smartphone, laptop, tablet and/or handheld device (Office of National Statistics, 2019).

Patient expectations

Patients' expectations have changed dramatically over the years. Thankfully gone are the days when we sent the patient out of the door with a pill and advice to come back and see us in 'x' number of months. Primary care remains the gateway to secondary care, and with the help of technology we are now in the position to influence healthier lifestyle choices and improve patient education. In the long term, this can only result in improved health and well-being and better management of the demand for care services.

The focus on prevention encompasses not only improved patient awareness, but also more responsibility to self-manage more effectively through education and empowerment. The clinician/patient relationship then becomes more a partnership to support patients to maximise their health, rather than the typical paternalistic clinician/patient dynamic of the past (NHS England, 2016a).

Some clinicians are fearful that technology may damage or dilute the relationship of trust that they have with their patients. When deployed correctly, technology can enhance a patient's relationship with his or her clinician and enable more helpful conversations, if, for example, a patient has a technology resource to support his or her learning. Ultimately, if technology is leveraged appropriately, patients will be better able to manage their conditions, resulting in public health benefits at scale and reduced pressure on health services.

Shared care

To encourage patients to successfully manage and take responsibility for their own health and LTC or adverse lifestyle habit, a true partnership or shared responsibility between professionals and the public (patient) is needed. The NHS England Leading Challenge, Adding Value framework emphasises that 'the use of technology and informatics by clinicians is vital to enhance practice, address unwarranted variations and enhance outcomes' (NHS England, 2016b). The NHS England national Ten Point Plan for General Practice Nursing emphasises a focus on TECSs to 'embed and deliver a radical upgrade in prevention' that is demonstrated by the GPN nursing team (NHS England, 2017). Improving health outcomes and reducing inequalities allows clinicians to maximise the impact they have with patients and incorporates proactive work to prevent illness, allowing patients to make informed choices about their health. TECSs can help clinicians respond to both individual and local population needs, allowing people to take more responsibility for their care (NHS England, 2017).

Introduction of digital tools in health care

Most people are often very receptive of using TECSs in their own health care because they already use such modes of technology in their daily lives. Digital technology tools allow patients to take responsibility for and control of their LTCs or adverse lifestyle habits through increased self-awareness and self-management of condition(s) via self-education. This increases patients' personal knowledge and control of their condition(s), allowing them to take a more central role in managing their condition. Most people are keen to be educated about their condition and how they can manage it more effectively, and trust a referral from their clinician to a suitable source of information. Clinicians can offer tools that patients to access for information and advice when they require it. Patients can then access advice at a time convenient to them; it is up to them to use these resources as and when needed. Access is easy once the app has been downloaded to a patient's personal mobile or tablet, and often presents information in an interesting and engaging format that is easy for the patient (or his or her family carer) to absorb.

Engagement and communication can be improved between clinicians and patients through the incorporation of digital tools, as engagement becomes two-way. This approach also allows clinicians to engage with cohorts of patients who are hard to reach through traditional means such as mail drops or telephone calls or who are unable or unwilling to attend face-to-face appointments. (This could be for several reasons – accessibility, language barriers, mobility, etc.) Digital tools can offer alternative solutions to the traditional face-to-face appointments and reach a wider audience when sharing information. Using digital tools to share and cascade information is often more efficient than traditional methods of sharing information via leaflets in practice, as the promotion of best practice can reach a wider audience quickly and with less manual involvement. Whole cohorts of patients can be contacted with a click of a button. In general, the use of TECSs for sharing health messages is less intrusive and more engaging, and allows clinicians to target specific cohorts of patients when required, including hard-to-engage cohorts of patients and carers. The introduction of digital tools can aid clinical consultations, as it provides another tool for the patient to use in their self-care. This can create a positive improvement in patient and clinician relationships, as it quickly becomes routine to discuss and use digital tools in consultations. Demonstrations of use of digital technology and tools in consultations allow patients to feel comfortable with various modes of TEC and to be confident in using them as required.

Using digital technologies such as selected trusted apps, social media, video consultation and telehealth to support patients with key LTCs creates a focus on preventative clinical and self-care interventions. Patients are more engaged in their own health, which can be a double-edged sword, as the internet is awash with information that has varying degrees of reliability and accuracy. However, when supported with the right technology, patients can be supported to harness their engagement and enthusiasm to learn more about their condition from trusted resources. GPNs have a responsibility to ensure that patients safely and appropriately use the technology promoted to them.

Health apps

Health apps are a great introductory way to engage patients in their health care. They allow clinicians to signpost patients to safe and trusted sources of information about their conditions or general health. Health apps can provide quality and relevant information for specific conditions, and for health and well-being in general, in an engaging and creative way (Clintecs, 2017). The NHS and Public Health England have app libraries or stores where trusted, safe and secure apps can be accessed. Apps on the NHS library undergo rigorous testing by the NHS Digital Team to ensure they meet a specific set of standards before they can be published on the NHS Apps Library (NHS Digital, 2018). Health-related apps are often bought by individuals and uploaded directly onto their mobile phone or tablet, and can enhance a person's understanding of his or her health condition, as well as provide specific information regarding conditions. Recommended and trusted apps can promote healthy living and lifestyle choices and empower people to manage their health and be more aware of their lifestyle habits. Signposting patients to safe, secure and trusted apps allows patients to access information about their condition as and when they need it, and reiterates the advice given to them by their clinician, helping to improve patient experience and medicine adherence.

Introducing health apps into a care plan creates a customised approach to care, as patients are able to choose and access what is best suited for their needs and have on-demand access to the information as and when they need it, which can increase engagement and adherence to their care. Health apps often incorporate detailed information in easily digestible chunks, and many include avatars which provide visual examples of how to take medication or perform procedures correctly and safely because this is often easier for the patient to understand and learn than just descriptions or texts.

Social media

Social media can be used to engage with patients and to create peer support groups, encouraging individuals to care for themselves better. Using social media can be an effective way of communicating with people who often ignore other forms of communication or who cannot be reached via traditional health care promotion (Clinitecs, 2017).

Social media (e.g., a public Facebook page directed towards the public and to patients and their relatives) can provide information about both the practice and the wider health economy, and can also be used to share health campaigns or population health messaging and to target hard-to-reach patient cohorts. Instagram and Twitter can be used to reach the younger population, sharing health campaigns and messages such as breast cancer awareness or cervical screening, in a simple but informative and effective way.

Closed Facebook groups can be used to connect patients for peer-to-peer informal support, offering guidance from others who have experienced the same illness or condition. Disclaimers can be used to ensure that the function of the group is clear (e.g., that it is not a forum where individualised clinical advice will be given, but a 'safe space' for people to access to discuss their concerns, share stories, offer advice or ask for help from others in a similar position). Signposting to trusted information sites or apps can be shared in this space. The Nursing and Midwifery Council (NMC) have produced a social media guidance underpinned by The Code, which covers the need to use social media and social networking sites responsibly (NMC, 2019). The guidance sets out the broad principles to enable clinicians to act professionally and ensure public protection at all times (NMC, 2019).

Animations

Animations provide a creative and visual way to communicate important health issues to patients. They allow succinct health messages to be shared across several platforms in simple, engaging and understandable ways. Important messages such as information about how to manage illnesses, when to contact clinicians, vaccines, flu vaccinations, cervical screening, etc. are presented in a clear and easy-to-digest format. Animations can reach and engage a wider audience than can be achieved using traditional ways of communicating health information, for example by uploading animations onto social media platforms. The animations are bright and colourful and appeal to young people and those who cannot read or understand English. Subtitles can be added so these can be shared in general practices on TV screens in the waiting rooms, and these can be written in any language required to reach specific cohorts of patients. A suite of animations made by GPNs to communicate simple health messages is available to download for free at: www.clinitecs.uk.

Video consultation

Video consultation (where clinicians and patients meet virtually through the use of video calls) allows patients to attend a consultation and to be seen by the clinician in a booked appointment without the need for physical attendance. This can help to reduce 'did not attends', because a patient can attend a short follow-up appointment via the use of video consultation from their home or other private location, which is less time-consuming than attending at the clinic. This allows people who are unable to take time off work or who cannot travel to the practice to attend their appointment and can offer an alternative to home visits. It allows the clinician to evaluate, diagnose and treat patients efficiently and effectively. The benefits to remote consultations include minimising travel (for patients or clinicians), reducing the spread of infections, reducing stress (particularly for patients who feel pressure to attend a clinic) and encouraging self-care, as this can also be linked to self-monitoring. Suitable patients include (but are not limited to) those who need a follow-up appointment to review a change in medication, those who need a follow-up appointment for asthma review and patients who are suffering from an LTC where accessing GP services is difficult.

Video conferencing can also be used for clinician to clinician interactions, for example, for a remote peer professional meeting or between practitioners in different settings or locations (such as colleagues working between different sites or multidisciplinary team meetings which include colleagues from a number of settings, such as general practice, acute hospitals and local authorities). This can encourage and increase attendance at the meetings, as only the meeting time needs to be set aside, and there are no travel implications and costs.

Barriers in practice to the adoption of technology-enabled care services

There is a need for the clinicians to be aware of potential barriers – particularly those around clinical governance, information governance, privacy and accessibility concerns from members of the wider practice team. Ensuring that these questions or concerns are addressed early in the process of establishing TECS will ensure that implementation runs smoothly. There are codes of conduct, standard operating procedures, privacy impact assessments that can be completed in advance of introducing digital technology and consent forms for the patients to sign to state that they agree for digital tools to be included as part of their care (National Data Guardian for Health and Care, 2106).

The role of a digitally operative GPN can come with challenges because nurses are often working alone; however, the development of online nurse forums allows for both sharing of knowledge and troubleshooting amongst professionals. Although these forums are not new, clinical supervision is now being promoted in specific localities, and the use of video call capabilities can mean easier, more flexible access to support from colleagues. Many clinicians belong to small WhatsApp groups that provide informal methods of staying in contact. Further information and resources for clinical supervision have been produced as part of the General Practice Nursing Ten Point Plan and are available on the FutureNHS Collaboration Platform: www.future.nhs.uk.

To push technology forward it is crucial to normalise the idea that delivery of care should be digital by default. Ambassadors for TECSs in individual GP practices could consider introducing technological and digital discussions in surgery meetings or locality gatherings, or could look at other good practices locally to understand the kinds of solutions that are available.

Technology is not a silver bullet and will never replace nurses or other clinicians; but it does have the effect of enhancing and extending the support on offer and ensuring that clinicians can spend their time where it is most required.

Digital readiness

For GPNs to be able to confidently share the digital modes of technology available to their patients, it is crucial that they are digitally ready themselves and understand what is available, how to use it and the safety and security of what they are advocating to their patients. GPNs must be able to assess their current levels of digital confidence, competence and capability and recognise if these need to be improved to promote the digital tools that can help patients to better care for themselves and manage their health condition(s) and adverse lifestyle habit(s) more efficiently. If GPNs are not able to do this, then they will not be able to encourage patients to adopt digital technology effectively and efficiently, and more importantly, safely. Patients trust their clinicians to guide them to safe information, as they often already use digital technology in their personal care, but feel more reassured when this is signposted by a clinician.

The '7Cs' (Chambers et al., 2018) listed in Box 13.1 describe the elements required to achieve this:

Benefits of introducing digital health care

The main benefits to clinicians and patients in introducing digital health care fall into five main areas: (1) improved communication and engagement with

Box 13.1 The '7 Cs'

Competence: nurse, manager and patient/carer/citizen – ability in relation to personal use of range of modes of delivery of technology-enabled care services (TECSs) for agreed purpose and feeding in information or acting on advice and information

Capability: nurse, manager and patient/carer/citizen – actual best practice in use of range of modes of delivery of TECSs for agreed purpose and feeding in information or acting on advice and information in daily professional/everyday life

Capacity: nurse has protected and prioritised time for initiating and participating in remote delivery of care that is regarded as key element of work role (practitioner or manager) or personal life (patient/carer/citizen), and the information technology infrastructure and equipment is available and easily accessed by all service providers and users

Confidence: nurse and manager confident that organisational infrastructure is in place and in line with code of practice, including reliability and validity of equipment and its outputs; patient/carer/citizen confident that usage of TECSs is an integral part of clinical best practice as agreed with clinician, and that their responsible practitioner will access or act on relay of TECSs messages or interchanges

Creativity: nurse or manager able to adopt and adapt agreed TECSs for different purpose or patient/carer group in line with code of practice

Communication: the sharing and dissemination of digital modes of delivery and associated clinical protocols and evaluation of applications/outcomes/challenges, etc, with a team or organisation working together and sharing what has worked well and what has not worked so well

Continuity: at least one nurse or other practitioner/patient able to interact via TECS mode along one pathway for long-term condition/lifestyle habit; if practitioner not at work, cover arranged as appropriate and preagreed with patient in line with agreed shared care management plan.

From Chambers, R., Schmid, M., Al Jabbouri, A., & Beaney, P. (2018). *Making digital healthcare happen in practice*. Otmoor Publishing.

patients; (2) increased education and knowledge for patients (and clinicians), which enables patients to look after themselves and control their condition better; (3) patient empowerment by giving ownership and responsibility back to patients, resulting in improved compliance; (4) increased accessibility, resulting in improved relationships; and (5) increased safety – signposting patients to accurate and secure trusted information, ensuring that patients can access this information and ensuring that patients are not obtaining incorrect information from unreliable sources.

Wider practice team support is a necessity to keep the momentum going and to ensure succession planning for the future of primary care delivery. Having TECS protocols in place makes both the patient and clinical team members feel more comfortable.

Given the conveniences that technology affords us in so many areas of life, it is vital that GPNs, as the foot soldiers of the wider health system, are ready to support the health system's technological transformation. With an ageing population, demands on the health system are only going to increase – so there are few missions that are as important as ensuring that GPNs can manage demand and support patients to manage their conditions.

Digital technology is accessible for all and allows for effective and efficient information-sharing in an interesting way – it is engaging for all, allows for two-way interactions in consultations, opens conversations and allows signposting to safe, up-to-date and reliable health information. The NHS needs to 'move with the times' – TECS is part of most people's daily life, and most people are happy to embrace that in their health care.

Person-centred technology-enabled care services

We expect TECSs to help individuals live healthier lives, better manage their own health and well-being and reduce demand on local services so that the majority of the population can be supported in efficient ways, leaving traditional and increasingly scarce face-to-face resources focused on those with complex conditions. Many patients appear interested in taking more responsibility for their own health and well-being, but many lack the motivation, information and knowledge to adopt a healthy lifestyle and practise self-care. GPNs have a very important role in encouraging and supporting patients' self-care, and TEC is likely to help in making this happen at scale. The extent to which remote care effectively supplements, underpins or replaces face-to-face care remains to be seen, so GPNs should be willing and able to evaluate new ways in which they deliver person-centred patient care via technology.

Person-centred care is central to digital delivery of health and social care. It needs to be:

- The right care for the person's (or carer's) needs and preferences, delivered with dignity, compassion, sensitivity and respect, at the right time and place and with due regard to the person's age and any cognitive impairment
- Holistic care that includes physical, mental, emotional, spiritual and social aspects and person's own perspective and experiences, as appropriate
- Shared care: informed, value-based, preference-sensitive, agreed between person (and carer or family if appropriate) and care professional
- Safe: with informed decision-making balancing potential benefits and risks where there are options for different routes and modes of delivery of care
- Designed and evaluated with public and patient input and feedback
- Proactive and inclusive of health promotion, as well as primary, secondary and tertiary prevention
- Integral to a quality-improvement culture in health and social care.

This requires eight distinct elements in any organisational approach to ensure that nurses can deliver patient-centred TEC:

1. Promoting nurses' skills in person-centred care
    i. Behavioural change
        The National Institute for Health and Care Excellence (NICE) recommends a solution-focused approach by care professionals that includes:
        - Self-monitoring by patient or service user of behaviour and progress (with agreed shared care management plan or goals)
        - Goal setting (mutually agreed by care professional and person (and carer))
        - Encouraging social support
        - Problem solving (with patient or service user encouraged to report issues)
        - Assertiveness–encouraging patients and carers to be assertive
        - Cognitive restructuring by patient or carer (modifying thoughts)
        - Reinforcement of changes (in behaviour/treatment/interventions by patient and carer)
        - Relapse prevention/individualised strategies (NICE, 2014).
    ii. Self-management, self-care
        Nurses should consider shared management plans between them and their patient with an LTC or patients whose lifestyle habit(s) may adversely affect their health. They (one or all members of their practice team) should be able to help patients (and their carers) understand their condition(s), suggest options for interventions which support the person to choose and maintain the right treatment for them and self-manage their condition(s) on an ongoing basis, taking into account their ability, cognition, skills and motivation. They should be able to supply and engage a person with an appropriate decision aid (matching their values, preferences, knowledge and skills). Thus, it is important to sign up to a culture of shared decision-making and gain the skills needed to communicate evidence and its limitations in ways that people understand, using their preferred modes of delivery of decision aids (paper-based, online, individualised, generic, etc). The shared management plan should be accessible to all other health and care professionals involved in delivery of care for a particular patient, in line with the patient's informed consent about sharing personal data and details of their care.

2. Generating, collating and acting on patient feedback
    There is a United Kingdom – wide push to continuously invite individual patients' feedback – comments, complaints, suggestions – whether directly from a person or from his or her carer. Try to understand patients' or service users' perceptions to minimise barriers and provide person-centric care.

3. Engaging the public and service users of health and social care in service development and service redesign
    General practices should be actively engaging patients, service users and the public in shaping the services they use and provide (or should provide),

overcoming system 'inertia' and NHS/local authority 'know best' attitudes. This might be as a 'partnership' model with coproduction of service redesign with the practice participation group members, so that the person is at the centre, rather than fitting patients into services that are a convenient way for the practice to operate.

4. Sharing of a person's medical records

   Nowadays, online access in general practice to a person's medical records, appointment booking and repeat prescription ordering is usually available to individual patients who have signed up. The integrated care record (in place or expected, depending on progress in the area you work in) should enable all those working in health and social care to identify the individual person in the same way, with a view to sharing personal data in valid, reliable and safe ways.

5. Empowering service users of health and social care about their own care

   Empowered individual patients with good access to their health and care information should have opportunities to use these resources to better manage their own health. They should be enabled (supported and educated) to gain the knowledge, skills and confidence they need to effectively manage their symptoms and condition(s) themselves so that they are able to make informed decisions and adhere to their medicines and treatment plans to achieve the best possible outcomes. The culture of the health or social care front line should be one that welcomes and encourages people's commitment to change and improve their health and well-being (e.g., patients may wish to use an appropriate app to link their own generated health information to their medical records or care plan).

   A self-management plan or other care plan should be in an accessible format and include:

   ● Start and review dates
   ● A description of condition(s)/lifestyle habit(s) that are being managed
   ● Current treatments, including frequency of use, flexibility in doses of medicines and any restrictions
   ● Arrangements for follow up with a responsible care professional if their condition deteriorates, or there are side effects from medicines, etc.

6. Providing patient decision aids and clinical decision support tools

   NICE emphasises that putting people at the centre of decisions about their care can enable them to use the medicines that they are prescribed safely and effectively and to achieve the best possible outcomes and mode of care that align with their values (NICE, 2015). Shared decision-making is central to the delivery of evidence-based health or social care. Everyone should be offered the opportunity to be involved in making decisions about the delivery and scope of their care. Where there is more than one reasonable option, each with potential benefits and harms, the use of a high-quality patient decision aid can facilitate patient engagement and empower patient input into selecting an option.

A patient decision aid should describe the options available in a way that the person is likely to understand, and help the patient make an informed, value-based, preference-sensitive decision with the care professional after weighing the specific risks and benefits of the various options (NICE, 2014; Stacey et al., 2017). As a GPN you should feel confident about the content and appropriateness of the chosen decision aid, and the balanced way that risks and benefits are described.

7. Ensuring patient safety

Patient safety from the person's perspective includes:

- a holistic care plan
- medicine reconciliation – for comorbidities and when an LTC is diagnosed, treatment is changed, etc., or when provision of a person's health or social care changes setting or extends across multiple settings
- learning from past patient safety incidents to minimise the likelihood of similar incidents occurring in future.

8. Performing patient-centred evaluation

Patient-reported outcome measures (PROMs) are commonly used in health economic evaluation to evaluate outcomes of health interventions, in economic evaluation of medical technologies and to compare the performance of health service providers (Agoritsas, 2014). PROMs might be condition-specific, focused on a specific aspect of health. Generic PROMs measure health-related quality of life generally, enabling comparisons of health across conditions and health services. Person-centred evaluation should focus on the elements of care and support and treatment that matter most to a patient, family and carer:

- dignity, compassion and respect
- coordination of care, support or treatment
- personalised care, support or treatment
- support for people to recognise and develop their own strengths and abilities to live an independent and fulfilling life (Health Foundation, 2014).

Best practice for technology-enabled care services at the front line

TECSs are gaining increasing recognition for their potential roles in supporting delivery of health and social care at the front line and across organisational boundaries. TECSs include video consultation/Skype/telemedicine, telehealth (information-giving or interactive texting), apps, social media (e.g., Facebook, WhatsApp or Twitter), assistive technology/telecare, online resources (e.g., specific websites) or GP Online.

A single, integrated care record across a health economy will enhance interoperability between different health care settings and facilitate the use of TECSs by multidisciplinary teams. Data security frameworks, assurance schemes and standards already exist. Data security standards for every organisation handling health or social care information will support rather than inhibit data sharing (DOH, 2013).

Each GPN conducting a non–face-to-face consultation with a patient is responsible for ensuring that the mode and quality of the TECSs for that consultation are of sufficient standard and scope for safe practice in relation to the patient's health care needs. If not, he or she should discontinue the consultation and arrange an appropriate mode of clinical consultation to be delivered by himself or herself or by another practitioner within a safe timescale.

Selecting a particular mode of consultation will depend on the need for shared decision-making and shared management between patient and practitioner; availability and accessibility of TECSs (in relation to NHS and patient/carer ownership); patient's/carer's preference(s); self-care and/or continuity of care recommended; established relationship, trust and understanding between the patient/carer and practitioner; whether the appointment is a follow-up or a first presentation; severity and urgency of clinical management or prevention of disease or deterioration; availability of the right type or level of clinician; appropriate risk management; working across organisational boundaries; making the best use of technology; whether the chosen TECS mode is affordable and sustainable; quality, safety and efficiency; expected outcomes being clear and reasonable; quality and safety of the TECS mode; and the competence and confidence of practitioner(s) involved and the patient/carer to use preferred mode(s) of TECS(s).

There should be formal risk management procedures in place in a general practice to identify, report, document and investigate all incidents in relation to delivery of all types of clinical consultation. In parallel there should be a benefits analysis to assess how effective the use of TECSs is and if it improves or impedes productivity of the practice team, to inform future implementation of digital delivery and aid its sustainability.

All clinical consultations should be recorded in the patient's medical records in the usual way, whatever the mode of delivery. Clinicians must use all forms of spoken, written and digital communication responsibly, which includes social media and networking sites. Nurses and other health care professionals must stay objective and have clear professional boundaries at all times with people in their care, especially with the use of social media. The standards expected of clinicians communicating with patients via social media, telephone or email are no different than those applied to face-to-face consultations (e.g., confidentiality, maintaining professional boundaries) (Academy of Medical Royal Colleges, 2016). The NMC have produced The Code – professional standards of practice and behaviour for nurses, midwives and nursing associates (NMC, 2018).

Good nursing practice in determining the type of delivery of care offered to patients

It is the responsibility of each GPN, working closely with his or her general practice team, to select patients for an appropriate mode of consultation depending on their symptoms, signs, cognition, support, confidence and preferences. Selection criteria should be modified to take account of their experience and special interests and expertise.

1. Telephone consultation

   Telephone consultation is defined as an 'in-depth clinical assessment of a patient via the phone and…when patients or carers communicate with someone in a healthcare profession about a health problem or enquiry'. A telephone consultation may be initiated by the patient or by the clinician prebooking the consultation, or can be used for a follow-up review rather than a face-to-face consultation.

   Telephone triage is used in the NHS to identify what is urgent, what can wait and what needs to happen next; if the patient needs to be seen and if so by whom and where. This can lead to more effective skill mix, for example by establishing whether a subsequent face-to-face consultation can be safely provided by a nurse rather than a doctor.

   Potential benefits are: immediate access to care, easier and more convenient access, patient empowerment to self-care and improve compliance with treatment, possibly avoiding the need for face-to-face consultation, cost-effectiveness, cost savings (e.g., saving travel time and costs of patient/carer/clinician) and prioritisation of delivery of care (Pygall, 2017).

   Potential risks: nurses might make assumptions that the patient understands the information they relay; a lack of visual clues might lead to clinician uncertainty or inappropriate outcomes; the success of the consultation relies on the telephone caller (his or her comprehension of his or her symptoms and signs, as well as his or her memory or communication skills); and a third party relaying the patient's symptoms may overplay or underplay the description. Clinicians must use 'active listening' skills and concentrate on the conversation to appreciate the patient's tone of voice, the inferences that are used and what information is emphasised.

2. Face-to-face consultation

   This differs from remote modes of consultation, as the nurse's assessment includes the patient's or carer's body language and nonverbal communication such as facial expressions. That can be vital in diagnosing and treating a patient in a balanced way.

3. Email communication

   Email communication is used increasingly between clinicians in different settings as a good way of communication when their access is limited to be able to arrange, for example, telephone communication at a time when both parties are available.

4. Social network site set up for patients with a long-term condition by a nurse
   There should be no confidential information about any individual patient(s) on any social media site set up and managed by a health professional; this includes identity, personal life, health or circumstances. Any information posted on such a site is generic and in the best interests of service users, with no commercial component.

5. Video consultation
   A GPN might offer a video consultation for a patient's follow-up review for their LTC in the patient's own home or a private area at work. The practice will need to have an agreed protocol attached for undertaking video consultation. They will need to make sure that they have clinical indemnity cover for those clinicians undertaking video consultations, explaining to their medical defence organisation that this is instead of, and not as well as, a face-to-face consultation between clinician and patient. Here are some example selection criteria for an appropriate and safe mode of video consultation between a GP or GPN and a patient in his or her own home, chosen setting or nursing/care home:

Inclusion criteria

- Children aged between 13 and 15 years with written and recorded parental consent
- Patients 16 years of age and above
- Routine review by practice nurse or GP of any chronic health condition or adverse lifestyle habit (e.g., smoking)
- Medication review
- Low-risk patients requesting a consultation for any symptom.

Exclusion criteria

- Children aged 12 years and under (unless the responsible clinician wishes to modify the age of children who can be included, with parental consent and presence)
- Acute deterioration of the discussed chronic conditions
- Any condition requiring face-to-face clinical assessment or clinical examination
- Intermediate- to high-risk patients for specific symptoms
- Someone who is distinctly unwell and/or has raised temperature (and, for instance, will need clinical assessment of heart/lungs)
- High-risk patients where it is not possible to monitor vital signs.

Table 13.1 captures a way of thinking through whether a follow-up video consultation is an appropriate mode of consultation for a GPN to offer a patient, for example with cognition difficulties.

Table 13.1 Range of levels of risk for patient selection for video consultation between clinician and patient

Low risk	Intermediate risk	High risk
0–2 comorbidities; comorbidities that are present must be of low significance in terms of patient longevity, e.g., osteoarthritis	≥3 comorbidities of any significance Comorbidities present should not be directly related to presenting complaint	≥3 comorbidities of any significance Comorbidities that could be related to presenting complaint Current or previous diagnosis of cancer Age >90 years Dementia

National standards and good practice relating to technology-enabled care services

All general practice teams need to be aware of the local TECS Code of Practice to which they must adhere, as well as when and where they are responsible for delivery of patient care, how to encourage patients to practise self-care and how agreed shared care management underpins the patient's health and well-being.

The general practice team must agree to endorse and adhere to national requirements relating to information technology security, clinical safety, data quality, use of patient data, data protection and privacy and information standards. These include:

1. Information governance – defining standards, engaging staff, building professional capability (Department of Health, 2013; Department of Health, 2014; NHS, 2017)
2. Clinical governance (NHS, 2019)
3. Legal and regulatory obligations and compliance with standards, that is, Privacy Impact Assessment and Standard Operating Procedure (NHS, 2019; ICO, 2019; Gov.uk, 2017)
4. Procurement of technology and equipment for TECSs, such as medical devices; third-party contracts relating to delivery
5. Health and safety (NHS, 2013)
6. Quality management (RCGP, 2015)
7. Care Quality Commission – information security and governance (Care Quality Commission, 2016)
8. NHS England requirements and priorities (The King's Fund, 2016a)
9. Identification of patient by NHS number
10. Upskilling staff (clinicians, managers, administrators) to raise competence and confidence in TECSs within their own organisation and promote networking with others in connected ways; oversight of staff members' professional and manual competence in line with agreed responsibilities (The King's Fund, 2016b)

11. Shared care management between clinicians and selected/signed-up patients and citizens, with synchrony between all organisations in health economy for shared care management plans for all relevant care pathways and delegated authority and responsibilities on organisation and individual patient levels. Valid, trustworthy, relevant and up-to-date data must be available when and where needed, and accessible swiftly and securely for staff, as well as within and between organisations (Care Quality Commission, 2016)

12. Patient consent/opt-out if or when it is proposed that patients' personal confidential data is being used for purposes beyond their direct care (unless there is a mandatory legal requirement or an overriding public interest) (Care Quality Commission, 2016)

13. Patient safety, reinforcing adherence to preagreed interventions between clinician and patient with underpinning delivery protocols focused on specific selection criteria for involving patient groups that avoid unintended consequences of TECSs which might otherwise have put patients at risk (Powell-Cope et al., 2008)

14. Medical and other clinical or social care provider indemnity for clinician/social care workers delivering care via TECSs instead of alternative modes of delivery of care (Digital Health, 2016)

15. Security of transmission of care via TECSs underpinned by a protocol describing patient selection criteria, setting, patient consent, etc.

16. Measuring and demonstrating impact; collating evidence of positive outcomes (e.g., improved clinical outcomes, avoided health care usage such as hospital admissions, enhanced patient convenience, improved patient satisfaction, enhanced safety for vulnerable patients, increased independence of patients or citizens) and unintended consequences (safety risks, extra costs from, e.g., more workforce input) (Campbell et al., 2014)

17. Reliable infrastructure for everyday relaying of TECSs and associated equipment needed, such as for bodily measurement by patients

18. Involving patients, citizens and carers in the type and remit of TECSs that are commissioned or provided by the organisation

19. Being aware of and sustaining cybersecurity (Department of Health, 2014; NHS, 2017)

20. Security standards for NHS mail in line with ISB 1596 (PRSB, 2015).

Incorporating diverse modes of delivery of care into the usual service you provide – adapting to adoption of digital delivery of care

GPNs need to reflect on and capture their insights about how they adapt to new ways of working, such as providing TEC as usual practice. They will need digital technical or functional competence, organisational competence, autonomy or independence, stability and sustainability of modes of digital delivery, a creative approach, a purpose (from their and/or the patient's perspective), pure challenge and the ability to adapt to their new workplace habits. Such reflection

Table 13.2 Analyse your strengths, weaknesses, aptitudes and values from your personal and nurse perspectives

	How does this match with your current work situation? (score out of 10)	How important is this aspect of your career to you? (score out of 10)
Digital competence		
Organisational competence		
Autonomy or independence		
Stability or sustainability		
Creative approach		
Purpose of technology-enabled care services for a cause		
Pure challenge		
Workplace change habits		

Table 13.3 Plan ahead as a digitally ready nurse

What might you change?	How? When?	Can you foresee any risks?

should help nurses define their self-image in terms of what kind of nurse they appear to be or actually are and come to understand more about their talents, motives, resistance to change and values – and which of these is so important to them that they would not give up those facets of themselves if forced to make a choice. You can interpret these for yourself in relation to the adoption of TEC as your usual practice in delivery of care that you provide. These are listed in Table 13.2.

What are your conclusions? Is there a mismatch? Are you well suited to adopting TECSs as a norm in your current work role? Should you change elements of your current work role? Complete Table 13.3.

Conclusion

The NHS has evolved from its creation in 1948 and now serves a much larger population (of approximately 61 million in England). To continue to deliver the health care that patients deserve in sustainable ways, the NHS must adapt and embrace new ways of working, and this includes the adoption and implementation of digital tools for both patients and clinicians. This use of digital tools will improve patients' education and knowledge of their health or health condition(s) and will help to encourage them to be more involved in the management of their own health care, taking more responsibility for their LTCs and adverse lifestyle habits.

Genuine person-centred care is central to the digital delivery of health and social care, creating an efficient and safer way to share management of patients' health and LTCs with their responsible clinicians. The culture of the health or social care front line should be one that welcomes and encourages a person's commitment to change and to improve his or her health and well-being. The use of digital tools for TECSs, and digital inclusion of patients in delivery of their care, can drive this, resulting in improved adherence to medication and other treatments through better interactive communication and enhanced patient empowerment whereby patients take more responsibility for their own health and well-being. Embedding a range of digital tools as part of usual health service delivery results in more efficient, effective and productive working across the whole general practice team. Understanding patients' and service users' perceptions (and those of their carers', where appropriate) can help to minimise barriers and result in person-centric care.

Clinicians have the responsibility of advising and introducing patients to the most appropriate mode of consultation for their needs and capabilities, depending on their symptoms, cognition, confidence and preferences, and therefore they need to be digitally ready, that is, confident and able to use available and accessible digital tools themselves.

With their substantive direct interactions with patients in relation to their health conditions and lifestyle habits, GPNs are the key to this successful implementation and the future of primary care.

References

Campbell, J. L., Fletcher, E., Britten, N., et al. (2014). Telephone triage for management of same-day consultation requests in general practice (the ESTEEM trial): A cluster-randomised controlled trial and cost-consequence analysis. *The Lancet, 384*(9957), 1859–1868.

Care Quality Commission. (2016). *Policy statement on information security and governance.* http://www.cqc.org.uk/.

Chambers, R., Schmid, M., Al Jabbouri, A., & Beaney, P. (2018). *Making digital healthcare happen in practice.* Otmoor Publishing.

Clinitecs. (2017). *TECS in use.* http://www.clinitecs.uk/category/TECS-in-use/.

Department of Health. (2013). *The information governance review.* https://www.gov.uk/government/uploads/system/uploads/attachment_data/file/192572/2900774_InfoGovernance_accv2.pdf.

Digital Health. (2016). *Doctors need guidance on mobile technology use.* http://www.digitalhealth.net/news/22744/doctors-need-guidance-on-mobile-technology-use.

Gov.UK (2017). *Guidelines for standard operating procedures (SOPs).* https://www.gov.uk/government/uploads/system/uploads/attachment_data/file/98034/standard-op-procedure.pdf.

Health Education England. (2019). *The Topol review: Preparing the healthcare workforce to deliver the digital future.* https://topol.hee.nhs.uk/the-topol-review/.

Health Foundation. (2014). *Person-centred care made simple. Quick guide.* Health Foundation.

Information Commissioner's Office. (2019). *Privacy impact code of practice.* https://ico.org.uk/media/for-organisations/documents/1595/pia-code-of-practice.pdf.

The King's Fund. (2016a). *A digital NHS.* https://www.kingsfund.org.uk/sites/files/kf/field/field_publication_file/A_digital_NHS_Kings_Fund_Sep_2016.pdf.

The King's Fund. (2016b). *Transforming our healthcare system.* https://www.kingsfund.org.uk/publications/articles/transforming-our-health-care-system-ten-priorities-commissioners.

National Data Guardian for Health and Care, (2016). *Review of data security, consent and opt-outs.* https://www.gov.uk/government/publications/review-of-data-security-consent-and-opt-outs.

NHS. (2013). *Workplace health and safety standards.* http://www.nhsemployers.org/~/media/Employers/Publications/workplace-health-safety-standards.pdf.

NHS. (2017). *Information governance toolkit.* https://www.igt.hscic.gov.uk.

NHS. (2019). *The main components of clinical governance.* http://www.uhb.nhs.uk/clinical-governance-components.htm.

NHS Digital. (2018). *How we assess health apps and digital tools.* https://digital.nhs.uk/services/nhs-apps-library/guidance-for-health-app-developers-commissioners-and-assessors/how-we-assess-health-apps-and-digital-tools.

NHS England. (2016a). *Putting patients first.* https://www.england.nhs.uk/wp-content/uploads/2013/04/ppf-1314-1516.pdf.

NHS England. (2016b). *Leading change, adding value – A framework for nursing, midwifery and care staff.* https://www.england.nhs.uk/wp-content/uploads/2016/05/nursing-framework.pdf.

NHS England. (2017). *General practice – Developing confidence, capability and capacity – A ten-point action plan for General Practice Nursing.* https://www.england.nhs.uk/wp-content/uploads/2018/01/general-practice-nursing-ten-point-plan-v17.pdf.

NICE. (2014). *Obesity: identification, assessment and management.* www.nice.org.uk/guidance/cg189.

NICE. (2015). *Medicines optimization: The safe and effective use of medicines to enable the best possible outcomes. NICE Guideline 5.* www.nice.org.uk/guidance/ng5.

Nursing & Midwifery Council. (2018). *The Code – Professional standards of practice and behaviour for nurses, midwives and nursing associates.* https://www.nmc.org.uk/standards/code/.

Nursing & Midwifery Council. (2019). *Social media guidance – Our guidance on the use of social media.* https://www.nmc.org.uk/standards/guidance/social-media-guidance/.

Office of National Statistics. (2019). *Internet access – Households and individuals, Great Britain: 2019.* https://www.ons.gov.uk/peoplepopulationandcommunity/householdcharacteristics/homeinternetandsocialmediausage/bulletins/internetaccesshouseholdsandindividuals/2019#almost-two-thirds-of-households-now-have-mobile-broadband-access.

Powell-Cope, G., Nelson, A. L., & Patterson, E. S. (2008). Patient care technology and safety. In R.G. Hughes (Ed.), *Patient safety and quality: An evidence-based handbook for Nurses.* Agency for Healthcare Research and Quality (US). https://www.ncbi.nlm.nih.gov/books/NBK2686/.

Professional Record Standards Body for Health and Social Care. (2015). *Faster, better, safer communications using email in health and social care (in England) for patients and healthcare professionals.* www.theprsb.org.

Pygall, S. A. (2017). *Telephone triage and consultation*. RCGP.

RCGP. (2015). *Quality improvement for general practice.* http://www.rcgp.org.uk/clinical-and -research/our-programmes/~/media/Files/CIRC/Quality-Improvement/RCGP-QI-Guide-2015 .ashx.

Stacey, D., Legare, F., Col, N., et al. (2017). Decision aids for people facing health treatment or screening decisions. *Cochrane Database Syst Rev, 4*(4), CD001431.

Index

Page numbers followed by *f* refer to figures, by *t* to tables and by *b* to boxes